The Roadmap for Diagnosis

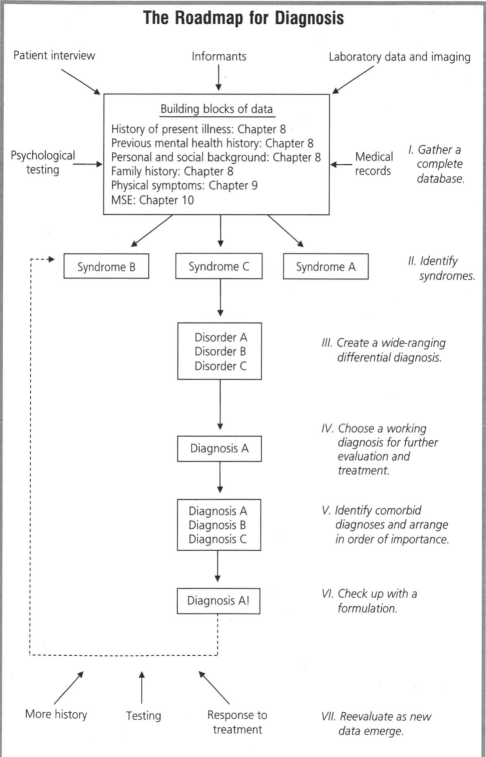

Patient interview

Informants

Laboratory data and imaging

Building blocks of data

History of present illness: Chapter 8
Previous mental health history: Chapter 8
Personal and social background: Chapter 8
Family history: Chapter 8
Physical symptoms: Chapter 9
MSE: Chapter 10

Psychological testing

Medical records

I. Gather a complete database.

Syndrome B

Syndrome C

Syndrome A

II. Identify syndromes.

Disorder A
Disorder B
Disorder C

III. Create a wide-ranging differential diagnosis.

Diagnosis A

IV. Choose a working diagnosis for further evaluation and treatment.

Diagnosis A
Diagnosis B
Diagnosis C

V. Identify comorbid diagnoses and arrange in order of importance.

Diagnosis A!

VI. Check up with a formulation.

More history

Testing

Response to treatment

VII. Reevaluate as new data emerge.

Diagnosis Made Easier

Diagnosis Made Easier

Principles and Techniques for Mental Health Clinicians

James Morrison

The Guilford Press
New York   London

© 2007 The Guilford Press
A Division of Guilford Publications, Inc.
72 Spring Street, New York, NY 10012
www.guilford.com

Printed in the United States of America

This book is printed on acid-free paper.

Last digit is print number: 9 8 7 6 5

Library of Congress Cataloging-in-Publication Data

Morrison, James R.
   Diagnosis made easier : principles and techniques for mental
health clinicians / James Morrison.
       p. ;   cm.
   Includes bibliographical references and index.
   ISBN-13: 978-1-59385-331-0
   ISBN-10: 1-59385-331-9
   1. Mental illness—Diagnosis.   2. Mental health services.
I. Title.
   [DNLM: 1. Mental Disorders—diagnosis.   2. Interview,
Psychological.   3. Physical Examination—methods.   WM 141
M879di 2006]
   RA469.M67 2006
   616.89′075—dc22

                                                           2006011629

For Chris, who makes everything easier

About the Author

James Morrison, MD, earned his BA at Reed College in Portland, Oregon, and obtained his medical degree and psychiatric training at Washington University in St. Louis. With an extensive work history in both the private and public sectors, he is currently Professor of Clinical Psychiatry at Oregon Health and Science University in Portland. Dr. Morrison's other books for professionals include *The First Interview, DSM-IV Made Easy, When Psychological Problems Mask Medical Disorders*, and *Interviewing Children and Adolescents*. He is also the author of *Straight Talk about Your Mental Health*, a comprehensive guide for consumers.

Contents

Introduction

When I set out to write about the diagnostic process, I envisioned a text that could both complement classroom teaching and provide a guide for independent study. That was before I undertook a completely unscientific survey of practicing health care professionals, to learn how *they* had learned about mental health diagnosis. What I found surprised me.

For most of the practitioners I surveyed, training in the refined art of diagnosis was—well, no training at all. Most of the professional schools at which my interviewees trained presented no formal course material on diagnosis, and still do not do so. Even in medical schools, students and residents are expected to know the current diagnostic criteria, but they receive little if any exposure to a method for making diagnoses. Almost to a person, my sample endorsed the sentiment "I learned diagnosis through on-the-job training." Similarly, chapters and books that strive to teach clinicians how to perform a competent clinical evaluation focus on the product, while largely ignoring information about the process.

That process is neither simple nor intuitive, and I'd certainly never describe it as easy. But after decades of experience and months of consideration, I believe it can be explained it in a way that is straightforward and comprehensible—in short, to make diagnosis easier.

In this book, I present a way of thinking about diagnostic problems. The material doesn't depend much on the vagaries of the latest diagnostic standards or code numbers. Instead, I focus on the essential characteristics of mental disorder, which have been recognized for decades. What's imperative to learn is the scientific method—yes, and the art—of evaluating patients and arriving at logical diagnoses consistent with the facts.

Part I focuses on the process of diagnosis. Learning how to diagnose well involves systematically applying logical, easily understood principles to information of several different types, assembled from a variety of sources. Although real life requires us to confront many diagnostic issues at once, for convenience I've divided the tasks into chapters. By the end of Part I, you'll see how seasoned clinicians unite their experience with new information to create a working diagnosis.

The three chapters of Part II explore the social and other background data you need to understand each patient's mental health diagnosis. Of course, this is the stuff you need to have *first*, so you can make the diagnosis. But when learning new material, you have to start somewhere, and I have judged that many (probably most) of my readers already have some familiarity with interviewing and information gathering. That's why I've gone ahead and presented the diagnostic method first.

Finally, in the chapters of Part III, we'll sift through a great deal of clinical material to see how the Part I methods and the Part II data apply to various clinical disorders. We won't consider every disorder, or even all the varieties of the main disorders; other manuals (including my own *DSM-IV Made Easy*) handle that chore. Rather, we'll concentrate on the issues and illnesses that mental health clinicians confront every day.

To illustrate the diagnostic methods, I've included over 100 patient histories. Before you read my analysis of each clinical example, I recommend that you try working through the decision trees and writing up your own list of relevant diagnostic principles. It has been amply proven that we all learn far more efficiently by actively thinking about the solution to a problem, rather than just passively reading something printed on a page. I think you'll benefit from the practice of thinking about the histories and determining how their clues direct you to the diagnosis.

You may wonder why each decision tree endpoint reads "Consider . . ." Why not just name the disorder and move on? After much thought about these diagrams, I have decided that the more tentative wording is safer. Without being too prescriptive, I want to encourage you to avoid a trap that any clinician can fall into: rushing headlong into diagnostic closure before you have all the necessary facts.

Figure 1.1 of this book (which is also printed on the front endpaper) provides a roadmap that shows the diagnostic process graphically. The Appendix (which is also printed on the back endpaper) lists the diagnostic principles I consider important to apply in making a mental health diagnosis. In the interest of space and economy, I've put quite a lot of information relevant to currently recognized major diagnoses into tables in Chapters 3 and 6. Table 3.2 provides a differential diagnosis for each major diagnosis; Table 6.1 lists the illnesses that are commonly comorbid.

If I haven't covered every question you have about diagnosis and the diagnostic method, I urge you to consult my website (http://mysite.

verizon.net/res7oqx1). There I've archived some of the queries I've received over the years. And to try to repay, in some small way, the debt I feel I owe to my profession, I'll continue to answer questions from readers and others on the site.

Finally, every writer owes an unpayable debt to many unseen hands who provide inspiration, guidance, and courage. For my most recent effort, I owe special thanks to my wife, Mary. Though she has midwifed each of my books, for this one she provided prenatal checkups in the form of careful reviews of the manuscript. I salute my collaborators at The Guilford Press, especially my long-time friend and editor, Kitty Moore, who worked closely with me to develop the concept of this book. Through her superb copyediting, Marie Sprayberry added immeasurably to the readability of the text, whereas our production editor, Anna Brackett, had the patience to hold my hand through the final stages to make this book possible. These people are the best in the business. I am indebted to the fine writing and teaching of George Staley. And innumerable clinicians and countless patients have, however unwittingly, furthered my own education and helped show me the way.

PART I

The Basics of Diagnosis

1 The Road to Diagnosis

Carson

Years ago I evaluated Carson, a 29-year-old graduate student in psychology. He had always lived in the town where he was born, among numerous relatives and friends. Through a long history of repeated depressive episodes, he had taken antidepressant medications on and off for a decade. At one time or another he had complained of trouble concentrating on his studies, of worries that he wouldn't be able to find a job, and of fears that he would become chronically depressed like his maternal grandmother.

When Carson was at his worst (usually in the late fall), he had trouble sleeping and eating, so he was pretty thin by the time Christmas rolled around. Each spring his mood picked up, and he invariably felt well the entire summer and early fall, though he admitted that he was prone to be "sensitive to the minor vicissitudes of life." What he meant, his wife told me, was that he sometimes felt down when things weren't going well.

A typical teenager, Carson had experimented with both alcohol and drugs. Once, when withdrawing from a 3-day run of amphetamine use, he had briefly become depressed, but his mood had lifted spontaneously within a few days. His girlfriend had agreed to marry him only on the condition that he "clean up his act"; now he swore he had been completely clean and sober for the 4 years they had been together. He had never had symptoms of mania, and he thought his physical health was excellent.

Medication had helped Carson get through college, after which he had spent the summer searching for a graduate fellowship. Finally, though the economy was depressed and few positions were available in the social sciences, he was offered a graduate fellowship with a generous stipend in a good department. Despite the triumph, his celebration was muted: His new university was nearly 2,500 miles away, in a part of the country where he'd never lived before.

On a Friday afternoon in late June, at his regular clinician's request, Carson appeared for an emergency evaluation. He sat slumped uneasily in his chair, with one knee jumping up and down, and his gaze drooping. He complained of terrible anxiety: His wife was pregnant with their first child; the following day they would start driving across the country to the site of his new job, in a city he'd never even visited. The previous afternoon he had become "almost panicky" when he was asked to sign a routine extension of his student loan.

As Carson described his fears for the future, his eyes reddened and he brushed away tears. Though he didn't think he felt depressed, he confessed that he "couldn't go through with it"—that he felt abandoned and alone. "I'm falling apart," he said, and broke down in sobs.

A Roadmap for Diagnosis

As you can imagine, a lot rides on an evaluation like Carson's. If you were his clinician, you would need to answer a lot of questions. What's wrong? Is it the same as his previous problems with depression? Does he need treatment at all? If so, what's most likely to help? Should he have more medicine, or a different antidepressant, or psychotherapy? What should you tell Carson and his wife—should they postpone their move? What should Carson tell his new boss? The answer to each of these important questions would depend on your assessment of his condition. To be helpful, it must be based on information that will assist you in finding a road to the future. Reaching an initial destination on that road—we can call it a diagnosis—is what this book is all about.

The ancient Greek term *diagnosis* means "distinguishing" or "discerning." Beyond the word itself, the concept of distinguishing one disease from another is crucially important to patients and medical scientists alike. As British psychiatrist R. E. Kendell wrote a generation ago, without diagnosis our journals would print only case reports and opinions.

When a person goes to a medical doctor with a physical complaint, in most cases the diagnosis conveys three sorts of information: the nature of the problem (symptoms, signs, and history), its cause, and the physical changes that consistently occur as a result. Any disorder that clearly meets these criteria can be called a *disease*. Take pneumonia, for example. This term tells us that the patient feels weak and tired, and that the person suffers from the symptoms of shortness of breath, fever, and a cough that produces sputum. But only after we learn the results of sputum cultures and other tests do we learn that the cause of the pneumonia is bacteria growing in the patient's lungs, causing the air sacs to fill with fluid and cells, producing shortness of breath. Then we can say that the patient has the disease of pneumococcal pneumonia.

The clinical symptoms and other information establish coordinates on the roadmap a doctor follows in prescribing treatment and predicting outcome. I'm somewhat geographically challenged, so whether I visit the automobile club or log onto Mapquest.com, I like to have both driving directions and a graphic depiction of the route for my trip. Having both verbal and pictorial guidance is a belt-and-suspenders approach that helps reassure me I'll arrive on time at the right place. In the list below, we'll take a brief overview of the "driving directions" for mental health diagnosis. I've indicated the page numbers where you can find discussions of these parts of the evaluation. (In Figure 1.1, I've drawn them as a map so you can see just where we're going. For convenience, you'll find the same graphic inside the front cover.) Don't worry if some of the terms seem unfamiliar— we'll define them as we go.

- *Level I.* Gather a complete database, including history of the current illness, previous mental health history, personal and social background, family history, medical history, and mental status examination (MSE). Obviously, you must first have material that describes your patient as fully as possible. Most of it will come from interviews with the patient and, very often, with other informants. You'll read a lot about these building blocks in the Part II database quarry. Pages 87–123.
- *Level II.* Identify syndromes. *Syndromes* are collections of symptoms that go together to produce an identifiable illness. Major depression is a syndrome; so is alcoholism. Page 9.
- *Level III.* Construct a differential diagnosis. *Differential diagnosis* is just a term for all of the disorders you think that a patient could have. You don't want to overlook any possibilities, however unlikely, so at first you must cast a very wide net. Page 14.
- *Level IV.* Using a decision tree, select the most likely provisional diagnosis for further evaluation and treatment. Page 19.
- *Level V.* Identify other diagnoses that might be comorbid with your principal diagnosis. Arrange multiple diagnoses according to the urgency of their need for treatment. Page 56.
- *Level VI.* Write a formulation as a check on your evaluation. This brief statement of your patient summarizes your findings and conclusions. Page 79.
- *Level VII.* Reevaluate your diagnoses as new data become available. Page 81.

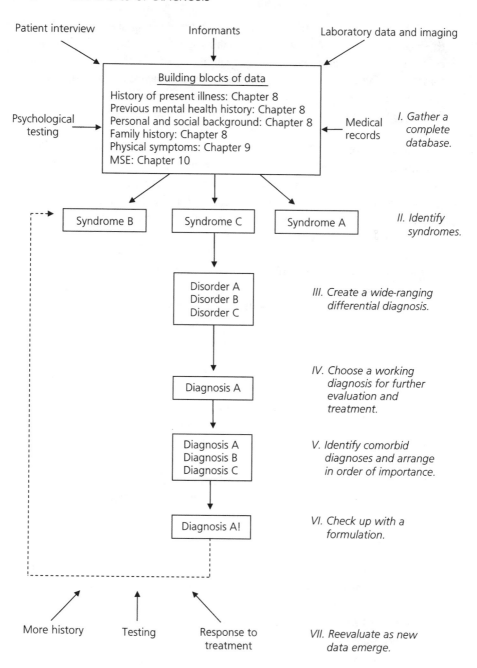

FIGURE 1.1. The roadmap for diagnosis.

2 Getting Started with the Roadmap

Most often, the information the patient provides at the initial interview starts you on the road to diagnosis. As with Carson (see Chapter 1), relatives can provide additional details. I cannot emphasize enough the importance of collateral information to the overall clinical picture. Patients don't usually mislead us on purpose, but often they lack the advantage of perspective on their own situations. I have frequently found that friends, relatives, and other clinicians provide information crucial to my appraisal. At the very least, such information adds color and depth to the emerging portrait of a new patient. When available, old records can sometimes save hours of digging for background information; at times they've saved me from a calamitous misdiagnosis.

The clinical history usually begins with the problem that was immediately responsible for bringing the person to clinical attention—the *history of the present illness*. Perhaps this was an acute episode of depression, the recent onset of hearing voices, a heavy bout of drug use, or conflict within a personal relationship. Woven through will be information that helps you understand how the lives of patients, relatives, and close associates have been affected. You'll also begin to pick up *previous mental health history*, which includes information about other mental or emotional problems, or earlier episodes of the current problem, which can also be important in determining what's currently wrong.

In the movies, in novels, and on the stage, far more is involved in storytelling than a simple narrative. Any but the simplest Dick-and-Jane story implies information about the main character's surroundings, culture, family, and social milieu. Sometimes this material is called the *back story*, and it provides texture and layers of meaning that illuminate the motives, actions, and emotions of the characters. So it is with patients—all of whom have their back stories, too, which clinically we call *personal and social history*. For the same reasons that a play is more compelling when we understand what motivates its characters, this information is not just interesting but often highly relevant, even vital, to diagnosis. I consider this information to be so important that Chapter 8 is devoted to discussing childhood background, current living situation, and *family history*, especially of mental disorder. Medical background (Chapter 9) is another important part of your evaluation. Finally, you'll make use of the *MSE* (Chapter 10)—though perhaps not quite as much use as you'd initially think. Throughout Part I of this book, we'll be examining these various parts of the mental health evaluation and how we can use them to create a diagnosis.

In the real world, patients, like Shakespeare's sorrows, tend to come not as single spies, but in battalions. As a result, you may not have enough time to gather all the material you need for a complete initial evaluation. That's OK. The task here is to learn how the job is done when conditions are ideal; with practice, you will later become able to accomplish the same thing in the course of a busy office day or frantic emergency room evening.

Symptoms and Signs

In Chapter 3 we'll discuss the basic plan for making a sound diagnosis. But before we get there, we need to define some terms that relate to the raw materials for any health care diagnosis. Technically, *symptoms* are what patients complain of, whereas *signs* are what clinicians notice. The patient with pneumonia described in Chapter 1 has complained of several symptoms, including a cough, shortness of breath, and feeling tired. Symptoms are the indicators of disease that are perceived by patients or their friends and relatives; they are the issues that patients mention when they talk to their care providers. In the mental health field, symptoms can include a tremendous variety of emotions, behaviors, and physical sensations. At one time or another, Carson's symptoms included feeling depressed, trouble concentrating on his studies, panicky feelings, trouble sleeping, and poor appetite. Hallucinations and delusions are symptoms. So are "nervousness," fear of spiders, and ideas of suicide.

Of course, circumstance and degree play important roles in determining what is and is not a symptom: Many people don't care for spiders, and doctors normally wash their hands frequently, so as not to spread germs from one patient to another. So we can see that symptoms are always more or less subjective; they depend on a person's perspective. Signs, on the other hand, are far more objective clues to illness. Usually patients and informants don't complain of signs; rather, the clinician identifies them from a patient's appearance or behavior. The patient with pneumonia would probably show the signs of fever, increased heart rate, and perhaps altered blood pressure, and a physician with a stethoscope would hear crackling sounds of fluid in the lungs. Carson's signs of mental illness included tearfulness and slumped posture.

The sets of signs and symptoms sometimes intersect. At times in this book, I may talk about a sign that could be a symptom (see the sidebar "Symptoms and Signs"). You'll have to put up with that ambiguity; it's part of the clinical mystique. So why, you may want to know, do we need to note that there is a difference? The reason is that because signs are more objective, we can rely on them more than symptoms. In fact, one of the diagnostic principles that we'll use later on is that "signs trump symptoms"—not always, but often enough that it justifies paying attention to the differences between signs and symptoms. For example, despite his doubt that he felt depressed, Carson's tearfulness and slumped shoulders told another story.

Symptoms (and signs) are useful in two ways. First, like Carson's panic attack, they signal that something is wrong. In the same way, suicidal thoughts, poor appetite, or hearing voices can indicate the need for a mental health evaluation. The second use of signs and symptoms is to set us on the path to an appropriate diagnosis: Repeated public intoxication suggests alcohol dependence; an arrest for shoplifting should prompt an evaluation for kleptomania; and an anxiety attack when watching a war movie might motivate a combat veteran to seek attention for posttraumatic stress disorder (PTSD).

> **Symptom:** A subjective sensation, discomfort, or change in functioning that a patient or informant complains about. Examples include headache, abdominal pain, itching, depression, and a tickling sensation in the nose.
>
> **Sign:** An indication of disease that can be noticed by others. Examples include a lump on the head, abdominal tenderness to touch, skin rash, weeping, and sneezing.

Why We Need Syndromes

Signs and symptoms by themselves aren't enough to make a usable diagnosis. Our physical medicine patient with cough, shortness of breath, and weakness could have pneumonia, but the same symptoms could indicate

Symptoms and Signs

Mental health doesn't have a lot of signs, but here are a few of them: weeping, sighing, pacing, weight loss, tattered clothing, and poor hygiene. Some indicators can be either a sign or a symptom, depending on who notices. Carson wouldn't have complained about his own slumped posture, but his wife or a next-door neighbor might notice it and mention it to a clinician. Depending on circumstances, nearly any behavior that can be observed by others and that is usually treated as a sign could be a symptom instead.

Until about 1850, clinicians didn't discriminate between signs and symptoms; now whole books are devoted to the concept. Recently, however, there have been a few indications that we may once again be blurring the boundary, at least in the United States. In the late 1990s, concern that medical people too often ignored patients' pain led to calling pain a "fifth vital sign." The intent of this was that pain would be documented at every clinical visit, along with the four classical (and undeniable) vital signs—temperature, blood pressure, pulse, and respiration rate. Technically, however, pain is a complaint that can only be a symptom, because of its innate subjectivity.

Sometimes we clinicians get careless in our speech and forget the very real difference between signs and symptoms. After decades of experience, I've decided that there's no winning this battle. But we should never forget that there is a difference, and that we can use it to help us evaluate our patients.

---

lung cancer—or nothing more than a simple cold. To make a diagnosis that we can use to make predictions, we must consider the circumstances surrounding the signs and symptoms we have identified.

Although many normal people worry about what lies in the future, worry can also be a symptom of an anxiety or mood disorder. If you buy a handgun, you are probably only interested in improving your marksmanship for a shooting competition. But if a depression has you believing that life's no longer worth living, the purchase becomes ominous. If I break down in tears during a professional meeting, it could mean that I am depressed and need treatment. But suppose I've just received a text message that my sister has died unexpectedly; then I'm only reacting normally in the context of appalling news.

And so we come to the *syndrome*, a Greek term first used nearly 500 years ago that means "things running or occurring together." More than just a collection of symptoms and signs, it should be more fully understood as symptoms, signs, *and events* that take place in a recognizable pattern and imply the existence of a particular disorder. Thus a syndrome includes such diverse features as rapidity of onset, age at onset, occurrence of precipitants, history of previous episodes, duration of current episode, and the extent to which a person's work or social life is disrupted. Each of these features restricts the meaning of the syndrome and helps identify a uniform group of patients. An obvious feature of Carson's recurring depression was that it regularly began and ended at a certain time of year. The combination of this one piece of historical evidence with his mood symptoms defined the syndrome of seasonal affective disorder.

A syndrome is an excellent starting point for disease identification, but we mental health professionals still have a long way to go

> *Syndrome:* Symptoms, signs, and events that occur in a particular pattern and indicate the existence of a disorder.

before we reach a diagnosis. Internal medicine categorizes illness according to its cause. Pneumonia, as we've noted, can be caused by bacteria (a great variety of them), viruses (many to choose from here, too), or even chemicals (someone who has swallowed gasoline can develop breathing problems that are very similar to better-known types of pneumonia). The virtue of a cause-based diagnosis is that it accurately directs the clinician to the best treatment. Unfortunately, we've managed to identify very few mental health diagnoses by cause. Indeed, current diagnostic schemes remain proudly "atheoretical," using criteria written so as not to force clinicians to choose among competing hypotheses about how and why mental disorders develop. Perhaps this facilitates communication between clinicians endorsing different schools of thought—for instance, a behaviorist and a psychoanalyst could amicably discuss Carson's diagnosis—but it wouldn't help them agree about treatment.

Creating a collection of symptoms, signs, and other features that *reliably* identifies homogeneous groups of patients is only a part of disease identification. The next phase is to see whether the selection process can help predict the future—that is, whether it is *valid* (see the sidebar "Validity and Reliability"). Here's how it is done. Researchers follow up patients from the group being studied to learn their outcomes: After several years, do they continue to have similar symptoms and respond uniformly to treatment, or do different diagnoses become apparent with time?

An excellent example occurred during the middle years of the 20th century, when the term *hysteria* was still in common use as a diagnosis. By tracking down patients who had been diagnosed with hysteria, researchers learned that years later some were completely well, whereas others now had a physical illness that could explain the symptoms that their doctors had once thought to be emotional in origin. Oh yes, and quite a few still seemed to have symptoms that were, well, hysterical in origin. These researchers concluded that hysteria is not a valid diagnosis because it does not predict a uniform outcome. From this realization sprang the concept of somatization disorder, which is far better than hysteria at predicting the outcome for patients.

Because we know that many and perhaps most mental illnesses run in families (Carson's mother also had depression), another check on the validity of a diagnosis is to learn how likely relatives of the patient are to have had the same or similar illnesses. We'll discuss this more fully in Chapter 8.

A meaningful diagnosis for Carson's mood disorder would help you as his clinician decide whether to treat him with antidepressants, mood stabilizers, or cognitive-behavioral therapy—or possibly all three. Accurate labeling would also help avert the harm that ineffective treatments might cause Carson by delaying the use of effective ones. In addition, you would anticipate the course of Carson's illness and advise him whether to use a treatment that would help protect against future episodes, whether to obtain additional health care insurance, and whether his siblings and children might develop a similar illness. Finally, carefully defined syndromes facili-

Validity and Reliability

Validity and *reliability* are two words often used to describe findings in all fields of health care. They have meanings that are quite distinct and different, yet they are sometimes used interchangeably in everyday speech and writing. Here is the important distinction: A *valid* finding has been proven through scientific study to be sound or well-established. A *reliable* finding is one that, regardless of its basic truth, can be replicated from one time or individual to another.

Take weapons of mass destruction, for example. If politicians and journalists repeatedly state that that some country (let's say Iraq) is making them, the reports might seem reliable. But such a claim would only be valid if investigators verified it, perhaps by actually finding such weapons during an inspection. If severely depressed patients repeatedly complain that they awaken early in the morning and cannot get back to sleep, we can say that early morning insomnia is a reliable characteristic of depression. But not until double-blind sleep studies, possibly using electroencephalograms (EEGs), affirm the observation would we call it validated.

tate research into new treatments. And the more narrowly defined the syndromes are, the better the predictions based on them will be.

Ultimately, we would like to know that a syndrome can be supported by laboratory or imaging findings that are similar to those for pneumonia. But so far, almost no objective laboratory tests have been devised in the mental health field. Without definitive testing, it is hard to attribute causes, without which we cannot really say that we have identified a mental *disease*. *Syndrome* remains the dominant conception of mental disorder, and it is likely to stay that way for many years into the future. But that's OK—the concept works well, and there is simply no good alternative.

Of course, there's a lot more to diagnosis than just identifying syndromes. Otherwise, you'd now be finishing a pamphlet rather than beginning a book. In Chapter 11 you can find a fuller discussion of Carson and his problems, which turned out to be a little more complicated than they first appeared. Now, however, we'll move on to a discussion of a diagnostic method that many experienced clinicians use, though few realize it.

3 The Diagnostic Method

Even an experienced clinician sometimes stumbles when making a mental health diagnosis, so where does that leave a trainee? Fortunately, a number of scientific studies have confirmed the value of two important clinician behaviors. The first of these is to consider alternative diagnoses right from the first meeting with a new patient. When clinicians formulate a number of hypotheses early in their diagnostic decision making, they are more likely to reject those that are incorrect in favor of those that are right. The second behavior is to sift systematically through all the possible diagnoses early on.

In this chapter we'll talk about two devices that can help us generate and evaluate alternative hypotheses. The differential diagnosis is the best way I know to ensure a comprehensive listing of all the possible causes of a patient's condition; we'll discuss it just below. The decision tree is a systematic method for sifting through the possibilities in that list. Regardless of our level of experience as clinicians, all of us can exploit these two keys to thinking about the diagnostic process.

> Two behaviors are vital for accurate diagnosis:
> 1. Beginning early in the process, consider all alternatives—think differential diagnosis.
> 2. Systematically sift through all possible diagnoses. Climb the decision tree.

The Differential Diagnosis

The *differential diagnosis* (this term is often shortened to *differential*) is a comprehensive list of conditions that could account for a patient's symptoms. For example, the possible diagnoses for a 23-year-old who hallucinates

would include psychotic depression, medication toxicity, mania, schizo- .
phrenia, alcohol misuse, and some medical conditions (such as epilepsy or
a brain tumor). If you've had little experience with the symptom at hand,
you'll need some help with creating such a list; in Part III of this book, I've
provided many examples. If you are an experienced clinician, you'll have
encountered dozens of patients who hallucinate, and you'll be able to rattle
off many possible disorders that could be responsible. However, even highly
experienced clinicians occasionally need to be reminded of the possibilities
in difficult or unusual cases. From my own experience, I know how important it is at least to glance at a list of differential possibilities. As an example,
I once encountered a patient with a baffling case of dementia.

> For several months, 58-year-old Alvin, a certified public accountant, had
> been having problems with his memory. At first he couldn't recall the lat-
> est changes in tax law; later he forgot appointments and blanked on the
> names of clients. Eventually he had to take leave from his job with a na-
> tional tax preparation firm. Within a few months, the ages of his children
> had escaped him; eventually he couldn't even remember *their* names.
> Now he could no longer care for himself, and his wife had to employ a
> practical nurse several hours a day just to cope with his bathing and feed-
> ing.
>   Alvin's doctor had diagnosed Alzheimer's disease, and was on the
> verge of recommending nursing home placement, when Alvin was hospi-
> talized for pneumonia. There a consulting neurologist put together sev-
> eral important observations: his relatively young age, a negative family
> history for Alzheimer's, his shuffling gait when he walked, and the unmis-
> takable odor of urine that clung to his clothing. The problem with walking
> and the loss of bladder control were the classic symptoms of normal-
> pressure hydrocephalus (NPH), a potentially correctable condition. When
> imaging studies confirmed the diagnosis, a shunting procedure was un-
> dertaken.

Had Alvin's first doctor worked through a careful differential diagnosis
of dementia, a nightmarish gradual deterioration might have been avoided.
Started soon enough, effective treatment for NPH can restore much of a
person's lost cognitive ability. Although it accounts for as many as 10% of
all dementia cases, NPH is much less common than other causes of
dementia—including Alzheimer's disease and cerebrovascular accidents
(strokes)—so it is often overlooked or forgotten.

The Safety Hierarchy

Alvin's tragedy illustrates that even experienced clinicians sometimes must be reminded about unusual conditions that may be treatable. There is more to creating a differential list than simply collecting syndromes; it makes a big difference how we arrange them. Think of it as you would a list of home repair jobs—paint the porch railing, sweep the garage, mend the pipe that's just burst in the basement. You don't just select a job at random to do first. Rather, you prioritize: "Hmm, maybe I really ought to deal with my flooded basement first."

So at the top you place emergencies, such as the burst pipe or a fire on the stove. In the middle will be those matters that are important but less urgent, such as mending a hole in the roof or exterminating the carpenter ants. Toward the bottom are the jobs that can wait until the other, higher-up tasks have been attended to—the patching, plastering, and painting that are all aspects of general maintenance. Note that what we put at the top won't necessarily be the most likely to occur: Defective pipes are pretty rare, especially compared with the amount of painting and plastering any house requires. In effect, we've created a *safety hierarchy* for home repairs.

And this is exactly what we need for our differential diagnosis—a way to list the possible diagnoses so as to expose our patients to the least possible risk of such perils as inadequate or downright erroneous treatment, inaccurate prognosis, social stigma, and inappropriate placement. A safety hierarchy places at the top those conditions that are most urgent to treat, are most likely to respond well to treatment, and have the best outcome. For me, a safe diagnosis is one that I'd prefer to have for myself or for a member of my family. Such a diagnosis, if it turns out to be correct and treatment is effective, could restore sanity, cure a threatening physical illness, or even save a life.

At the bottom go conditions that treatment seems unlikely to help—that have a terrible prognosis. Everything else goes somewhere in the middle. We'd probably get pretty good consensus among experienced clinicians as to what belongs in the top and bottom categories, but the exact order for what goes in the middle could be debated forever (and probably will be).

> *Diagnostic Principle:* Arrange your wide-ranging differential diagnosis according to a safety hierarchy.

Now our list has become a tool with which we can wring some sort of order out of the chaos that confronts us every time we evaluate a new patient. And with the safety hierarchy, we arrive at our first diagnostic

Diagnostic Principle: **Physical disorders and their treatment can produce or worsen mental symptoms.**

principle: List the items of your differential diagnosis according to a safety hierarchy, such as that in Table 3.1.

I need to mention one other thing here—well, two, really. The safety hierarchy sets us up for a couple of additional diagnostic principles. Notice what's right at the very top of the safety hierarchy: disorders that are due to a physical disease (you'll find quite a number of them listed in Table 9.1) or that are due to the effects of substance use (Tables 9.2 and 9.3). I'll have quite a lot more to say about these in Chapter 9, but for now let's just note that these two classes of conditions belong at the top of every differential diagnosis we create.

Diagnostic Principle: **The use of substances, including prescribed and over-the-counter medications, can cause a variety of mental disorders.**

TABLE 3.1. Hierarchy of Conservative (Safe) Diagnoses

Most desirable (most dangerous, most treatable, best outcome)
    Any disorder due to substance use or a medical illness
    Recurrent depression
    Mania or hypomania

Middle ground
    Alcohol dependence
    Panic disorder
    Phobic disorders
    Obsessive–compulsive disorder
    Anorexia nervosa
    Adjustment disorder
    Substance (other than alcohol) dependence
    Borderline personality disorder

Least desirable (hard to treat, poor outcome)
    Schizophrenia
    Antisocial personality disorder
    AIDS-related dementia
    Alzheimer's dementia

Note. Adapted from *Boarding Time: The Psychiatry Candidate's New Guide to Part II of the ABPN Examination* (3rd ed.) by James Morrison and Rodrigo A. Muñoz, 2003, Washington, DC: American Psychiatric Press. Copyright 2003 by the American Psychiatric Association. Adapted by permission.

More about Carson

To see a differential diagnosis in action, let's revisit Carson, whom we met at the beginning of Chapter 1. For the moment, we'll limit ourselves to the possible causes of his depression. Even an abbreviated list would include mood disorders (bipolar, major depressive disorder, and dysthymia); depression due either to a physical illness or to substance misuse; seasonal affective disorder; adjustment disorder with depressed mood; and some sort of personality disorder. As I have indicated above, we don't just write down what we consider *likely*, but also the "barely possibles." We include them all because every so often a real long shot comes in first, and we want to be alert and receptive when that happens. Even so, some of the conditions on this list appear a bit far-fetched. With a previous history of good health, the risk that Carson's depression was due to a physical illness such as a brain tumor or endocrine disorder would be pretty small. On the other hand, though we haven't read any evidence that suggests a personality disorder, there's no proof of its absence, either.

Although as Carson's clinicians we would have to contend with quite a long and complicated list of mental disorders, we'll use the safety hierarchy to create some order.

Depression related to a
   medical illness

Substance-related depression
} Treatable disorders that can quickly have a profound effect on a patient's health

Bipolar depression

Major depressive disorder

Seasonal mood disorder

Dysthymic disorder
} Disorders that are serious, but a little less urgent to treat

Adjustment disorder

Personality disorder
} Disorders that are chronic, have no specific treatment, or have a poor prognosis

In Table 3.2 I've listed differential diagnoses for the more common mental disorders. That is, in the row for each mental disorder listed in the left-hand column, I have indicated with an "×" each diagnosis in the column heads that should be considered in the differential for that disorder (the other mental disorders or conditions with which the index disorder shares at least one criterion or characteristic). The degree of similarity is strong in many cases (e.g., dysthymia and major depression); in others, the similarity is weak (e.g., schizophrenia and major depression, the latter of which includes psychotic symptoms only in extreme cases). Nonetheless, the purpose of a differential diagnosis is to list all possibilities, however remote. I've included physical and substance use causes everywhere—a reminder whenever you use the table to consider first these important causes of mental symptoms.

Of course, diagnoses on a list are only part of the battle; to do you and your patient any good, you must discriminate among them. To that end, the differential lists I've included in most of the chapters in Part III contain brief definitions for each disorder. The second issue is that the diagnoses in such a list aren't usually "ready to wear"; you can't just lift one off the rack and tell your patient to slip it on. This is especially true when someone has symptoms in several classes (depression, mania, psychosis, etc.). Your differential list could grow to include quite a lot of possibilities, and you may need to explore more than one decision tree, which we'll discuss next.

The Decision Tree

A *decision tree* is a device that guides the user through a series of steps to arrive at some goal, such as a diagnosis or treatment. On paper, it does look something like a tree, if you think of trees as growing upside down. You use it by answering a series of yes–no questions; each answer determines which branch to take next. The word *algorithm* is another way that this concept is commonly expressed.

I first ran across decision trees in biology, where they are used to identify unfamiliar plants. Whole books are devoted to keying out grasses, bushes, and other wild life from various parts of the world. Perhaps without realizing it, you have used a similar device to help make commonplace life choices. For example, let's consider a decision about where to have supper:

> "For a big occasion, and depending on my financial health, I'd like to have a really nice meal—the Ritz, if I can get a reservation, or Figaro's, which just opened, so it isn't crowded. Otherwise, I might go to the Sea Grotto, unless Mom comes along—she hates fish. Then we could try Chiquita's for tacos (unless it's Monday, when they're closed). But if this sneezing fit turns into the flu, my fall-back position is to fix veggie burgers at home."

TABLE 3.2. Differential Diagnosis by Diagnosis

Use these → diagnoses in the differential diagnosis for these disorders ↓	Physical causes	Subst. intox./withdr.	Delirium	Dementia	Schizophrenia	Schizoaffective dis.	Schizophreniform dis.	Delusional dis.	Shared psychotic dis.	Major depression	Dysthymia	Mania (bip. I)	Hypomania (bip. II)	Cyclothymia	Panic dis.	Agoraphobia	Specific phobia	Social phobia	OCD	PTSD	GAD	Somatization dis.	Pain dis.	Hypochondriasis	Body dysmorphic dis.	Any anxiety dis.	Dissoc. amnesia	Dissoc. fugue	Dissoc. identity dis.	Depers. dis.
Delirium	×	×	—	×	×	×	×	×		×		×														×				
Dementia	×	×	×	—	×					×																				
Subst. intox./withdr.	×	—																												
Schizophrenia	×	×	×	×	—	×	×	×	×	×		×										×								
Schizoaffective dis.	×	×	×	×	×	—		×		×		×										×				×				
Schizophreniform dis.	×	×	×	×	×	×	—	×	×	×		×										×								
Delusional dis.	×	×	×	×	×		×	—	×	×		×							×					×	×					
Shared psychotic dis.	×	×			×	×	×	×	—	×		×																		
Major depression	×	×			×	×	×	×		—	×	×	×	×								×								
Dysthymia	×	×									—											×								
Mania (bip. I)	×	×			×	×	×					—	×	×								×								
Hypomania (bip. II)	×	×								×	×	×	—	×								×								
Cyclothymia	×	×								×	×	×	×	—								×								
Panic dis.	×	×								×					—	×	×	×	×	×	×	×				×				
Agoraphobia	×	×													×	—	×	×	×			×								
Specific phobia	×														×	×	—	×				×		×						
Social phobia	×														×	×	×	—				×								
OCD	×	×						×							×	×			—			×		×	×					
PTSD	×	×																	×	—										
GAD	×	×														×		×	×	×	—	×								
Somatization dis.	×	×			×	×	×			×	×	×	×	×	×	×	×	×	×	×	×	—	×	×	×	×	×	×		
Pain dis.	×	×																				×	—							
Hypochondriasis	×	×						×									×					×	×	—	×					
Body dysmorphic dis.	×							×									×					×			—					
Dissoc. amnesia	×	×	×	×																		×					—	×	×	×
Dissoc. fugue	×	×																									×	—	×	×
Dissoc. identity dis.	×	×			×	×	×			×												×					×	×	—	×
Depersonalization dis.	×				×										×		×	×				×								—
Paraphilias	×	×		×																										
Gender identity dis.	×																													
Anorexia nervosa	×									×	×															×				
Bulimia nervosa	×									×																				
Intermitt. explos. dis.	×	×	×	×								×																		
Kleptomania	×	×	×									×																		
Pyromania	×	×	×									×																		
Path. gambling	×																													
Trichotillomania	×																		×											
Adjustment dis.	×	×																		×										
Paranoid PD	×	×			×	×		×																						
Schizoid PD	×	×			×			×																						
Schizotypal PD	×	×			×			×																						
Antisocial PD	×	×										×																		
Borderline PD	×	×								×	×	×																		
Histrionic PD	×	×																												
Narcissistic PD	×	×																												
Avoidant PD	×	×														×		×												
Dependent PD	×	×								×	×					×														
Obsess.–compul. PD	×	×																												

Note. OCD, obsessive–compulsive disorder; PTSD, posttraumatic stress disorder; GAD, generalized anxiety disorder; PD, personality disorder.

Use these → diagnoses in the differential diagnosis for these disorders ↓	Sexual dysfunctions	Paraphilias	Gender identity dis.	Anorexia nervosa	Bulimia nervosa	Intermitt. explos. dis.	Kleptomania	Pyromania	Path. gambling	Trichotillomania	Adjustment dis.	Paranoid PD	Schizoid PD	Schizotypal PD	Antisocial PD	Borderline PD	Histrionic PD	Narcissistic PD	Avoidant PD	Dependent PD	Obsess.–compul. PD	Personality change	Factitious dis.	Malingering	Normal decline	Mental retardation	Bereavement
Delirium																						×	×	×			
Dementia																						×	×	×	×		
Subst. intox./withdr.																											
Schizophrenia												×	×	×													
Schizoaffective dis.																											
Schizophreniform dis.												×	×	×													
Delusional dis.												×															
Shared psychotic dis.																											
Major depression									×																		×
Dysthymia																											
Mania (bip. I)																											
Hypomania (bip. II)																											
Cyclothymia																×											
Panic dis.																											
Agoraphobia																											
Specific phobia																											
Social phobia																			×								
OCD							×																				
PTSD											×													×			
GAD											×																
Somatization dis.	×			×	×										×	×							×	×			
Pain dis.																							×	×			
Hypochondriasis																											
Body dysmorphic dis.			×	×																							
Dissoc. amnesia																								×	×		
Dissoc. fugue																								×			
Dissoc. identity dis.																								×	×		
Depersonalization dis.																											
Paraphilias		—	×																				×			×	
Gender identity dis.		×	—																								
Anorexia nervosa				—	×																						
Bulimia nervosa				×	—																						
Intermitt. explos. dis.						—									×	×								×			
Kleptomania							—								×									×			
Pyromania								—							×											×	
Path. gambling									—						×												
Trichotillomania										—													×				
Adjustment dis.											—																×
Paranoid PD												—	×	×	×	×	×	×	×			×					
Schizoid PD												×	—	×					×			×	×				
Schizotypal PD												×	×	—		×		×	×			×					
Antisocial PD												×			—	×	×	×				×					
Borderline PD												×		×	×	—	×	×		×		×					
Histrionic PD															×	×	—	×		×		×					
Narcissistic PD												×		×	×	×	×	—				×					
Avoidant PD												×	×	×					—	×		×					
Dependent PD																	×	×	×	—		×					
Obsess.–compul. PD												×		×				×			—	×					

21

To work through these choices, you could set up a decision tree, which would look something like Figure 3.1. Of course, once you've made a decision, as a successful diner (or clinician) you should always remain alert for new information that could suggest the need for a last-minute change of plans.

Decision trees are somewhat like training wheels: useful when you're learning, but something you remove and store in the garage later on. If you want to see how the decision tree is used for a patient, you can skip ahead to Chapter 11, where we'll employ one to explore Carson's diagnosis further.

Before moving on, let's take a break (maybe we'll have a plate of nachos at Chiquita's—let's hope this isn't Monday) and recap our diagnostic method so far. We've learned to aggregate symptoms and signs into familiar groups, called *syndromes*. Because they can have many causes, we gather the syndromes a patient might have into a list, called a *differential diagnosis*, which we arrange into a *safety hierarchy*. Perhaps aided by the use of a *decision tree*, we'll find our working diagnosis at or near the top of that hierarchy.

Pass the salsa, *por favor.*

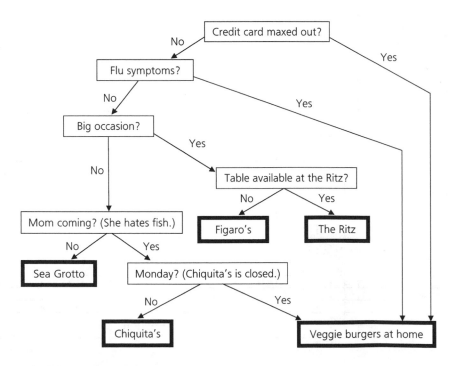

FIGURE 3.1. A decision tree for dining.

4 Putting It Together

And now you have the chance to put together all the material you have gathered for your patient and create a diagnosis that will guide treatment and predict outcome. The chapters of Part III focus on specific areas of diagnostic interest; this chapter covers the basics of how you can weave together the various threads of information to create an initial diagnosis. The first big issue is judging the relative value of the pieces of information you have assembled.

Sometimes, of course, everything points in the same direction:

> Nedra was a 78-year-old widow whose daughter-in-law and son related that over the past 2 years her memory had gradually worsened. At first, she only seemed to misplace things; with time, she progressively forgot conversations she had just had, could not remember how to prepare certain favorite foods, and several times forgot to turn off a burner on the stove. Always a cheerful, positive person who had never had a word to say against anyone, now she appeared morose and angry. Her only family history of mental disorder was in her own mother, who, after a lengthy period of decline, had been diagnosed as "senile" by the family doctor a year before she died in a nursing home. When examined, Nedra refused to shake hands and would only respond, "Damned foolishness," when asked to identify her son. When a nurse's aide walked into the room, Nedra began to curse and mutter racial epithets.

Nedra's diagnosis of Alzheimer's is suggested powerfully by three data sources: the recent history, the family history, and the current MSE. There's nothing to suggest a different diagnosis, though data from a routine physical exam and laboratory screening would have to be obtained.

Such unanimity among sources isn't always the case. Consider the history of Rusty.

When he was 23, and again at 28, Rusty had been clinically depressed. Despite the fact that his father had for many years been "a hopeless alcoholic," as Rusty's mother put it, with each episode Rusty had been treated with antidepressant medication and responded rapidly and completely each time. For several years between episodes, he had seemingly required no medication. Now he was 36, had just gotten remarried, and had become depressed for the third time. This time, however, there was a difference: Whereas during his two previous episodes he had complained of rather severe terminal insomnia, this time he felt "forever tired" and slept 12 hours a day. His clinician referred Rusty to an internist, who determined that his thyroid was severely underperforming. Within a week of starting thyroid replacement hormone as his only medication, Rusty was on his way back to normal.

Rusty's past history told one story; his family history told another. And then along came a third episode—with a subtle difference in symptoms. When one line of information contradicts another, determining what weight to give the various lines of evidence can pose problems.

When Information Sources Conflict

Fortunately, a number of diagnostic principles can help sort out the confusion that can result from conflicting information sources.

History Beats Current Appearance

Clinicians need to keep reminding themselves that accurate diagnosis depends heavily on the previous history of mental illness. Take delusions as an example: What does it really mean when Jerome reports feeling that a scanning radio has been implanted in his brain? Of course, he could have schizophrenia, which is what we usually (sometimes mistakenly) think of first when considering any psychotic symptom. But delusions can also take place in the context of a substance use disorder, dementia, or even antisocial personality disorder. In particular, they may characterize severe depression and mania.

Five years earlier, Dick had been hospitalized when he became acutely excited and psychotic. Believing that he had the divine power of healing, he had wandered the streets, placing his hands on the head of any person using a wheel chair he met and praying. He was hospitalized for several months, during which he received antipsychotic drugs. Subsequent to his discharge, he developed what was called a "postpsychotic depression"; in its depths, he left his position at work and isolated himself almost completely from his family life. He later reported that several times during this period, he had nearly killed himself.

Eventually, however, Dick recovered completely and took a better job than the one he had resigned. Reunited with his family, Dick prospered for 3 years until once again, while attending an out-of-town convention, he became acutely confused and began entering the homes of strangers, where he would inform the startled residents that he was the "literal brother of Christ." Again hospitalized, this time he was diagnosed with bipolar I disorder and treated with antipsychotics and lithium. He recovered within 10 days, after which he was successfully maintained on lithium alone.

Dick's MSE suggested schizophrenia, but the historical information conveyed a far different picture: abrupt onset (the onset of schizophrenia would be gradual) and complete recovery (with schizophrenia we'd expect some residual symptoms). Patients with schizophrenia sometimes have extremely severe and long-lasting depressions, but these are far more typical of bipolar I disorder. In other words, for Dick, as for many mental health patients, the longitudinal history suggestive of bipolar I disorder far outweighed the MSE that seemed to say "schizophrenia." Using the course of illness as the basis for diagnosis was first described in 1852 by French psychiatrist Benedict Morel, who also coined the term *dementia praecox*, an early name for schizophrenia.

Sorting out a delusion's true meaning requires us to focus on many elements from the patient's history, including the presence of physical health

> **Diagnostic Principle:** A patient's history often provides better guidance for diagnosis than does the cross-sectional appearance (MSE).

problems, family history of mental illness, or severe depression or mania. How long have they been present? Do drugs or alcohol seemingly cause them to appear? Do they regress only with medication, or do they come and go spontaneously? These historical considerations, of course, apply to hallucinations and to many other symptoms that the patient presents. We'll discuss them more fully in Parts II and III.

Recent History Beats Ancient History

Here we pay homage to the fact that symptoms reported early in the course of a patient's illness may carry far less diagnostic information than later evidence may.

> When I first saw Nancy as an office patient, she was just 16 and none too delighted to be there. Her mother had insisted on the appointment, however, because of Nancy's problem with appetite. "Her weight just keeps going down," Mom said, "and she picks at her food. I'm so afraid that she has anorexia, like Julie down the street." But Nancy denied thinking that she was too fat. "I guess I do look kinda skinny," she confided, in what was just about the last complete sentence she would speak before dropping out of treatment. She told her mother that she'd try to eat more and not to bug her, and that seemed to be the end of it.
>
> At the time, I realized that Nancy could have anorexia nervosa or another eating disorder, but that depression and schizophrenia were also possibilities. It could even turn out that her symptom was just an expression of the problems nearly all adolescents experience while becoming adults. I didn't learn the answer until one afternoon 8 years later, when Nancy returned on her own, again with loss of appetite—and a 15-pound weight loss. This time, she admitted that her mood was so low she was having trouble performing on her job as a bank junior officer. To the consternation of her fiancé, her sex interest had dropped to near zero, and she was even having thoughts about suicide. Her diagnosis this time was clearly severe depression; I suspected that, in attenuated form, this had also been her problem as a teenager.

Diagnostic Principle: **A patient's recent history often more accurately indicates diagnosis than does older history.**

Clinicians of long experience have had similar encounters with anxiety symptoms (will they become generalized anxiety disorder [GAD], panic disorder, or a mood disorder?) and depression (will it become bipolar I or II disorder, dysthymia, or an adjustment disorder?). When older symptoms are clarified, newer ones can change diagnosis and inform treatment.

Collateral History Sometimes Beats the Patient's Own

Let's not go overboard here. Of course, what drives diagnosis is largely what your patient tells you. But some patients lack perspective on their own difficulties. An elderly widow who lives alone may not realize how forgetful she has become; a teenage boy may grow up unaware of how troublesome his gang affiliations have been. Occasionally, someone just plain lies. Even patients who try their best to provide accurate, complete information may simply lack access to family history or early social history, with its sometimes crucial influence on diagnosis.

A biology student at a local college, Jack complained about "indecision and lack of direction." He told me that he feared he was developing schizophrenia, the diagnosis for which his father had been institutionalized years ago. When later (with Jack's permission) I met privately with his mother, she told me that Jack was not their biological child, but the product of a brief relationship her younger sister had had with her boss. The older sister and her husband had adopted Jack at birth and had never told him the truth about his origins. Her husband's diagnosis thus had no biological bearing on Jack's own illness.

> *Diagnostic Principle:* **Obtain collateral history whenever possible; it is sometimes more accurate than the patient's own.**

Signs Beat Symptoms

Here we need to insist on the technical definitions of signs (what you observe about the patient) and symptoms (what the patient tells you seems to be wrong). The trouble with symptoms is that they can carry two different interpretations—yours and the patient's. Some patients may not understand your interpretation; others may even misconstrue your meaning as they report it to others. In other words, signs are more objective and can sometimes more reliably indicate a patient's true diagnosis.

You've probably encountered the phenomenon yourself—perhaps when an office patient, with eyes filling quietly with tears, denies feeling hurt when abandoned by a lover. More striking denials are those of the gaunt patient with anorexia nervosa who claims to look fat, or the patient with schizophrenia who denies hallucinations but keeps glancing uneasily around the room.

Imogene was a patient with somatization disorder who lay on a gurney in the urgent care center, immobilized by "complete paralysis" from the waist down, yet nonchalantly chewed gum and discussed with a nurse the just-played Super Bowl game. This sort of disconnection between the sign of her emotion and her physical symptom of paralysis was a classic example of *la belle indifférence*, or emotional insensitivity.

> *Diagnostic Principle:* Signs (what you observe about a patient) can be a better guide to diagnosis than symptoms (what the patient tells you).

Be Wary of Crisis-Generated Data

When people are acutely troubled, it can affect how they view the world and their place in it. If your patient has just been fired, bereaved, or jilted by a lover, the resulting mood can color the tone of the story you hear, even to the point of affecting the patient's perspective on experiences that occurred long ago.

> The day after her apartment was burglarized, Jill complained that she was the unluckiest person in the world: "I *never* catch a break!" she moaned. Her therapist, who had known her for some time, decided it was time to institute a course of cognitive-behavioral therapy, in an effort to help her deal with the negative stereotypes she held of herself.

> *Diagnostic Principle:* The stress of crisis can color how a patient perceives life's experiences.

The flip side is that a positive experience like the joy of new love can also distort a person's understanding of reality.

Objective Findings Beat Subjective Judgments

Here's a reminder that clinicians' intuitions, while sometimes uncannily accurate, should never outrank verifiable information. The "schizophrenic feel" you might experience when talking to a new patient should only prompt due diligence in your hunt for signs and symptoms. My own favorite *bête noir*, borderline personality disorder, is a diagnosis that clinicians often make without full evaluation.

> Or take 19-year-old Henry, whose slow, quiet speech, level gaze, and sad smile created instant sympathy in his interviewer. Although he claimed not to know what triggered his anxiety attacks, just a few minutes' conversation made it seem likely that he had panic disorder. Perhaps it covered a pretty severe major depressive episode. These predictions were

shattered when more history was obtained from his older sister, who accompanied him to his appointment. She reported that he had been increasingly distressed by his feelings about his own sexual orientation. Confusion, shame, and fears that his homophobic father would become enraged had caused him to confide only in her. With the sister's additional information, adjustment disorder moved closer to the top of the differential diagnosis.

> *Diagnostic Principle:* **Resist the allure of the hunch—embrace objective data as the bedrock of diagnosis.**

Consider Family History

For decades, we've known that mental disorders run in families. Indeed, during the last half of the 20th century, a great deal of work established the fact that there is a strong genetic component to many (perhaps most) of the syndromes we confront every day. In Chapter 8 we'll consider the issues surrounding family history in greater detail, but for now we'll just note an example:

> Although Grant had always been a quiet, thoughtful boy, his behavior became erratic not long after he turned 15. For several months his family endured verbal outbursts over minor disappointments. He became belligerent, several times on the street accosting total strangers who he thought had "looked funny" at him. One afternoon after school, he actually picked a fight with a policeman—who escorted him to the emergency room, where he talked to himself in apparent response to auditory hallucinations. Twice he masturbated openly in the ward day room. After a week on antipsychotic medication, he was not much better, and the staff wondered whether he had schizophrenia. However, a consultant noted that years ago Grant's uncle (his mother's brother) had had an acute psychosis, and had subsequently been successfully maintained on lithium. With the addition of a mood stabilizer, Grant's psychosis rapidly resolved.

Although it would be unwise to base your entire therapeutic strategy on a single piece of data, family history can establish a useful signpost on your diagnostic path. I will qualify this point somewhat (and will provide a revised version of the following diagnostic principle) at the end of Chapter 8, but for the moment let us state the principle as follows:

> *Diagnostic Principle:* **Family history can guide diagnosis.**

Simplify with Occam's Razor

William of Occam, a 14th-century English philosopher, stated a law of economy that applies in many fields beyond health care. Now a mainstay of
medical diagnosis, it advises that if something has two possible explana-
tions, you should choose the simpler one. Because it "shaves away" concepts that are not necessary, it has come to be known as *Occam's razor*, or
the principle of parsimony.

When he was 47 years old, Jakob appeared at the emergency room complaining of two problems: He felt terribly depressed, and he had been
hearing voices. The depression had so plagued him for several months
that he felt "at the end of [his] tether." He feared he was close to committing suicide—the fate of his older brother, Hans, only 2 years earlier.
Jakob admitted that his appetite had been depressed; he slept poorly; he
had little interest in his usual activities (he was an avid collector of old
guns and usually haunted antique shows); and his concentration at work
was so poor that his boss had ordered him to take time off to "get straight-
ened out." Jakob believed he had let everyone down, including his boss
and his family, and he felt enormously guilty and deserving of death.

The voices had troubled him for only a few days. He heard them just
behind his left ear and, though he didn't know their cause, they seemed
terribly real. At all hours of the day and through much of the night, two
strangers, a man and a woman, shouted that he was "a real bum" and told
him that he should use one of his weapons "for the purpose God intended
them"—that is, to kill himself. Tears welled in his eyes and his lip trem-
bled as he stammered, "I feel really terrified."

Although Jakob resisted talking about it, he did admit to drinking "a
little too much, now and again." Close questioning revealed the following:
Whereas for 20 years he had consumed nearly three fifths of hard liquor a
week, over the past 6 months his alcohol intake had nearly doubled. A
week earlier, "stomach flu" had caused him to vomit so often that he
couldn't keep anything down, not even alcohol. It was shortly afterward
that the voices began their insistent clamor.

A novice diagnostician might consider Jakob to be suffering from three
different mental disorders: major depression, an acute psychotic disorder,
and alcohol dependence. Occam's razor, however, pares the problem to its
essentials: As is quite common in alcohol dependence, Jakob's heavy alcohol use eventually induced a severe depression. When he became physically ill (was it really flu, or did his system finally rebel at so much alco-

hol?), he went into alcohol withdrawal and heard voices. The auditory hallucinations a person with alcohol dependence experiences upon withdrawal closely mimic those of schizophrenia. Occam's razor thus allows us to propose that Jakob had one basic illness upon which many other symptoms and two additional mental diagnoses were built.

Such parsimonious thinking is important in part because it helps us understand what not to do. For example, Jakob's depression would probably abate once he stopped drinking. Antidepressant medication would both burden his system with yet more chemicals and reinforce the idea that his depression was an independent illness that could be dealt with chemically, without facing the issues of his alcohol dependence. The diagnosis of a psychosis due to alcohol use would militate against the long-term use of antipsychotic agents: Once Jakob was off alcohol, his hallucinations would surely disappear within days.

> *Diagnostic Principle:* **Use Occam's razor: Prefer the diagnosis that provides the simplest explanation for your data.**

Zebras and Horses

The healing professions have a saying, taught to generations of students: "If you hear hoofbeats in the streets, think of horses, not zebras." In other words, be aware of the not-too-surprising fact that you are more likely to encounter common disorders than uncommon ones, and adjust your diagnostic thinking accordingly. This highly useful adage is also a diagnostic principle, but it can be used in a right way or a wrong way.

The wrong way is to make it the mainstay of your diagnostic strategy, as I've seen happen, especially in regard to depression. We clinicians so often encounter what appears to be major depressive disorder that it tends to crowd out competing possibilities. Because it is readily reimbursed by insurance, clinicians often feel pressured to use this term instead of other, less well-compensated diagnoses, such as personality or adjustment disorders. Some writers have quite seriously suggested that a purely statistical approach to diagnosis (that is, always diagnose major depression, which is encountered in over 50% of mental health patients, especially in the outpatient arena) could be a winning strategy more than half the time. Of course, what you want for your patients is to be right *all* the time, or as nearly so as possible.

The apparent rarity of any condition depends on the population you typically work with. If you are employed in a mental hospital, psychotic patients with schizophrenia and bipolar disorders may constitute the bulk of your practice. If you only see outpatients, you'll probably encounter many who have anxiety disorders or mild to moderate depression. Similarly (no surprise), you'll find a lot of people with drug-induced disorders in substance use treatment facilities, and persons with PTSD in Department of Veterans Affairs (VA) hospitals. It's seductive, isn't it, to think that if you see a regressed patient in a nursing home, Alzheimer's dementia will be the diagnosis? Alas, you can't rely for your diagnosis on the popularity of a given condition in your own patient population. I've encountered depression in veterans (who often have PTSD); bipolar disorders in schoolboys (who typically have attention-deficit/hyperactivity disorder [ADHD]); and many, many instances of depression (and mania too) in geriatric patients.

A better way to use the "horses, not zebras" principle is always to consider common diagnoses, but not to the point of ignoring other possibilities. For example (as we'll discuss in Chapter 10), when formulating a differential diagnosis I often include mood disorders, though they may not make the final cut.

When Irwin came to the mental health clinic, he had felt depressed for nearly 6 months. His symptoms were pretty typical, the clinician thought—trouble sleeping, loss of appetite (though his weight had actually increased a few pounds), feelings that he was a failure, and inability to focus on his work as a designer of kitchen remodels. He emphatically denied any thoughts about suicide. It was his boss who suggested the appointment, because Irwin seemed to be suffering so much. At age 38, he had never had previous emotional difficulties; he neither drank nor used drugs.

The weight gain puzzled his clinician, who wondered whether, in the face of reduced appetite, the depression could have a physical cause (such as hypothyroidism or another endocrine disorder). To be on the safe side, Irwin agreed to a checkup from his family practitioner, whom he hadn't seen for "almost longer than I can remember." In the meantime, recognizing that a physical cause for a mood disorder like Irwin's was a long shot, the clinician started cognitive-behavioral therapy with him.

The diagnosis of a rare disorder is so attractive that it can seduce you into ignoring more common causes for whatever mental symptoms the patient has. Making (and reporting) such a finding is a coup; the clinician achieves instant hero status. Whereas it is vital always to keep in mind that such a thing is possible, a measured approach that also em-

Diagnostic Principle: Horses are more common than zebras; prefer the more frequently encountered diagnosis.

ploys Occam's razor melds the benefits of accurate diagnosis with speedy treatment. (In the event, the concerns of Irwin's clinician were set to rest when a workup revealed no evidence of a physical cause for depression.)

Evaluating Your Data for a Differential Diagnosis

Putting the principles discussed above to work in the service of an everyday diagnosis may seem daunting. However, if we follow the steps below, we'll end up with a viable differential list that leads to a working diagnosis, which will help us formulate a prognosis and recommend treatment. I've never met a patient whose condition required that I use all the diagnostic principles at once, but the somewhat more detailed case vignette that follows will serve to illustrate several of them.

Edna

Edna had recently become engaged, yet she had begun having anxiety episodes that she was afraid would make her lose her scholarship. "Could I just have a few Valiums to get me through finals?" she begged the counselor who saw her. "Maybe we should try to understand the whole picture first," came the reply. The story was too complicated for a few tablets to fix.

Edna had been a cheerful, somewhat roly-poly baby born to first-time parents when they were in their 40s. Her mother juggled a professional career and obsessive–compulsive disorder (OCD), which limited the time she spent with baby Edna. Her father traveled on business; when home, he spent much of his free time attending Alcoholics Anonymous (AA) meetings to maintain his rather tenuous sobriety. As a result, Edna was reared by a succession of housekeepers whose principal duties weren't child care. Left largely to her own devices, she grew up with books and television for friends, and not much in the way of social graces. She was a moody child to begin with, and her disposition didn't improve when her menstrual periods started at age 13.

Edna reported that she had been "unnaturally shy." In fact, throughout high school she had had only one date, and that was with a second-string football player who had tried to have sex with her after the movies. "He got me down to my underwear before good judgment grabbed hold, and I got dressed." Throughout high school and her first 3 years of college, she immersed herself in study and not much else. By the fall of her senior year, she was on track to graduate a semester early, *summa cum laude* in political science.

Near Christmas, she met a young man. Always persuaded that she would never marry, she hadn't bothered much with her looks, but this year a roommate had taught her how to fix her hair and burned the tacky pair of jeans she wore to class nearly every day. Perhaps the new clothes and lipstick did the trick; her young man, himself a perpetual wallflower, had pursued her vigorously and proposed on the second date. On the spot, she accepted him. "I guess I was so grateful that I just said 'Yes,' " she commented to the clinician. "It was the happiest night of my life, to coin a cliché." It was also the last truly happy day she'd had.

In the week since, Edna had spent many anxious hours. "I feel afraid—though of what, God knows—and I get short of breath and my heart beats too fast. It makes my chest hurt." In 2 days she would introduce Geoffrey to her parents, and she felt nauseated at the prospect. Now she stayed up at night, trying to study, worrying that she would fail her final exams and have to remain in school an extra year. She also worried about how her parents would regard Geoffrey. Most of all, she worried about the prospect of getting married and perhaps having the responsibility of a family. Edna's facial expression was lively, though concerned; once or twice she became appropriately tearful, but otherwise she spoke pleasantly enough, showing good command of her facts and speaking logically in complete sentences.

Toward the end of the evaluation, Edna mentioned that her roommate wanted to speak with the clinician. Ann's information was brief, but important: Edna seemed just fine when she was with Ann. It was only when she was with Geoffrey, or was about to see him, or sometimes was even talking about him, that she seemed flooded with anxiety.

Here's how I'd go about mining Edna's history to create a broad-ranging differential diagnosis:

1. As in any differential diagnosis, I would first question whether there was a medical or substance use problem (two diagnostic principles that I've already mentioned, and that we'll cover further in Chapter 9). Of course, I consider medical disorder causes first—not because they are so terribly common, but because of the considerable potential for causing mischief to the patient and for being effectively treated. Either the current use of or withdrawal from substance use commonly causes anxiety, and Edna had asked her doctor for Valium.

2. Because Edna's chief complaint was anxiety, I'd then review the full spectrum of anxiety disorders, summarized in Table 12.1. She could have an incipient panic disorder or GAD, though the course of her symptoms had been very brief. The history of her present illness informs many of the choices in our differential diagnosis.

3. The family history diagnostic principle strikes! Edna's mother was at one time treated for OCD, which runs in families. Its presence suggests potential diagnoses for Edna. Genetic studies have told us repeatedly that a patient with an anxiety disorder is likely to have relatives with a variety of other anxiety disorders, not just the one.

4. What wouldn't I include from the anxiety disorders list? I'd agree there's no evidence for agoraphobia, and Edna said nothing about phobias, other than whatever might be implied by the prospect of growing old without a mate. Although Geoffrey's sudden proposal preceded Edna's symptoms, it would be a real stretch to frame her story as a stress disorder (PTSD or other).

5. Among the other items of information from the initial assessment, we note Edna's somewhat isolated childhood, which suggests the possibility of avoidant personality disorder. (However, later on we'll note a diagnostic principle that cautions us to be wary of diagnosing a personality disorder in the face of an active Axis I disorder.) And by the way, I'd certainly want to rule out somatization disorder for any young woman.

6. I don't mean to slight the MSE; however, its components often serve best to guide an interviewer to fertile fields for evaluation. Edna's tearfulness did show some evidence of depression, which I nearly always include in a differential diagnosis.

7. This vignette also demonstrates the important yet often ignored principle that collateral history can help frame the discussion of diagnosis. The information from Edna's roommate provided something that Edna seemingly could not—perspective on timing and precipitating events. The "horses, not zebras" diagnostic principle reminds us that we should especially consider those diagnoses that occur commonly in the general population, among which are situational problems (also known as problems of living).

Considering all of the points made above, I'd want to consider the following differential diagnosis in evaluating Edna's problem (I'll leave it as an exercise to arrange these items in a safely hierarchy and determine the best diagnosis overall):

- Adjustment disorder with anxiety symptoms (problems of living)
- Anxiety disorder due to medical problem
- Avoidant personality disorder
- Depressive disorder
- GAD
- OCD
- Panic disorder without agoraphobia
- Somatization disorder
- Substance-related anxiety disorder

Dealing with Contradictory Information

When clinicians with years of experience face contradictory information, the appropriate diagnosis often seems to emerge almost by instinct. As I'll try to show with another fairly detailed vignette, this apparent intuition is usually just a matter of noticing when clues from the history conflict with one another, or when cues from the MSE don't match up with the usual course of a mental disorder. Resolving contradictory information is not a matter of spiritualism but of practice. I feel strongly enough about this to call it a diagnostic principle.

> *Diagnostic Principle:* Watch for contradictory information, such as affect that doesn't fit the content of thought, or symptoms that don't match the usual history of a disorder.

Tony

Tony was only 45, but as he related his complicated history, he looked a good 10 years older. Homeless and severely depressed, he suffered from poor concentration and appetite, punishing insomnia, inability to work, and recurrent death wishes and suicidal attempts. During one such attempt, he parked his car in a remote area and ran a hose from the exhaust into the passenger compartment, started the engine, then settled down to die. That attempt failed when the gas ran out before he even lost consciousness. More recently, he pointed a borrowed pistol at his head. Because several friends intervened to take it away from him, he fired all five shots harmlessly into the ceiling.

That episode prompted his admission to a VA hospital, where he was treated with medications. (Of all the antidepressants he had tried over the years, he felt that Prozac helped him the most.) While in the hospital, Tony applied for housing assistance, which was ultimately denied—he didn't know why. Subsequently, he apparently checked himself out of the hospital; 4 days later, he found himself 200 miles away, in yet another VA hospital. He didn't know how he traveled from one city to the other, and he could not recall what happened during the lost time. At first he couldn't even dredge up personal information such as his Social Security number, though he was always able to state his name.

Besides depression, Tony stated that for many years he had intermittently heard several different voices. There was his mother's voice, which laughed at him, and the voice of his dead brother. A stranger he knew only as "Cathy" pronounced his name so clearly that every time he heard it, he turned to see who might be there. He had heard none of these voices for several days prior to the current evaluation. From time to time he also had visual hallucinations of a man who stands about 12 inches tall, whom he had seen for the first time many years ago on Okinawa when serving in the army. He also sometimes saw his mother (who is alive) in a scene "so real I could touch her." From time to time he felt that she and other people were "laughing behind my back."

During his interview, Tony's mood appeared to be about medium in quality and appropriate to the content of his thought. His affect, normal in its lability, became tearful when he was discussing his failed marriage. This story was that two decades ago he had married a woman from Colombia, taking pains to ensure that she, her children, and her mother all became legal U.S. residents. As the result of his wife's unfounded accusations and legal chicanery, he ended up living in a hotel room while she and her family continued to occupy his house. He eventually abandoned all his property and moved on to become a security guard at a casino. He claimed never to have used alcohol or street drugs intemperately.

As a child, Tony was always depressed. Nearly friendless, he had concocted his own playmates, including a rubber lizard he called "Tonto" and a number of imaginary playmates. He had a clubbed foot that was treated with a cast, which he remembered kicking through the boards of his crib, even when he was just a small baby.

Analysis

Some of Tony's data conflicted either with one another or with common sense. For example, the repeated suicide attempts that had gone badly (though fortunately) awry seemed exaggerated and possibly insincere. In answer to his devastating marriage, he stoically shouldered his fate and moved on. The visual hallucinations of his mother were more vivid than is usual for psychosis. Seeing Lilliputian people is characteristic of delirium tremens, yet he denied the use of alcohol. He had named one of the voices he heard, which is unusual in psychosis. Whereas psychotic people try to ignore their tormenting hallucinations, he invariably turned to see who was talking. While in a purported fugue-like state, he traveled with apparent purpose to another VA hospital, where he was not known. Although he could have been recounting what others had told him, some of his statements about his own childhood seemed extravagant: He had "always" been depressed; he could recall kicking his crib. Finally, despite his many afflictions and sorrowful history, his mood on interview was comfortable, not depressed.

Taken one at a time, these characteristics might seem unimpressive, but in aggregate they would create a reasonable suspicion of a patient trying to present himself as sicker and needier than he really was. This clinical picture, which would also fit with a motivation for the secondary gain of being housed, would place a duty upon the clinician to reject the story's face value and to investigate further before making a diagnosis and recommending treatment.

Malingering

I hate it when I have to diagnose malingering. Of course, if I refuse, I can't fulfill my duty as a diagnostician—but once someone's been labeled as a "malingerer," the cat's among the pigeons, and it's hard ever again to regard that individual as anything but a liar. If someone admits to inventing a story, and if I can be absolutely sure of my ground, I will limit my statement to that one piece of behavior: "History of fugue state was fabricated." In other words, I label the behavior as "malingering" rather than the person as a "malingerer."

My reluctance to use these terms stems from the twin facts that, especially for mental events, malingering is terribly hard to prove, and there are no valid criteria. A patient series that demonstrates my concern was reported from Israel in the journal *Military Medicine* in 1996. Of 24 individuals diagnosed as "malingerers" in the course of a year, the authors rediagnosed nearly all as having serious psychopathology, including psychosis, mental retardation, and mood disorders. All but 3 of the 24 were judged unfit to serve in the military.

The manufacture of physical symptoms is relatively easy to spot: Careful observation will reveal that the patient claiming to have a kidney stone drops grains of sand into a urine specimen, or that an apparently persistent fever has been augmented by stirring coffee with the thermometer. Much more difficult to detect is emotional fakery, which can include amnesia, PTSD, psychosis, eating disorders, bereavement, depression, mania, and even stalking. I've discussed some of the warning signs in the sidebar "Recognizing Red Flag Information."

Besides the prospect of obtaining money—think insurance fraud—a variety of motives can encourage the reporting of false symptoms. Some patients want to avoid social responsibilities (such as work or child support) or dangerous assignments (especially in the military). Many clinicians have encountered patients who fake pain to obtain prescription drugs they can sell or misuse. An occasional person may minimize actual mental symptoms, "faking good" to win release from a mental hospital or win custody of a child. And a well-known motive is to avoid punishment for a crime, through a plea of reduced capacity or insanity.

One of the most notorious (and nearly successful) instances of blatant malingering was that of Kenneth Bianchi, one of two men who carried out the Hillside Strangler murders in the 1970s in Los Angeles and Washington State. A charming, lifelong chronic liar, Bianchi had previously set himself up as a psychotherapist with fake diplomas and credentials, including a "doctor of psychiatry" from a nonexistent institution. When caught, Bianchi produced a second personality, Steven, who brazenly claimed responsibility for the murders ("Killing a broad doesn't make any difference to me"). So persuasive was this performance that several clinicians who were experts in multiple personality disorder (MPD, now referred to as dissociative identity disorder) pronounced him psychotic and thereby not accountable for his crime. But Bianchi met his match when the prosecution brought in psychiatrist Martin Orne, who told him (falsely) that all cases of MPD have more than two personalities. Within hours, a third personality obligingly emerged. One of the clinicians who had been taken in, after becoming a prison psychiatrist and learning that he had "no reason to believe anything they said," later recanted belief in Kenneth's MPD.

There are degrees of malingering. In the most blatant cases, patients simply make symptoms up; others exaggerate actual symptoms. Still others may falsely attribute their symptoms to something they know is not actually the cause; for example, a patient may claim that anxiety symptoms, actually of long standing, arose after a minor industrial accident.

Whether history and behaviors are merely augmented or are made up out of whole cloth, clinicians must consider a rather substantial differential diagnosis. Besides malingering, it includes factitious disorder (most famously, persons with Münchausen syndrome, who obtain admission to a succession of hospitals) and, as seems probable in the case of Kenneth Bianchi, antisocial personality disorder. You may encounter unconsciously augmented or made-up symptoms in patients with various somatoform and dissociative disorders.

Recognizing Red Flag Information

A variety of characteristics raise the red flag of warning that a patient's data cannot be accepted at face value. Before fully trusting information, you must compare it with interview data from informants, with previous medical records, with laboratory tests, or perhaps you should test it by the simple means of further frank discussion. Especially revealing among such items of history and behavior are the following, listed in no particular order:

Memory loss in the absence of cognitive disorder. A poor memory, readily fabricated and difficult to verify, can prove irresistible for patients who have something to hide or to gain.

Spotty amnesia. Someone may claim not to remember personal information, but can converse about contemporary issues of the day.

Extreme language to describe symptoms. Examples of such descriptions include "I lost 20 pounds in 3 days," "I sometimes go a whole week without a wink of sleep."

Criminal behavior in a hospitalized patient. This may include assaults, sex with staff or other patients, and dealing drugs.

Repeated unsuccessful suicide attempts. Although many patients make multiple, sincere efforts to end their lives, others seem to be play-acting in an effort to attract attention or sympathy. The danger is that it isn't always easy to tell one from the other.

Unusual symptoms. By unusual, I mean symptoms that are excessively dramatic, rare, or severe—beyond the usual range of psychopathology. One example was Tony's behavior on hearing voices (he turned to confront them every time he heard them). Others would be claims to have schizophrenia characterized by delusions that begin or end suddenly, visual hallucinations of foot-high people, or hallucinations that are continuous rather than intermittent. The onset of symptoms may be more sudden that is usual for the given diagnosis (e.g., delusions that appear full-blown overnight). Symptoms of many disorders at the same time can sometimes be a tip-off. Of course, some patients read enough textbooks to know something about typical presentations of mental illness.

Absence of typical symptoms. For example, most depressed people will have problems with sleep and appetite; the absence of such problems should raise suspicions.

A story that keeps changing. People who make up or exaggerate material may find it hard to keep their stories straight.

Multiple personalities. Genuine MPD has been well documented for decades, but so has the fabrication of "alternates" by some people to avoid detection or punishment for criminal or otherwise unwelcome behavior.

Secondary gain. Symptoms that help a person gain money or avert loss require thoughtful evaluation.

History that conflicts with the usual course of a mental disorder. For example, if a patient who has worked steadily for a decade claims a long history of schizophrenia, this should arouse suspicions.

Poor cooperation. Patients who evade or outright refuse to answer questions during testing or the interview may have something to hide.

Incongruous affect. Bland or even cheerful affect that doesn't match a person's serious circumstances, such as paralysis or blindness, is called *la belle indifférence*; it is often encountered in patients with conversion disorders. However, a silly or otherwise incongruous affect can also be encountered in schizophrenia, disorganized type.

Interpersonal manner. Some researchers have documented our tendency as clinicians to believe assertive individuals who have pleasant facial expressions and dominate the conversation. We need to be alert lest these characteristics overwhelm our judgment of a patient's essential truthfulness.

Performance below chance on standard tests of memory, cognition, or intellect. Even random answers should yield performance at chance levels; to score below chance requires planning. Some patients give blatantly false answers: "2 times 2 is 5," "Santa's suit is green," "There are 30 hours in a day."

Hospitalization in many locations. In what is classically referred to as Münchausen's syndrome, patients move from one caregiving institution to another.

Normally adequate treatment that doesn't help. A patient who remains depressed after treatment with five different antidepressants, cognitive-behavioral therapy, and a course of electroconvulsive therapy deserves a complete reevaluation rather than yet another medication trial.

Internal inconsistencies in the patient's history. For example, if a patient who talks about business deals receives welfare checks, this should prompt more careful examination of other areas.

5 Coping with Uncertainty

When I was still a medical student, several of my teachers, in agreement rare among psychiatrists, pointed out that a well-trained mental health clinician can make a valid diagnosis after a single interview about four times out of five; on the fifth, however, the clinician could talk for 3 hours and still be uncertain. Over the intervening decades, that figure hasn't changed much, if at all. The result is that if you evaluate several new patients a week, you'll have to learn to cope with diagnostic uncertainty. This chapter presents some ideas on dealing with uncertainty when it arises, and explains why the concept itself is so valuable to the pursuit of accurate diagnoses.

Why Aren't We Certain?

You may think that someday all the uncertainty will be gone from the diagnostic process, but *I* think that this happy state will be a very long time in coming. The main reason is as obvious as it is inescapable: We can hardly avoid patients for whom we lack adequate information. Although patients with cognitive deficits such as Alzheimer's dementia may want very much to cooperate, they will have difficulty remembering important facts. Relatives may have been out of contact with such patients too long to have essential information to contribute. Someone who is paranoid or who has previously had unhappy experiences with health care may be afraid to reveal facts pertinent to diagnosis.

> When Nigel first consulted his new caregiver, a young woman still in training at the university clinic, he felt suddenly embarrassed about the cause of his anxiety and depression. It required most of the first session before he finally disclosed that he had been repeatedly impotent with his fiancée, who had suggested the evaluation.

Other patients may try to shield themselves or others from possible prosecution.

> Accused of destroying his neighbor's home in a futile search for money and drugs, Trevor was interviewed in jail. He alleged that he had a bipolar disorder, and he said that he was "blacked out" for the events in question. He refused to allow clinicians to contact family members for additional information that could validate—or, of course—refute his claim of a potentially exculpatory mental disorder.

Still other patients who seek to restrict information about their histories include those who have factitious and paranoid disorders. And some, for a great variety of reasons, just plain don't tell the truth.

It happens more often than we sometimes realize that a patient's database simply will never be complete until we've obtained collateral information—usually from a relative, but sometimes from old charts or previous clinicians.

> Jeff gave a history of bipolar illness, with manic and depressive mood swings. Although he denied that he had ever used alcohol heavily, Louise, his ex-wife, left me a voice mail message that she had often seen him in a stupor. It wasn't until I went to his house one evening, after a neighbor had called Louise to express concern about a raucous disturbance, that I saw him acutely intoxicated on both alcohol and cocaine. I persuaded him to be admitted to a hospital; the following day, he finally confessed that his mood swings had all occurred while he was under the influence.

Sometimes the clinician must bear the responsibility for insufficient information. If I omit questions about anxiety symptoms in the rush to complete an evaluation, I risk overlooking an important diagnosis. In the middle of the night, a sleepy clinician who doesn't dig through a thick chart may fail to note that a psychotic patient had an abnormal EEG the year before and was successfully treated with anticonvulsants. I believe that many missed and incorrect diagnoses stem from failure to collect and use all the relevant data, although I have no data other than my years of observing interviewer performance to support this belief.

On the other hand (wouldn't you know?), sometimes extra information confuses the diagnosis. The situation can be something rather simple, as when a patient with a long history of psychosis has symptoms that are not typical for schizophrenia—terrific insight and well-modulated affect, perhaps. Or consider a patient with somatization disorder who gives positive answers to such a broad array of questions that you can't rule out anything. Then it's a matter of sifting through the facts and deciding which are most relevant to your diagnosis. I've already described in Chapter 4 how contradictory information sources can lead to diagnostic confusion.

An issue we don't often mention is the clinician who fails to keep up to date with the explosive growth of knowledge. I've encountered any number of mental health professionals who base diagnoses of schizophrenia on their clinical intuition, rather than on the best practices informed by scientific studies. Such irresponsible behavior represents the sort of nightmare that drives most of us—almost from the moment we complete training and embark on independent careers as health care providers—to read journals, attend conferences, and accumulate continuing education credits, all in the effort to stay current with the latest developments in diagnosis and therapy. Keeping current has become institutionalized for medical professionals, whose board certifications are now good only for a limited time (usually 10 years), after which they must sit for a recertification exam.

Of course, the myriad combinations of symptoms individual patients present can confuse even the best-trained, most up-to-date practitioners. Some examples are well recognized and are even written into established criteria. A commonplace example is *atypical depression*, in which appetite and sleep may be increased, not decreased as you'd expect in the usual case of depression. However, other instances get less attention and can cause a practitioner who sticks too closely to established criteria to miss a diagnosis.

> A rare example would be the case of Corrine, whose magnum of red wine every day never caused her problems. Single all her life, she lived on inherited wealth. A companion managed her affairs and saw to it that she got proper nutrition and health care. If you required the exact criteria for alcohol dependence, Corrine might not qualify.

The point is that established criteria don't cover every possible manifestation of mental disease, and plenty of patients have symptoms that don't conform to conventional notions of a given disorder.

> Arvin recently moved west from Indiana, where he had attended college. At 35, he had a long history of mood disorder, beginning at the age of 10 when he attempted suicide by drinking Lysol. Fortunately, before he could get much of the liquid down, he gagged and suffered no lasting ill effects. At about that time he also took his first drink of alcohol, and thus began a

long downward spiral of substance use (marijuana and amphetamines when he was 12) and depression. Because he was bright and could take tests easily, he finished high school with his class, but when he was 19 he suffered his first episode of mania.

Arvin's depressions had always been brief, lasting 10 days at most, and about half the time they were interwoven with bursts of mania. Both his lows and his highs met official criteria for major depression and either manic episode or mixed episode (a mixture of depressive and manic symptoms). However, because his depressive episodes were so brief, a doctor recently refused to diagnose him with bipolar I disorder. "He told me that I had 'mood disorder not otherwise specified,' " Arvin reported in some consternation when a medical student presented his case. "What does that mean?"

Despite his diagnosis, Arvin's moods leveled out when he started taking a mood-stabilizing medication. Every experienced clinician has seen countless patients like Arvin who in some way or other don't quite fit official diagnostic criteria. Mostly therapy proceeds just as though the criteria had been fully met, and mostly it works out just fine. I echo the view of many expert clinicians, enshrined in the easily overlooked statement in the fine print of official criteria sets: Criteria should be viewed as guidelines, not straitjackets, and clinicians should use them with judgment that takes all the individual circumstances into account.

We must also acknowledge that some behaviors can resemble mental illness at first glance, but are actually more or less "normal" (see the sidebar "What's Normal?" on page 54). Sometimes these are termed *mental illness confounds*. For example, many people will respond to a variety of situations with emotion that is more intense than average. What I'm trying to warn against is overinterpreting behavior that may differ from what our own might be in a similar circumstance. Here are a few examples:

- Francine is a senior in college. Her anxiety could signal GAD, but it might reflect a normal response to the divorce of her parents and the impending Graduate Record Examination. Often anxiety is perfectly normal, even expected.
- Do Oscar's feelings of intense sadness indicate mood disorder or a response to breaking up with his fiancée? Personal unhappiness isn't necessarily abnormal.
- At 16, Winnie repeatedly shoplifts from several stores in the mall. She could have kleptomania, but might she be responding to a

schoolmate's threats to tell her religiously strict parents that she has had an abortion? Isolated bits of behavior can *suggest* a diagnosis, but they often don't *constitute* one.

- Gordon wore the colors of his school's arch-rival team on the day of the big game. He courted social disapproval and undoubtedly craved attention, but his behavior didn't qualify him for a diagnosis. A need for individuality and recognition is part of growing up, and of the human condition in general.
- Sandy drinks and uses drugs excessively, to the point of having declining grades and an arrest for drunk driving. Does this extremely common behavior foreshadow substance dependence, or is it simply going along with the gang?

Resolving Diagnostic Uncertainty

As I have noted earlier, only about 80% of new patients can be diagnosed on first interview. This section provides some techniques that may help you improve on that percentage.

It is natural that whenever we come to a stumbling block in the diagnostic process, our first impulse is usually to look for more information. Sometimes an additional patient interview, focused on the specifics of what we need to resolve our doubts, will succeed. At other times, information from another resource (such as a relative, friend, or former physician of the patient) or a review of previous health care records can make the difference. However, some histories are just plain confusing and will remain so well past the appropriate time to start treatment. Then we must look for clues that will help us arrange the possible diagnoses into a workable differential list.

Past Behavior

I've coopted as a diagnostic principle the truism that the best predictor of future behavior is past behavior. It applies to many areas of life in general, but it is especially valuable in making diagnoses. It suggests that any patient who has had a syndrome or set of symptoms for months or years is likely to remain the same far into the future. Here's an example:

Ned appeared to be in his mid-40s when the police brought him to the emergency room. That afternoon they had found him barricading the entry into a major shopping venue in the mall. Wearing a helmet made of aluminum foil, Ned was advising customers that a giant meteor was approaching the Pacific Northwest. When it struck, all life would be annihilated. He spoke rapidly, and his grandiose ideas (his ex-wife was a member of the Rockefeller family; he could control the outcome of the coming election) seemed to tumble after one another without logical connection. A telephone call to the number listed on a piece of paper in his pocket elicited the information that he had been chronically ill with psychosis for years. For the evaluating clinician, schizophrenia became the best working diagnosis.

> *Diagnostic Principle:* **The best predictor of future behavior is past behavior.**

More Symptoms of a Diagnosis

You'd think that a patient who has a lot of symptoms would fit a given syndrome better than someone with just a few symptoms, and you'd be right—to a certain extent. I would certainly vote for depression in someone who has seven or eight of the usual symptoms. But in using this diagnostic principle, remember that some symptoms carry far greater weight than others. For example, hallucinations and delusions strongly suggest schizophrenia, whereas pacing and muttering don't. Someone who stays up half the night pacing the room and muttering could be an aspiring author trying to punch through a writer's block (trust me!).

> *Diagnostic Principle:* **More symptoms of a disorder increase its likelihood as your diagnosis.**

And as a corollary, note that the mere fact of having *severe* symptoms doesn't necessarily mean that a given disorder is present. We'll see in Part II of this book that, for example, many people who have suicidal ideas don't necessarily have clinical depression as their primary diagnosis.

Presence of Typical Features

If your patient has symptoms or other features you usually expect to encounter in a given disorder, you'll want to consider it strongly for your working diagnosis. Loss of interest in work and leisure activities (including sex), poor concentration, and loss of appetite and insomnia point strongly to major depression. On the other hand, your diagnosis will be more secure if there aren't any symptoms that suggest other conditions. For example, if Serena complains of hallucinations, but you encounter a long history of multiple physical complaints or symptoms suggestive of mania, schizophrenia would seem a less attractive diagnosis.

> *Diagnostic Principle:* Typical features of a disorder increase its likelihood as your diagnosis; in the presence of nontypical features, look for alternatives.

Previous Typical Response to Treatment

Response to treatment can be tricky (a substantial number of patients with nearly *any* condition will improve, even on sugar pills—even if they *know* they are sugar pills!). However, sometimes the response to treatment can provide a clue to diagnosis. If you learn that Morton's earlier episode

> *Diagnostic Principle:* Previous typical response to treatment for a disorder increases its likelihood as your diagnosis.

of so-called schizophrenia resolved completely with a mood-stabilizing drug, you would strongly suspect that the actual diagnosis is a mood disorder.

The Value of the Term *Undiagnosed*

After you have recorded all the history you can find, pursued every clue from the MSE, interviewed relatives and friends, and consulted the available records, you still may not be able to come up with a definitive diagnosis. That's just fine. It is important to recognize that for some patients, no diagnosis will be possible immediately; for a few, you may not be sure for months or years. For all of these, you have at your disposal one of the most powerful descriptions in the book: *undiagnosed*.

I'm not kidding about this. *Undiagnosed* is my favorite diagnostic term of all time. I think of it as a safety valve. It allows us to acknowledge that something is probably wrong without rushing into closure—the point at which we usually stop thinking. It allows us to avoid making a diagnosis such as schizophrenia, Alz-

> *Diagnostic Principle:* Use the word *undiagnosed* whenever you cannot be sure of your diagnosis.

heimer's dementia, or antisocial personality disorder that could harm someone if it turns out not to be true. This is doubly important, now that insurance companies, employers, law enforcement bodies, and patients themselves increasingly exercise the right to review medical records.

Undiagnosed can keep you alert to data that don't quite fit. When you write it, you mean "This patient is probably mentally ill, though I'm not sure just how." By using this diagnostic principle, you keep yourself honest, and you demonstrate that honesty to others. Every time you see the *undiagnosed* label on a patient's chart or record, it forces you to think anew: "What additional information have I obtained since the last time? What I have learned about disease that might now be relevant to this patient?" If the answers continues to be "Not enough yet," *undiagnosed* stimulates further inquiry.

Some clinicians don't like to confess uncertainty: Could it reduce a patient's confidence in them? I think it far more likely that it will facilitate trust in a clinician candid enough to acknowledge that knowledge has its limits. Furthermore, by reducing unrealistic expectations, it could mitigate the likelihood of litigation if unforeseen difficulties should arise in the course of therapy. *Undiagnosed* can restrain you from rushing into unwarranted treatment that could be high-risk. (For example, if you admit you don't know what's wrong, you're unlikely to recommend electroconvulsive therapy.) It should certainly bar a patient from participation in any experimental treatment trial.

I've always considered diagnosis to be a team sport, not a vehicle for individual showboating. *Undiagnosed* alerts other clinicians on the team to think deeply about this patient. This is especially important in an institutional setting, where patients typically encounter many clinicians. Even in private offices, clinicians refer patients for specialized problems and take night and weekend calls for one another—more opportunities for a hasty, incorrect diagnosis to cause harm. Perhaps a fresh set of eyes will react to the *undiagnosed* label by uncovering information or making a connection that you have missed; additional symptoms may develop later that will allow a definitive diagnosis. *Undiagnosed* forces clinicians to confront uncertainty; without it, we could remain unaware that we are still in the dark.

Quite frankly, as I have gained experience with age, I have worried more about becoming too sanguine about my diagnostic ability. This is part of the reason I emphasize *undiagnosed* in my teaching and writing. One last note: *Undiagnosed* is somewhat like *not otherwise specified* (NOS), which is often cited as the official diagnostic expression. My concern is that NOS lends an aura of finality that tends to choke off further investigation. I try to avoid it.

Why Can't We Make a Diagnosis?

Managing uncertainty can be far more complicated than simply gathering additional information, though that's an excellent start. Here are several factors that can contribute to confusion about a given patient's diagnosis:

- Some people simply don't show enough traditional symptoms to make a diagnosis. Perhaps it is so early in the course of a patient's illness that the typical symptoms have not yet developed. Although time will sort out this one, it can still leave clinicians struggling to create a sensible treatment plan. It raises this question: How close to the ideal patient should we require a person's symptoms to be before making a diagnosis? Any illness close to the bottom of the hierarchy of safe diagnoses (Table 3.1) should require more symptoms and more typical symptoms before that diagnosis is made.
- Some patients have too many symptoms, promoting confusion. Although this should be simply a matter of further inquiry, sorting it out takes time and diligence. Resist the temptation to reach for the nearest likely approximation.
- Some features are unusual. Atypical features of depression have already been enshrined in their own special criteria, but a diagnostician who insists on the "letter of the law" could be perplexed by a patient who presents with unusual symptoms.
- Perhaps this patient has an illness that hasn't yet been identified. I admit that this is a long shot, but it's hardly beyond the realm of possibility. After all, textbooks of the early 1900s discussed only a few disorders, compared to the dozens of major ones (and hundreds of variants) we now recognize. Each of these relative newcomers came from somewhere, and there could still be other conditions out there waiting to be unmasked. Each edition of the *Diagnostic and Statistical Manual of Mental Disorders* (DSM) lists in an appendix research criteria for a dozen or more possible new disorders.
- Some emotional or behavioral characteristics may not lend themselves to being counted and lumped into categories. Perhaps dimensional criteria are needed instead. An example would be personality, for which various inventories have been devised that measure each individual (patient or otherwise) against a number of scales. Patterns of deviation on these scales constitute what we call *personality disorders*. The debate over dimensional versus categorical diagnosis has been raging for years, and it

is unlikely to be settled any time soon. But you should be aware that other diagnostic systems may better describe some aspects of psychopathology.

• Finally, some patients simply don't require a diagnosis. These are the folks who seek help not because they are sick, but because they fear they might be. When it's because they have a problem of living, it can be as vital to diagnose *no* mental disorder as it is for others to receive the correct diagnosis of a mental disorder. In short, the ability to rule a diagnosis in or out is one of the most powerful maneuvers in the clinician's toolbox. Even a condition that is fairly far down on the safety hierarchy can provide the comfort of no longer having to fear the unknown. Of course, for the clinician, nothing beats the shared joy of informing a patient, "I don't find any indication of an actual mental illness. You're only experiencing the sort of thing normal people experience from time to time, and we can work on that together."

> *Diagnostic Principle:* **Consider the possibility that this patient should be given no mental diagnosis at all.**

In the history that follows, look for evidence supporting the several reasons why I would choose to defer diagnosis.

Vickie

Though only 20 years old, Vickie complained of "lifelong depression." She had had two prior admissions to a psychiatric hospital for suicide attempts—the first one at age 10, when she overdosed on her mother's antidepressants. Now her husband's parents had just told her that they were moving to a retirement community, where they could no longer provide day care for her daughter.

Vickie had been under treatment for the past 3 years, during which she tried at least six antidepressant medications. Most recently, she took venlafaxine (300 mg per day); several weeks ago, when she was instructed to double the dose of this medication, her moods began to "fly up and down" and she was rediagnosed as having bipolar disorder. She then discontinued the drug because of hives. At interview, she described her moods as being depressed for up to a week, followed by 2 or 3 days of "high," by which she appeared to mean "approximately normal"—she denied grandiosity, rapid thoughts, or hyperactivity that would be typical of mania. Even when she was depressed, she reported feeling better when events distracted her ("I can be goofy at work").

She complained that her sleep had been terrible for years: "I go all night without any sleep at all, even when I take a double dose of medicine." Because her sleep was so poor, she had trouble concentrating on her usual activities, and she worried that she would be unable to keep her two jobs (both of which she needed for the money). Her appetite was down, though she had not lost weight.

For a long time Vickie had heard voices in her head that she didn't recognize; sometimes they said mean things to her, though often it was "just conversation." At times, as if watching a TV program, she could view herself "talking to someone else." As a result of these experiences, she had been tried on several antipsychotic medications, most recently ziprasidone. However, she denied ever feeling that she was being harassed, spied upon, followed, or otherwise persecuted.

Vickie had felt worse in the past 6 months. This decline was precipitated by current problems, including many bills to pay, some of which were the results of her multiple medical problems. She was also having disagreements with her husband, to whom she'd been married for 3 years. Some of this marital friction was due to her working two jobs; because their work schedules never seemed to match, they saw each other rarely. Moreover, Vickie despaired of finding another caregiver who would be as caring (and inexpensive) as her mother-in-law.

Besides her emotional difficulties, Vickie had been diagnosed as having fibromyalgia, hypothyroidism, and asthma. However, her physical symptoms weren't extensive enough for somatization disorder. When she was a child, her parents both drank heavily, and her father refused to seek help for an older sister who had mental retardation and problems with acting-out behavior. There was no other history of mental illness in her immediate or extended family. When she was 8, however, her mother's favorite brother got into bed with her when intoxicated and fondled her under her nightdress—an episode she had been forever afraid to reveal to her parents.

Vickie looked somewhat older than her stated age. Slightly overweight, she sat quietly during the interview. She was clean and neat, dressed casually in slacks and a brightly colored blouse. Her forearms were covered with red marks, which looked like healed-over scabs. She admitted that she picked at herself repeatedly "because I'm so nervous," and she showed thin white scars on her wrists where she had cut herself repeatedly during her early teens. She spoke clearly and coherently, and her mood seemed to be about medium, though appropriate to the content of her thought. She brightened visibly when she talked about the city in California where she was brought up ("I'd love to move back there some day"). Although the thought of suicide had been "my constant companion," she denied that she was having those thoughts now.

Analysis

Vickie presented a history of depression that she described extrava-gantly—it had been "lifelong," she went "all night without any sleep at all"—and with too few criteria to make any solid diagnosis. Although she claimed to be depressed, neither her mood nor her affect was currently de-pressed (we must invoke the diagnostic principle about contradictory infor-mation). Her symptoms of mania seemed too weak and too brief for bipolar disorder (in other words, she didn't meet the "typical features" diagnostic principle). She claimed some psychotic symptoms (hallucinations), but dis-played no other signs of schizophrenia, such as delusions or abnormalities of affect or speech. There was evidence that she and her husband had in-terpersonal problems; these, with a history of not providing care for her daughter and of cutting and picking at herself, would make me wonder about a personality disorder. However, as we'll discuss in the next chapter, I much prefer not to invoke a personality diagnosis so soon and in the face of a possible Axis I diagnosis. Vickie's multiple trials on antidepressants had been fruitless. Of course, this could simply mean that they weren't the right ones, but after several trials, you would begin to think how strongly Vickie's experience was contravening the diagnostic principle about typical response to treatment. On top of all this, she came to the clinic in the midst of a personal crisis—a diagnostic principle that we've already noted should make us careful in evaluating her information. In short, I can't get close to a concrete diagnosis for Vickie; for now, I feel we would be far better off with the *undiagnosed* label.

Comment

The term *undiagnosed* is hardly a recent invention. The *Oxford English Dictionary* notes its first appearance in 1864, but it wasn't until 1917 that it was first used to mean "psychosis not diagnosed" by the American Medico-Psychological Association, the forerunner of today's American Psychiatric Association.

What's Normal?

From my Internet correspondents, I repeatedly hear this complaint: "The textbooks and diagnostic manuals don't tell me what's normal."

It's a fair cop. We're so used to spelling out the abnormal that we sometimes end up defining what's normal by what we believe. That puts it into the dubious category of "I know it when I see it," as Potter Stewart, an associate justice of the U.S. Supreme Court, famously defined *pornography*. Derived from the Latin *norma*, meaning "carpenter's square," the meanings of *normal* include "average," "healthy," "usual," and "the ideal." There are problems with each of these; we might say that definitional problems are the norm. If we define *normal* as "average," then, it would mean some (if minor) degree of impairment, because so many adults are impaired by mental disorder. If it means "healthy," as in the absence of disease, then nearly half of Americans are mentally abnormal. If it's what's "usual," then those who drink no alcohol at all would be considered abnormal. And if it's "the ideal," then normality is a state to which we can aspire, but never attain.

We are left bobbing in a sea of ad hoc decisions concerning each illness or group of illnesses we encounter. For example, we must differentiate the misuse of substances from social drinking, recreational drug use (however normal that may be), and the appropriate use of prescription drugs. We've even coined special terms for some conditions that we regard as normal and must differentiate from illness: *adult antisocial behavior*, for common criminals who lack the cachet of antisocial personality disorder; *age-related decline*, for the not-quite-dementia experienced by each of us lucky enough to survive middle age; *bereavement*, which we all (mostly) hope never to experience ourselves, yet assume others will one day experience on our behalf.

Below I've listed some mental states and symptoms, along with the normal situations from which we must differentiate them. Note that we sometimes use the words *common*, *ordinary*, or *everyday* as code for *normal*. This brings up the interesting point that for some behaviors, the definition of what's normal is a little skewed. Consider, for example, ordinary shoplifting (as distinct from kleptomania), common criminality (vs. antisocial personality disorder), and everyday fire starting for profit (vs. pyromania).

Pathology	*Normal*
Psychosis	Dreams, imaginary playmates, déjà vu, and the hallucinations that occur when we are going to sleep or awakening
Depression, mania	Common sadness and joy experienced in daily life
Panic attacks	Adaptive fright that helps us avoid speeding trucks, raging torrents, and crashing bores

Phobias	Realistic concerns about being embarrassed (such as someone who stutters might feel) or unable to help oneself (as perhaps a paralyzed person might feel)
Social anxiety	Stage or microphone fright, and ordinary shyness that doesn't result in clinically important distress or impairment
Obsessions, compulsions	Superstitions and ordinary checking to see that the stove is turned off before we depart for the airport
Pathological worry	Legitimate concerns, such as paying the rent and putting the kids through college when we've just been laid off
Somatization, hypochondriasis	Concerns about demonstrable physical disorders
Dissociation	Daydreams, reveries, and fantasies
Compulsive gambling	Professional and recreational gambling
Rejection of gender identity	Tomboyishness, theatrical role playing, and any other cross-gender behavior that doesn't cozily fit our cultural stereotypes
Paraphilias	Ordinary use of fantasy to enhance sexual excitement
Deviant personality	Personality and character traits that are merely annoying (yours) or even endearing (mine)

6 Multiple Diagnoses

Among Aaron's complaints were severe depression, auditory hallucinations, trouble sleeping, bouts of drinking, and episodes of anxiety so severe that he couldn't focus on his day job as a computer programmer, let alone pursue the dream of forming his own rock band. We'll discuss his case in greater detail later on, but for now consider this question: As his clinician, how would you diagnose Aaron—with one illness or five?

Although you might think that multiple diagnoses would all have to be present at the same time to count, this isn't necessarily the case. And that's just one of the sometimes puzzling features of such diagnoses. Another is the fact that people with some disorders (a good example is social phobia) don't even appear for treatment until they develop symptoms of something else, such as depression or panic attacks. In this chapter, we'll sort all of this out and discuss what diagnosticians need to consider in making (or rejecting) more than one diagnosis at a time.

What Is Comorbidity?

When someone has multiple diagnoses, we speak of *comorbidity*. Some clinicians feel it should be applied to all patients in whom two distinct disorders occur together, but most would agree that truly comorbid diagnoses cannot cause one another. Just as you wouldn't say that coughs and sneezes are comorbid in a cold, the typical facial features of Down's syndrome cannot be comorbid with mental retardation (they both result from the same pathological process). Simi-

> True comorbidity occurs when a person has *independent* multiple diagnoses.

larly, because alcohol dependence and intoxication regularly occur together and derive from the same underlying process, we don't speak of them as being comorbid.

Although some illnesses appear to be highly comorbid, their relationship may simply be one of sharing many symptoms. For example, in recent years researchers have hotly debated the question of how social phobia and avoidant personality disorder are related. Some authorities argue that the two conditions are just statistical variations of one another; others insist that they are distinct conditions that often occur together. I could make a similar case for somatization disorder and histrionic personality disorder.

Even with narrow definitions, 21st-century patients with mental disorders have an enormous risk of comorbidity (see the sidebar "Comorbidity Rates"). For some individual diseases, the comorbidity is well over 50%. In the early 1990s, the U.S. National Comorbidity Survey of persons ages 15–54 found that a whopping 48% of the general population had at some time at least one disorder, and 27% had at least two; 14% reported three or more. A little math reveals that of those with at least one disorder, over half have at least one additional disorder. Of all mental illnesses diagnosed in adults, nearly half occur in just 14% of the overall population. This enormous burden of mental illness strongly suggests that every mental health professional should work diligently to rule in (or out) multiple diagnoses. Recognizing them all presents a challenge that often goes unmet; studies have repeatedly shown that professionals who employ an unstructured clinical interview make far fewer diagnoses than are identified by an interview that systematically covers all the bases.

Comorbidity Rates

Comorbidity rates for patients will yield estimates higher than those just given for a general population. It's easy to see why. Most people who appear for a mental health evaluation will have at least one disorder, with increased odds that one or more additional disorders will be found during the course of evaluation. Here's another factor that has increased comorbidity rates: Through the years, the DSMs have essentially eliminated all exclusionary rules. For example, most of the anxiety disorders can now be diagnosed along with a mood disorder—a practice that was not allowed earlier.

Why Look for Comorbidity?

Beyond the satisfaction of having the most complete picture possible of a patient's illness, searching out comorbid diagnoses has a lot to recommend it.

1. Comorbidity helps determine the scope of treatment. It seems obvious that if you are missing part of the diagnostic picture, you could also neglect part of the treatment. If Aaron's alcohol misuse goes undetected, he might not get substance use treatment that is vital to his overall outcome. Here's another wrinkle: I've repeatedly seen it happen that someone like Aaron with, say, schizophrenia and a substance use disorder gets bounced back and forth between treatment teams: The mental health team packs him off to the substance use folks, who throw up their hands because he's psychotic. With the remedy for each condition waiting on treatment for the other, Aaron's plight is a classic Catch-22. Obviously, he needs simultaneous treatment for both conditions, and this depends on an early, complete diagnosis. Here are two more wrinkles. First, the presence of one diagnosis may suggest the course of treatment for another, especially if drugs that interfere with one another are contemplated. Second, the patient may have a physical disorder as well (such as diabetes) that can be exacerbated by the drug prescribed for a mental condition.

2. This brings up the whole issue of prognosis. Patients who have, say, bipolar disorder comorbid with an anxiety disorder tend to get sick younger, stay sick longer, respond less well to traditional mood-stabilizing drugs, have an increased risk of suicide, and a quality of life that is less robust than someone with uncomplicated bipolar disorder. To successfully predict the interactions of multiple diagnoses, we must first realize that they exist.

3. Anticipating a second disorder can guard against future complications. For example, if your patient has bipolar disorder, you know to be extra vigilant for substance use, even though there's no current evidence for it. In a 2003 paper, several women with anorexia nervosa who were not drinking at the beginning of the study had developed alcoholism by the time they were followed up 7–12 years later.

4. Some writers have suggested that comorbidity indicates underlying common psychopathology. If research demonstrates this to be the case, we should begin to look for core underpinnings, rather than focusing on the separate diagnoses.

Identifying Comorbidity

Deciding when additional diagnoses are warranted isn't always easy. Such a decision relies on a complete set of data, to which the clinician must add the knowledge of diagnostic criteria and an understanding of cause and effect. The central question is this: After the principal diagnosis has been made, has anything been left unexplained? For an example, let's consider Aaron's mental heath history in more detail.

Aaron

When Aaron came to the clinic, he was in trouble up to his nose ring. His job as a computer programmer was being severely hampered by the worsening state of his mental health. Now 32, he had already suffered from one episode of acute psychosis 7 years earlier. Then diagnosed as having schizophrenia, he was treated first with Haldol and later with Risperdal. His symptoms had largely resolved, though he continued to have lingering fears that someone from "the government" might be watching to see whether he was creating computer viruses. He had nonetheless been able to hang onto his Silicon Valley job. At the suggestion of a new HMO physician, he had recently been backing off his medication "to see how little I could get by on." When he had been on half his usual dose for over a month, he once again heard voices saying, "You'd better watch yourself," and "Don't trust those doctors—they don't know what they're doing." His clinician immediately increased the dose of Risperdal to its former level, and the hallucinations began to abate.

Even as the psychosis lifted, Aaron's mood foundered. He remembered those weeks he had spent in a mental hospital long ago, and he feared a recurrence of medication side effects. Ruminations about the government interfered with his concentration, so that he could accomplish only a fraction of his daily work. He lost interest in his hobby (he collected the postage stamps of Denmark) and stopped attending meetings of his stamp club; professional and hobby journals piled up unread. Although he thought his appetite remained about normal, he lost weight.

Many nights, worries that a government agency was censoring his e-mail kept Aaron awake for hours. As he'd done before, he started to drink as a sleeping aid. "Mostly it was Bloody Marys—at least the tomato juice made them seem a little healthful—but lots of Bloody Marys," he confessed. Though he telecommuted from home, many mornings he was too hung over to start work on time. His parents told him how worried they

were about his drinking. Just before returning to his mental health counselor, he had begun to have thoughts that he "might be better off dead."

Analysis

The evidence supporting Aaron's diagnosis of schizophrenia was rock-
solid. He had had a long history (satisfying the diagnostic principle concerning past behavior) of both hallucinations and delusions (typical symptoms) that responded well to the dose of antipsychotic medication typically
used for this condition; once the dose was decreased, he relapsed (note the
diagnostic principle about typical response to treatment). But now other
symptoms appeared—low mood, the loss of concentration, problems with
eating and sleeping, and increasing thoughts about dying. His principal diagnosis of schizophrenia would not adequately cover this group of symptoms, so his working diagnosis should be expanded to include both schizophrenia *and* a depressive disorder; we shouldn't have to choose between
these two conditions.

Now let's consider Aaron's drinking, which had accelerated over the
time that his schizophrenia symptoms were increasing. The drinking had
been extensive enough that, all by itself, it alarmed both Aaron and his parents. Even if he didn't have schizophrenia, he would probably need help to
get sober and stay that way. Although substance use frequently accompanies many mental disorders, it appears nowhere among the symptoms of
schizophrenia. Aaron did not appear to have alcohol dependence (there's
no evidence that he had either developed tolerance for alcohol or suffered
from withdrawal), but he was clearly misusing the stuff. Some authorities
claim that patients with schizophrenia and mood disorders who use substances often do not develop dependence—social problems, yes, but not
tolerance or withdrawal. I'd diagnose Aaron as having alcohol abuse or, if
you prefer (personally, I don't), alcohol use disorder NOS. This diagnosis
would establish in my mind, as well as Aaron's, yet another issue for future
reevaluation and treatment.

But is that all? What about the possibility of yet another diagnosis—
say, a sleep disorder? Here the situation is a little less clear. Insomnia is a
diagnostic criterion for depression and also occurs in schizophrenia. But
the diagnostic manuals also include "insomnia related to another mental
disorder," which can be diagnosed when a sleep problem is serious enough
by itself to warrant clinical attention. Such patients usually focus on the
sleep symptoms to the extent that they downplay or ignore the underlying
illness, perhaps even blaming poor sleep for their other symptoms. In my

opinion, Aaron's sleep complaint didn't rise to this level, so I would not give him a fourth mental health diagnosis. The chances are overwhelming that this sort of insomnia will resolve once the other problems are brought under control.

Now let's summarize what we need to consider when making a comorbid diagnosis:

1. Are the symptoms covered by the principal diagnosis? If not, then consider the additional diagnosis.
2. What will be the benefits of the additional diagnosis? That is, does the diagnosis warn of a treatable disorder that threatens the patient's well-being?
3. Does the proposed additional diagnosis meet criteria for the comorbid disorder you have in mind?

> **Diagnostic Principle:** When symptoms cannot be adequately explained by a single disorder, consider multiple diagnoses.

Personality Disorder as Comorbidity

I'll discuss personality disorders further in Chapter 16, but right now I want to bring out one or two important points.

With a cooperative patient and some collateral information, personality disorder isn't too hard to diagnose—if it's the only issue at hand (admittedly, that doesn't happen often). However, it's often pretty hard to assess personality when your patient is acutely ill with an Axis I disorder. This will be especially true in the case of something serious like an acute episode of schizophrenia or a severe mood disorder. Depression, manic grandiosity, psychosis, overwhelming anxiety, and substance use are almost ideally suited to provide cover for the subjective and often subtle symptoms that point to a personality disorder diagnosis.

The flip side of this argument is that many acutely ill patients who have been diagnosed with a personality disorder eventually turn out *not* to have one; once the acute illness has resolved, the personality symptoms seem just to melt away. One study in 2002 found that of patients with major depressive disorder who had received a comorbid diagnosis of personality disorder, many no longer qualified for the personality disorder diagnosis once they had been treated with Prozac. My thoughts boil down to this: Be especially careful when diagnosing personality disorders in the face of other mental conditions. Wait until symptoms of other disorders have been reduced to their absolute minimum, when you'll more easily recog-

> *Diagnostic Principle:* Avoid personality disorder diagnoses when your patient is acutely ill with an Axis I disorder.

nize personality disorder symptoms and less readily misinterpret them. I feel strongly enough about this to enshrine it as a diagnostic principle.

Additional Factors to Consider in Comorbidity

A patient's demographic features can affect which disorders might be comorbid with others. For a man, give extra thought to the possibility of comorbid alcoholism, which is of course much more commonly found in men than in women. Similarly, anorexia nervosa and bulimia nervosa are more common in women. (Table 8.2 in Chapter 8 is a gender comparison chart.) And of course, you should be alert for any disorders that you've already identified as running in a patient's family.

Here's another caveat about dual diagnoses that include substance use. A 2002 study reported that Axis I comorbidity (such as mood and anxiety disorders) was substantially reduced once patients had been clean and sober for as little as 3 weeks. Although the finding needs to be substantiated, it suggests that we clinicians should not make hasty comorbid diagnoses in the face of substance use problems.

Imposing Order on Comorbidity

Once you have identified your patient's various comorbid diagnoses, does it make any real difference which you list first? It can, and often it does.

Clinicians are likely to pay special attention to the first diagnosis, under the logical though sometimes erroneous impression that it is the most important one—perhaps even the cause underlying whatever other pathology the patient may have. The order in which diagnoses are recorded can also have important implications for the treatment and prognosis. Any diagnosis listed on top also cries out for preference when the patient sees another clinician for further evaluation. So, if only for the purpose of signaling special attention, it makes sense to give some thought to the different ways you could impose order on your list of diagnoses.

One is to list first the diagnosis most important for the well-being of the patient. To demonstrate this strategy, let's return to Aaron—who, we eventually decided, should be given three separate diagnoses: schizophrenia, major depressive disorder, and an alcohol use disorder. Going by urgency of treatment, we would list his depression first, because at the time of his reevaluation dying had begun to look good to him. Next in order might come the schizophrenia, and finally his alcohol use disorder. An obvious drawback to this strategy would be the difficulty in knowing which diagnosis is the more urgent. Relevant to Aaron's situation, for example, is that suicidal behavior can also be associated with schizophrenia and substance use. Who could say that Aaron's growing suicidal ideas were related only to depression?

A second strategy is to list diagnoses in the order of your greatest confidence that they apply to your patient. That would put more speculative conditions lower on the list, below those that seem rock-solid. Of course, this strategy suggests a touching faith in your ability to rank-order the reliability of your diagnoses. In the case of Aaron, I would feel confident in my diagnosis of schizophrenia, but I'm pretty certain that he also had a mood disorder and, for that matter, an alcohol use disorder; I'm back to square one. All in all, listing in order of confidence is a strategy that probably works better for thinking about a differential diagnosis than for a group of comorbid diagnoses.

Another method would be to list first the diagnosis that appears to be the "prime mover," the underlying cause of the other disorders. This could work pretty well, if only we could be sure about cause and effect. For Aaron, we could probably agree that schizophrenia belonged on top; as is so often true, his alcohol use could be understood as self-medication of a chronic psychosis. But competent clinicians will often disagree about what causes, say, a patient's depression—is it stress, or a loss, or does it come out of the blue? In Aaron's case, did his psychosis cause the depression? This would be a tough sell for some clinicians.

On the other hand, it's a relative breeze to agree upon whether one illness began chronologically later than another. The one that arose first would be considered primary, whereas any that began afterward would be considered secondary and listed later. The question of whether a mood disorder is primary or secondary can also sometimes help direct patient and clinician to the quickest, most effective course of therapy. According to this strategy, Aaron's schizophrenia obviously would come first, followed by his depression and then his drinking.

Considering everything we've said above, I've written the diagnostic principle about multiple diagnoses to read that you should first address the diagnosis that is most urgent, treatable, or specific. (This reads a lot like the safety principle at the beginning of our diagnostic quest, but the point is well worth considering again near the end.) If possible, multiple diagnoses should also be listed chronologically. Here is a brief example:

> When she was only 16, Annie ran away from her home in a suburb of Chicago. After living on the streets of San Francisco for nearly 2 years, she applied to a crisis residence facility for a place to stay and for treatment for her deteriorated mental state. One clinician noted that she had heavily misused cocaine for over a year; another was concerned about her 2-month history of depression. Now she cried frequently and expressed hopelessness about the future, though she denied having suicidal ideas.

Because the depression had apparently started long after Annie began using cocaine (the control of which would probably address the depression), her two clinicians agreed to list the cocaine dependence first and the mood disorder second. They would withhold treating the depression with medication until they could reevaluate her mental state when she was drug-free.

> *Diagnostic Principle:* **Arrange multiple diagnoses to list first the one that is most urgent, treatable, or specific. Whenever possible, also list diagnoses chronologically.**

Relationships of Comorbidities

Here's a note about the strength of associations. Just because disorder A frequently accompanies disorder B doesn't mean that the reverse is true, so the table can be read only in one direction: You must start with a disorder in which you are interested from the left-hand column, then find the associations by reading across the row. The reason consists in the prevalence in the general population and the relative frequency of disorders. As you can see from the Venn diagram in Figure 6.1, most of the time when you find disorder A, disorder B will also be present, whereas B will often occur by itself.

Table 6.1 is a chart of which diagnoses commonly occur together. If I could, I'd have given percentages to indicate how often they are associated, but because the relevant studies often give such widely divergent figures, I decided to make do with "x" signs. Some disorders are so new or rare that they have yet to be carefully studied, which helps explain why some disorders have far fewer comorbidities than others. In Part III, I'll add comments about specific associations between disorders.

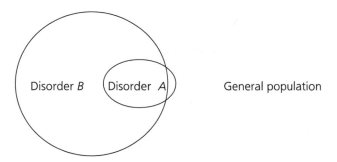

FIGURE 6.1. Relative frequencies and relationships of two mental disorders, *A* and *B*.

TABLE 6.1. Comorbid Diagnoses by Diagnosis

These diagnoses → are likely to be comorbid with these diagnoses ↓	Delirium	Dementia	Subst. intox./withdr.	Schizophrenia	Schizophreniform dis.	Delusional dis.	Major depression	Dysthymia	Mania (bip. I)	Panic dis.	Agoraphobia	Specific phobia	Social phobia	OCD	PTSD	GAD	Somatization dis.	Hypochondriasis	Body dysmorphic dis.	Any anxiety dis.
Dementia	×	—																		
Subst. intox./withdr.			—	×			×		×								×		×	
Schizophrenia			×	—						×				×						
Schizoaffective dis.			×																	
Delusional dis.						—	×							×				×		
Major depression				×			—	×		×				×						
Dysthymia				×			×	—												
Mania (bip. I)				×					—	×			×							
Hypomania (bip. II)				×						×			×							
Cyclothymia				×																
Panic dis.				×			×			—	×	×	×	×	×	×		×		
Specific phobia				×			×					—								×
Social phobia				×			×						—							×
OCD							×			×		×	×	—						
PTSD				×			×		×	×	×	×	×	×	—		×			
GAD				×			×	×		×		×	×			—				
Somatization dis.				×			×			×							—			
Pain dis.				×			×													×
Hypochondriasis							×											—		×
Body dysmorphic dis.						×	×						×	×					—	
Factitious dis.				×																
Dissoc. amnesia				×			×													
Dissoc. fugue				×			×								×					
Dissoc. identity dis.				×			×													
Depersonalization dis.				×			×	×										×		×
Sexual dysfunctions							×			×	×	×		×						
Paraphilias							×													
Gender identity dis.				×																
Anorexia nervosa				×			×							×						
Bulimia nervosa				×			×	×												×
Intermitt. explos. dis.				×			×		×											×
Kleptomania				×			×													×
Pyromania				×																
Path. gambling				×			×													
Trichotillomania				×			×							×						×
Paranoid PD			×	×		×	×					×		×						
Schizoid PD				×		×	×													
Schizotypal PD				×	×	×	×													
Antisocial PD				×			×										×			×
Borderline PD				×			×									×				
Histrionic PD							×										×			
Narcissistic PD				×																
Avoidant PD							×						×							
Dependent PD							×													×
Obsess.–compul. PD											×	×	×		×					

Note. OCD, obsessive–compulsive disorder; PTSD, posttraumatic stress disorder; GAD, generalized anxiety disorder; PD, personality disorder.

These diagnoses → are likely to be comorbid with these diagnoses ↓	Anorexia nervosa	Bulimia nervosa	Intermitt. explos. dis.	Kleptomania	Pyromania	Path. gambling	Trichotillomania	Adjustment dis.	Paranoid PD	Schizoid PD	Schizotypal PD	Antisocial PD	Borderline PD	Histrionic PD	Narcissistic PD	Avoidant PD	Dependent PD	Obsess.–compul. PD	Mental retardation	Tourette's dis.
Dementia																				
Subst. intox./withdr.												×	×							
Schizophrenia									×	×	×									
Schizoaffective dis.									×	×	×		×							
Delusional dis.									×	×					×					
Major depression	×	×											×							
Dysthymia													×	×	×	×	×			
Mania (bip. I)	×	×																		
Hypomania (bip. II)	×	×											×							
Cyclothymia																				
Panic dis.																				
Specific phobia																				
Social phobia		×														×				
OCD	×															×	×	×		×
PTSD																				
GAD																				
Somatization dis.												×	×	×						
Pain dis.																				
Hypochondriasis																				
Body dysmorphic dis.																				
Factitious dis.													×							
Dissoc. amnesia																				
Dissoc. fugue																				
Dissoc. identity dis.	×												×							
Depersonalization dis.													×		×		×			
Sexual dysfunctions																				
Paraphilias																				
Gender identity dis.																				
Anorexia nervosa	—												×							
Bulimia nervosa		—											×							
Intermitt. explos. dis.			—																	
Kleptomania		×		—																
Pyromania					—															
Path. gambling						—						×	×		×					
Trichotillomania	×						—												×	
Paranoid PD									—	×	×		×		×	×				
Schizoid PD									×	—	×				×					
Schizotypal PD									×	×	—		×		×					
Antisocial PD						×						—	×	×	×					
Borderline PD		×											—							
Histrionic PD												×	×	—	×		×			
Narcissistic PD	×								×			×	×	×	—					
Avoidant PD									×	×	×		×			—	×			
Dependent PD						×							×	×		×	—			
Obsess.–compul. PD																		—		

Note. OCD, obsessive–compulsive disorder; PTSD, posttraumatic stress disorder; GAD, generalized anxiety disorder; PD, personality disorder.

7 Checking Up

Before moving on to Parts II and III, let's pause to review the previous chapters with another vignette. It is a good deal more detailed than many of the previous case examples, so as to provide material for a sustained discussion of many of the points I've already raised.

Veronica

Just after spring break, her parents brought Veronica to the clinic for evaluation. Their visit had been occasioned by a chance encounter between mother and daughter one morning just after Veronica showered. "She always wears those baggy sweaters and pants, so I hadn't realized how much thinner she'd become," Mrs. Harper said. She dabbed at her eyes with a handkerchief. "She always promises to eat better, but she just seems to be wasting away. Now she only weighs 89 pounds, and she's five and a half feet tall."

"She looks like a stick figure!" Her father scowled and banged his fist on the arm of his chair.

Veronica flinched, but she didn't relent. "There's nothing wrong with me," she insisted. "Except maybe my weight."

"Now you're showing some sense, at least." Turning to the clinician, Mr. Harper added, "She belongs in the hospital."

"I mean, I'm pudgy and gross around the middle! Besides, I'm an adult. You can't make me go there." Her eyes filled with tears, and father and daughter each looked to the clinician for support. Veronica's mother frowned at her husband and encircled her daughter with a protective arm. The atmosphere in the room thickened with anger.

Veronica's peculiar eating behavior had begun in the ninth grade when she read a women's magazine article about cellulite. Suddenly fearful that she would become obese, from that time on she had dieted sporadically, though never before losing so much weight as now. At various times when she was in high school, both parents had noticed how she pushed food around on her plate.

Her mother had uncritically accepted her excuses—she wasn't hungry, or she was stressed by school, or she was having her period—but her father was concerned to a fault. When she was younger, he would insist that Veronica sit at the table until she'd eaten what was before her; once she had sat sulking until bedtime, her food undisturbed on her plate. With time, though, she'd learned to circumvent parental control by gobbling down what was required, then heading off to the bathroom, where she would cause herself to gag. At first this required a spoon or her finger, but later, she finally admitted, she learned to vomit at will. She masked the sound by flushing the toilet.

In 11th grade, Veronica tried amphetamines to control her appetite. Two girls who had dropped out of school the year before had introduced her to the practice. It had worked, but she stopped after just a few weeks because they "made me feel wired." She also briefly tried laxatives, but similarly abandoned them: "That was just plain yuck."

As a young child, Veronica had been very active and often inattentive—whether it was when listening to a story being read to her, or even watching a favorite TV show like *Sesame Street*. Despite high intelligence, she had trouble concentrating in class during her early school years. Her second- and third-grade teachers had each asked that she be evaluated for attention deficit disorder (as it was then called), but her father had refused. An attorney who specialized in malpractice litigation, he had declared, "No kid of mine is going to be drugged by some quack doctor," and that was that. Now even he admitted that something was desperately wrong. Strong measures seemed needed.

Off and on, Veronica had complained about depression. For several years she had felt worst right around Christmas ("Maybe it's because I'm an atheist, and I resent all the religious stuff"). She did note that she always seemed to improve again once spring set in. During these wintertime depressed periods, she would feel tired and sleep more than usual, and her concentration would suffer to the point of declining grades. Even her interest in working out would drop to the point that she found it hard to drag herself off to the pool. Strangely, she ate more and she noted with distress how she always picked up a few pounds when she was having "the winter blahs." "The depression must take her mind off dieting," her mother suggested.

Last winter, her doctor had put her on an antidepressant; within 3 weeks her sleep had returned to normal, and she was once again working hard in school—and avoiding food. She finished up her story by telling the clinician that she now felt "great" and was happy that with the return of her workout routine, her weight was settling back to what she regarded as normal. She denied feeling really hungry, just intensely interested in food. She rather proudly mentioned her file of hundreds of recipes, which she kept in a computer database. She didn't actually cook, but she enjoyed thinking about these dishes and used them to plan weeks' worth of menus.

Despite her profound weight loss, Veronica claimed to be in excellent health. She was fully active, swimming every day for 90 minutes before classes; earlier in the year, before becoming so busy with her studies, she had played on the women's volleyball team. An avid skier, she was impatient to get on the slopes—though, as her younger brother chimed in, "she looks like one of her poles." Her periods had stopped months earlier, and a trip to her family doctor the week before revealed that her thyroid was functioning at below-normal level. Besides her weight, the only other physical findings were that she had lost hair from her head (though not elsewhere, she admitted with a scowl in her brother's direction); what hair she had left seemed finer than it used to be.

After her initial rocky start in the early grades, Veronica had worked very hard throughout school to become an A+ student. She would rework any algebra problems she missed on an exam until she got them right, and she devoted countless hours to extra-credit work in biology. In her senior year, she was supposed to become the student coordinator of the science fair, but she ultimately turned it down because she feared the ridicule she'd experience if she "screwed it up." She agreed that for years she had felt insecure, and in part her diligence in high school served to avert criticism from her parents or teachers. Once she discovered that she could challenge her way up to be first chair in the school band, she had practiced her clarinet a full hour every day. She also sang in the choir and had leads in two school operettas. In one, she slit the skirt of her costume up the side, to acclaim from the boys in the chorus.

Veronica's older sister had been bulimic when she was in college; now married, she was currently pregnant and very careful about what she ate. Mr. Harper admitted having occasional periods of depression—but when he was in law school, he "sometimes felt so strong, so capable, so on top of the world that it seemed that if I gradually brought the tips of my index fingers together, sparks might jump between them!" Although he had never been evaluated for a mood disorder, his own father, depressed by business failure, had committed suicide in his early 40s. Mrs. Harper admitted that she liked things orderly and neat: "I guess I have OCD traits myself."

Now 19 and in her second year of college, Veronica admitted that she still had only one close friend, another young woman with a weight problem. "I don't feel comfortable with other people," she complained. "I get sort of, you know, anxious when I'm with people. For one thing, I think that they must be noticing how fat I am." She also denied any history of legal problems or of physical or sexual abuse.

In private, Veronica groused to the clinician about still living at home. "My parents didn't trust me to live on campus," she complained. She had had almost no boyfriends, other than Mitchell. For a time she had hooked up with him for sex, but he eventually dropped her—frightened off because she talked mostly about eating, yet seemed to be wasting away. His abandonment didn't bother her. She had never been especially interested in sex, which didn't even take her mind off food. "I'd just lie there and think of English muffins," she said, with the trace of a smile.

Discussion of Veronica

Note that Veronica's report draws on a wide variety of information: the history of the present illness; medical history; personal and social histories as far back as childhood; family history of mental disorder, as well as some family dynamics; and Veronica's current MSE. The resources used to develop this information included an interview with the patient herself and collateral information from her family, to which I'd add any available medical records and psychological information. Reports from school counselors, clergy, and social services would also be used when applicable.

Creating the Differential Diagnosis

First we'll evaluate Veronica's whole history for evidence of the syndromes we should initially include in a broad-ranging differential diagnosis. Of course, an eating disorder is high on our list. Anorexia nervosa is highly suspect, but because she indulged in some bingeing and purging, we'll add bulimia nervosa. She also had evidence of depression that would, depending on time course and other features, support a diagnosis of either dysthymia or major depression. Though the evidence is scanty, at times she was also irritable and overactive, so we should tack on bipolar disorder. Even a few somatic symptoms in a young woman suggest somatization disorder, which is attractive in part because it explains so many symptoms in one diagnosis—Occam's razor at work.

Shouldn't we mention substance use? At one time, Veronica did try amphetamines to reduce her weight. And we must consider that a medical condition can cause both mood and eating disorders. Although menstruation will stop with marked weight loss, could she have a primary endocrine disorder such as hypothyroidism? We'd better add that in, too. Severe weight loss due to a chronic disease would be only a dim possibility, especially inasmuch as Veronica had just been to her family doctor, but for completeness it needs to be mentioned. Because she thought about food a great deal and kept lists of menus, we should at least mention OCD. Scattered throughout the vignette were instances of difficulty in getting along with other people—so we need to add a personality disorder to the list of possibilities.

With only skimpy evidence supporting a number of the conditions on this list, including them might seem forced. However, it is a truism that you will never make a diagnosis if you don't think about it, and an extensive differential diagnosis doesn't mean that each possibility is likely. Rather, it should bring to mind even those disorders that may seem preposterous in context; occasionally one will turn out to be on the money. Because from the first we want to keep our options open, let us include even disorders that seem only remotely possible.

All things considered, then, Table 7.1 presents the differential diagnosis I'd consider for Veronica. Notice the five conditions at the top: According to the safety principle, they are not the diagnoses you or I might consider most likely, but those that would have the greatest immediate importance for the patient's treatment and overall well-being.

Winnowing the Differential List

The next step will be to eliminate many of the disorders from consideration. I've tried to explain in detail how an experienced clinician thinks about a complex patient. But by the time you've become experienced yourself, these steps will meld into a nearly seamless process that takes place within seconds, not the minutes it will take at first to puzzle through a diagnostic situation. Before reading on, you might want to work through Table 7.1 yourself, to see how your thinking compares with mine.

In our discussion, we could start with either depression or anxiety; indeed, the decision trees in Figures 11.1 and 12.1 could both come into play. Regardless of which we take up first, the top spot always belongs to the possibility that a medical or substance use problem could be causing the major symptomatology. Low thyroid functioning can cause depression and

TABLE 7.1. Differential Diagnosis for Veronica

Mood disorder due to hyperthyroidism

Mood disorder due to substance use

Weight loss due to a medical condition (e.g., AIDS, cancer)

Weight loss due to substance use

Amphetamine use disorder

Anorexia nervosa

Bulimia nervosa

Bipolar disorder

Major depressive disorder

Somatization disorder

Dysthymia

OCD

Social phobia

ADHD

Personality disorder of an unspecified type

low appetite; however, *seasonal* hypothyroidism would be a real novelty. Of course, one should always think of serious medical conditions when presented with profound weight loss, but I think we can take the word of Veronica's family doctor that, other than the weight loss itself, she was in pretty good health. Other than absent menses and low sex interest, she was apparently not complaining about multiple somatic symptoms, and somatization disorder would seem unlikely. Just to be safe, however, I'd review the symptoms of that condition (see Chapter 9, page 109).

Depression, anxiety symptoms, and anorexia are all famously associated with amphetamine intoxication and withdrawal (see Table 9.3), but the available information suggests that Veronica's substance use was (1) the result of a desire to lose weight, not the cause of it, and (2) no longer current. Furthermore, we have nothing to suggest that she used amphetamines only at specific times of the year (which might explain her mood changes), or that she only lost weight when using. Nonetheless, for the sake of completeness, she should have at least one blood or urine test for substances.

Having now dismissed medical and substance use etiologies in the depression and anxiety decision trees, let's further explore Veronica's numerous mood symptoms. Some were of the atypical type (increase in sleep and appetite), but atypical symptoms are often found in teenagers. Her response to previous treatment (that's a diagnostic principle, remember) would suggest an independent mood disorder. The fact that her mood symptoms recurred each year at about the same time also strongly indicates a seasonal mood disorder (another diagnostic principle: "The best predictor of future behavior is past behavior"). Listing it as such would remind future clinicians to watch for the recurrence of symptoms each winter and possibly supply prophylactic treatment. The relatively brief duration of her depressive symptoms would rule out dysthymia, which lasts unbroken for years.

Should we regard Veronica's activity level and bright affect as symptoms of mania? Even coupled with her father's possible hypomania, such an interpretation would seem pretty weak—though she and her family should certainly be alerted to watch out for possible future bipolar symptoms. (A 2005 study reported not only that women are more likely than men to have bipolar disorder, but that a woman's first episode was more likely to be one of depression.)

Although social phobia has been included in the differential diagnosis, Veronica wouldn't really qualify for it because she didn't avoid other people. There was no suggestion of panic attacks or compulsive behavior, moving other anxiety disorders lower on our list. She did have symptoms of ADHD when she was little, but she was never seen clinically at the time, and there is no suggestion that she currently had features of that disorder.

We must now strongly consider anorexia nervosa. Veronica herself hotly denied that there was anything wrong with her eating, so we must use two of our rules for evaluating competing information. First, the signs of her skeletal appearance and her activity level—both typical in patients with anorexia nervosa—would overrule her reported lack of symptoms. Second, her parents' statements about her eating and weight would beat Veronica's own history (collateral history wins again). Considering all the available data, we can make an excellent case for anorexia nervosa as one of Veronica's diagnoses.

Finally, what about personality disorder? Table 6.1 has indicated that personality disorders are commonly encountered with the eating disorders. At the time of the interview, Veronica had some symptoms that could suggest avoidant or histrionic personality disorder—but, as the diagnostic principle about personality disorders advises, these should be reevaluated after adequate treatment for her anorexia nervosa. For right now, a mention of personality *traits* is about as far as I'd care to go.

The Working Diagnosis

After careful and rather extensive pruning, we have left this list of diagnoses:

- Anorexia nervosa
- Major depressive disorder, seasonal affective disorder type (with atypical symptoms)
- Diagnosis deferred on Axis II; avoidant and histrionic personality traits

Arranging the order of Veronica's comorbid diagnoses shouldn't prove too difficult. We have only two principal diagnoses to consider, anorexia nervosa and major depression. From a variety of studies, we know that the outlook for most patients with anorexia nervosa is worrisome. About one-quarter recover, and half are much improved at 10-year follow-up; however, the rest become chronically ill, with some studies suggesting that the overall *mortality* rate is in the 15–20% range. Although major depression can also result in early death from suicide, Veronica's had been seasonal, she wasn't depressed at the time of the interview, and she had responded well to treatment. With plenty of time to work on her mood disorder later, it would be a safe second to the more urgent anorexia nervosa. Also, in all likelihood the anorexia nervosa antedated the depression by several years.

For nearly every patient, the Axis II stuff (mental retardation, personality disorders) usually comes last. With the information we have at this point, I see no reason to change Veronica's personality assessment from how it is stated above, which is only a little more precise than the ever-valuable term *undiagnosed*. However, her clinician would have to remain alert for additional information that would permit a more definitive diagnosis (or perhaps eliminate Axis II from consideration altogether).

Easily Overlooked Issues

Even with a working diagnosis in hand, you should still pay attention to these questions: "Do I still lack information [such as additional symptoms, family history; is there a gap in the history]? Have I overlooked any relatively uncommon, but still possible, diagnoses? Should I consider any additional comorbid diagnoses?" As an aid to memory, I've included in this brief section issues clinicians sometimes overlook.

• *HIV and AIDS.* Of course, plenty of infectious diseases can cause mental symptoms (see Table 9.1), but HIV and AIDS are prevalent now.

• *Substance use.* Alcohol, street drugs, and prescription drugs are probably not often overlooked when clinicians are evaluating most adult patients, but they can also present problems for geriatric, adolescent, and even child patients.

• *Schizophreniform psychosis.* The concept is simple: A patient's symptoms look like they might add up to schizophrenia down the road; during your investigation, however, not enough time has passed to be sure. I'll discuss this in greater detail in Chapter 13.

• *Mental retardation and borderline intellectual functioning.* Aside from borderline personality disorder (see below), we too often ignore Axis II. But when you think about it, at least 3 people of every 100 in the general population have some degree of limited intellectual functioning. Some of them pass through your office, and most of these will have other mental health disorders that require attention. And you might mistakenly attribute to other sorts of pathology some of the characteristics of people who have relatively low IQs: stiff affect, apparent lack of concentration, "hallucinations" that are somehow not quite psychotic, and chronic difficulty getting along at work and in society—all in the absence of a major mental disorder.

• *Somatization disorder.* Clinicians hardly ever consider it, yet it causes much misery. I've given it some of the attention it deserves in Chapter 9.

• *No mental illness.* Frankly, I don't know whether this "diagnosis" is over- or underused; you won't find a lot of research on the topic. But I do want to point out that it happens, if infrequently, that a person who comes for an evaluation truly has no mental disorder or even a relational problem—nothing, in short, that you can report on Axis I. Because the line that divides mental illness from normality isn't always clear and sharp, clinicians may mistake for illness a number of nonpathological features. Here are a few: conflict with a social institution (such as, for those with long memories, the conscientious objector vs. the draft); a poor fit with one's social role (remember when being a nerd was considered *un*cool?); and any emotion that a person feels intensely, such as plain old unhappiness. I've already enshrined "no mental illness" in its own diagnostic principle.

• *Undiagnosed.* Let me mention again this wonderful term, which implies the need for further thought and investigation without prejudicing the clinician as to the direction such inquiry should take.

• *Social and environmental issues.* Too often we forget that environmental or social problems can affect diagnosis or treatment. Most of these arise in the context of the personal and social history. They include the patient's family (e.g., can the parents help care for a person with schizophrenia?), immediate social setting (because of mental illness, does the patient face discrimination?), education, occupation, housing, financial support, access to health care, and criminal and civil legal issues. Of course, many people will have multiple problems—like Rupert, a once popular and wealthy dot-com survivor whose drinking cost him his business, health, and family support, leading to solitary living and financial ruin.

Most of these social and environmental issues will be negative ones—things that work to the individual's detriment, such as poverty, a ruptured personal relationship, or being arrested. However, occasionally an issue might seem quite the opposite.

> George III, King of England during America's Revolutionary War, required treatment for an acute psychosis. As you can see for yourself in the gripping film *The Madness of King George,* because he was Britain's supreme authority, it was difficult for his clinicians—let alone his servants—to detain him for treatment.

To a degree, lofty status could similarly hinder the care of a politician or corporate executive who enjoys a position of high power or authority. Whereas having advanced education in the mental health field would ordinarily seem to be a plus, a patient with a hypomania who has training in psychology might know enough about disease to enable the canny concealment of telltale psychopathology.

- *Strengths.* The flip side of stating your patient's environmental and social problems is stating the patient's strengths. For example, although Lennie has been experiencing a major bad patch—depression, death of both parents, and loss of his job to an overseas call center—he enjoys the advantages of a solid education, winning personality, and supportive family. The listing of such strengths is often honored in the breach, which is a shame, for it can help clinicians stay tuned to potentially valuable resources. Although assessment of strengths isn't a required part of diagnosis, perhaps it should be.
- *Global Assessment of Functioning (GAF).* Finally, there is the GAF, whereby we can assess the degree to which our patients' symptoms cause

distress or interfere with daily activities. This is the only part of adult diagnosis that uses a scale, and it is an irony that with it, we actually measure
nothing. Rather, we are supposed to make our best guess about a patient's
level of functioning and assign a number (from 1 to 100) to it. This is not a
measurement; it's an educated guess. Nonetheless, there is value in ascer-
taining, if with some imprecision, the degree to which our patients' illnesses affect their lives and the lives of those about them. The best use we
can make of the GAF score is to compare it to our own reassessments as
time progresses.

Overused Diagnoses

On the other hand, there are several conditions that clinicians tend to diagnose too often—when circumstances and criteria do not justify them, and
usually when another diagnosis entirely is warranted. I'll mention just
three of them here.

- *Schizophrenia.* This is (or used to be) notoriously overdiagnosed,
especially by North American clinicians. This was certainly the case a couple of generations ago, when a cross-national study found that American
psychiatrists were far more likely to diagnose schizophrenia than were European clinicians. Is it still a problem? Though studies show that American
clinicians have tightened up their practice, it still happens. At a meeting
several years ago, senior clinicians were reviewing the case of a young
woman who had hallucinations without delusions. Despite the fact that she
had been ill for less than a month and came from a culture where visita-
tions from spirits were common, the diagnosis of schizophrenia was mentioned freely and without objection. Because it carries a heavy prognostic
penalty, the diagnosis should depend on criteria based on careful research.
- *Dissociative identity disorder.* This also tends to be embraced most
enthusiastically by American clinicians. Formerly called multiple personality disorder or MPD, this condition has caught the eye of more than one
movie maker (*Sybil, The Three Faces of Eve*). It raises a question that every
clinician should keep in mind: Am I being overly influenced by my particular specialty or interests? We must beware the tendency to see our special
interests everywhere; otherwise, as time goes by, their boundaries expand
to encompass far too many patients. Long ago, I treated Emma, a college
student who was highly suggestible and easily influenced. During a summer vacation away from my watchful eye, she fell under the care of another

clinician—someone who had published many articles about patients with MPD. Sure enough, when Emma returned in the fall she had developed two new identities, for which she had spent her holiday in treatment.

• *Borderline personality disorder.* This continues to be diagnosed far more often than it is warranted. It has been well studied over the years, and from my own experience I am certain that it exists; however, I am equally certain that many (perhaps most) patients who receive this diagnosis don't deserve it. I'm afraid that too many clinicians use it as a sort of "wastebasket" category to cover their uncertainty when the term *undiagnosed* would do just fine. Sometimes they apply it to people they don't like—bosses and in-laws come to mind. As with all other personality disorders, the borderline diagnosis should be made only with a great deal of information from at least two sources, based on a thorough appraisal of the course of symptoms across the length of the patient's adult lifetime.

Checking Up with a Formulation

Once you've completed your evaluation and have the diagnosis well in mind, I would urge a quick reality check for logic and completeness, using a mental health formulation. This device can help ensure that you've covered all the pertinent facts and theories of disease development. It will be a brief statement (well, it could be of nearly any length, but I recommend brief) summarizing the history, significant symptoms (and pertinent negatives), possible causes, differential diagnosis, and the patient's important strengths. You can share this summary with the clinician who referred the patient for mental health evaluation, as well as with the patient. In fact, I strongly recommend this last step; it will let the patient in on your thinking and provide a chance to correct anything that could indicate a misunderstanding between the two of you. With the patient's permission, it could also help the family understand your evaluation. Finally, it will provide the rock from which to sculpt your treatment plan.

The traditional approach to evaluation and treatment prescription is the *biopsychosocial model*, which for every patient incorporates three sorts of information about possible influences on current symptomatology. The *biological* area includes data such as genetic heredity, physical development, childhood diseases, previous physical injuries and diseases, operations, and toxic factors in the environment. The *psychological* realm encompasses cognition, emotions, behavior, communications, and interpersonal relations, including methods for coping with adversity (or, sometimes, success). The *social* area describes how a person interacts with family, cultural groups, and various institutions (such as school, places of worship, and different levels of government), and the availability and competence of this support network.

Because each of these biopsychosocial areas is understood to interact with the others to produce the final mental disease state, each should be explored in your diagnostic formulation. Here is a sample, based on the evaluation of Veronica, whom we met at the beginning of this chapter:

> Veronica Harper, a 19-year-old college student, has a 5-year history of anorexia nervosa. At 89 pounds, she is at least 25% below the minimum normal body weight for her age and height; yet she believes she looks fat and fears gaining weight. She loves physical activity and participates in a vigorous swimming schedule. Her menses stopped 5 months ago. Although she briefly tried laxatives and amphetamines, for several years she has only restricted caloric intake to achieve low weight.
>
> For several years she has also had winter depression, beginning about December and spontaneously resolving each spring. Her symptoms include low mood, increased sleep, tiredness, improved appetite, loss of interest, and lack of concentration, but never suicidal ideas. Last winter, these symptoms resolved early with antidepressant medication. Other than low weight and mild hypothyroidism, her physical health has been good.
>
> Veronica is a painfully thin though lively and cheerful young woman who cooperates with the interview. Her speech is clear and coherent; she denies delusions, hallucinations, phobias, panic attacks, compulsions, and obsessions (other than an abiding interest in food, cooking, and recipes). Her mood shows normal lability and is appropriate to the content of thought. She has only fair insight—despite obvious wasting, she believes that she is overweight—and her judgment as regards her eating behavior is poor and dangerous to her health.
>
> Contributing to her principal disorder, anorexia nervosa, could be genetics (her mother may have some symptoms of OCD, and her sister has been bulimic), social factors (Western societies famously associate slenderness with beauty); and the psychological desire to thwart the attempts at control exerted by her father. Her seasonal major depressive disorder is in part accounted for by heredity (history of mood disorder, possibly bipolar, in her father), and in part by distress at feelings of rejection by her peers. Veronica's principal strengths are good intelligence; a strong work ethic; and parents who, though controlling, are also concerned and, in their way, supportive.

Following Through

Clinicians err and patients change—two reasons why we must always keep alert to the need for rethinking diagnosis. Yet readjusting diagnosis in the face of new information doesn't get talked about much. Although you should *always* consider the possibility of such a change, certain situations should set the rediagnosis machinery whirring.

1. Your new patient comes with a ready-made diagnosis. This situation, a walking trap for clinicians, often signals the need for a diagnostic reevaluation. Unhappily, not everyone practices scientific diagnosis, and the fate of many patients is still decided in the not-so-good old-fashioned way—by hunch or by prejudice. The start of therapy with a new patient is the ideal point to review the complete history and reassess the mental status. Once you've accepted the old diagnosis and begun treatment, it's much harder to backtrack.

2. Your own diagnosis leaves some symptoms unexplained. Examples might include an anxious patient who has depression, a depressed patient with delusions, and a psychotic patient who complains of anxiety. Although for each of these, a single diagnosis might embrace all the symptoms, each represents a situation I'd watch carefully to be sure that all symptoms respond fully to treatment.

3. A patient develops new symptoms not explained by current diagnoses. If you've treated depression in a patient who then develops symptoms of mania, you've obviously got some serious rethinking to do. But what about a patient with dementia who becomes depressed? Or someone with PTSD who stops eating? If the new symptom fits nicely into the current diagnosis, well and good. But if that isn't the case, try hard to resist the temptation to force new data into an old schema. Your patient needs you to maintain mental flexibility, so you shouldn't cling inappropriately to a diagnosis that is no longer appropriate.

4. Your patient remains mired in symptoms, despite treatment that seems appropriate. Of course, the therapy itself could be at fault, but have you unwittingly been treating for the wrong diagnosis? For example, perhaps the cocaine use for which the patient has faithfully attended Narcotics Anonymous has been hiding an underlying depression.

5. Despite improving symptoms, your patient's work or family situation deteriorates. Although behavior therapy had reduced Elisa's panic at-

tacks, she told of increasing fights with her husband and critical comments from her boss. A review of her history and reevaluation of her mental status revealed a supervening depression. In other patients, this might be the time to reevaluate for the presence of a personality disorder.

6. You finally meet the patient's relatives, spouse, or significant other. This can produce additional history, new family history, and other information that could revise your working diagnosis. At the very least, you'll have a new point of view with which to validate your previous diagnosis.

7. Laboratory data can add new clues. Occasionally an abnormal thyroid hormone level or an X-ray finding has triggered the reevaluation of a patient who might otherwise appear to be doing well.

8. A disease is born. OK, so new disorders don't appear all that often. But as an exercise, you might sometime scan the relevant appendix of the current DSM, just to see how many disorders are being studied for inclusion in future editions; last time I checked, there were over a dozen. And even more disorders are waiting in the wings. Recently proposed for consideration was body integrity identity disorder—an extremely rare condition in which a person becomes intent on having healthy body parts removed, such as the man who persuaded a surgeon to amputate his lower extremities. Such a disorder is sure to generate a lot of interest, but will it survive to posterity? (As they say in the movie business, will it have legs?)

9. On the other hand, perhaps just thumbing through a book about diagnosis (ahem!) reminds you of an existing disorder that you hadn't considered for a particular patient.

The Challenge of a Changing Diagnosis

When you obtain new information, or when other issues develop in the course of treatment, you may have to reconsider your working diagnosis or develop a new diagnosis altogether. The failure to do so if circumstances warrant it can be devastating (see the sidebar "False Positives" on page 84). Here are a few suggestions for finding your way through the swamp of an evolving diagnosis:

- Don't react hastily. Proceed with caution, especially if your patient is stable and doing well. Absent a true emergency, sudden moves can muddle rather than clarify. Even with great deliberation, you can come to grief.

> Candy, a young woman I once diagnosed as having a bipolar disorder, became increasingly psychotic despite mood stabilizers, lithium, and even a course of electroconvulsive therapy. After nearly 2 years, I reluctantly began to regard her diagnosis as schizophrenia. With antipsychotic drugs she improved somewhat, but she continued ill and incapable of maintaining a job; her husband divorced her. I eventually lost track of her, but several years later we met quite by accident and paused to talk. Using a newly available mood stabilizer, another clinician was treating her for bipolar disorder; she appeared to have recovered completely.

- Carefully reassess the new information. Considering both content and source, is it credible? How does it fit in with what you already know? The diagnostic principles we've already discussed can help evaluate breaking news.
- What are the possible consequences of a change in diagnosis? Before you leap, you should know where you might land. Of course, there may be a change in treatment, but what about prognosis? How will the family react?
- Get help. Mental health diagnosis can be a lonely occupation, and a consultant's fresh eye can sometimes stimulate new directions for your diagnostic thinking. Just having someone to discuss a difficult or confusing patient has helped me organize my thoughts. Of the meetings I attend, the most valuable are those where staff clinicians present their tough diagnostic problems to solicit new insights.
- Rethink any objective information that might help ensure a successful outcome. Psychological and medical tests are among the sorts of material to include.
- Share your thoughts. Fully inform your patient (and, if appropriate, the family) about the new findings, your opinion as regards the need to change diagnosis, and what all of this could mean for treatment. There is little you can do that will better ensure compliance than helping everyone to understand the situation, even (or especially) if that includes the degree to which you may be unsure of the diagnosis. I recommend candor, but of course it should be couched positively, so as to avoid inducing further emotional trauma.

False Positives

False positives—those diagnoses that turn out not to be accurate—are problematic enough that we ought to discuss them for a moment or two. (On the flip side, *false negatives*, in which diagnoses that should have been made aren't, can also be devastating; their consequences are pretty obvious.) There are a number of reasons to avoid false positives.

- One is the stigma of certain mental diagnoses. Antisocial personality disorder and schizophrenia are two that no one ought to be given without careful study and full confidence. Even without social censure, there is still the problem of loss in self-esteem and a diminished sense of personal responsibility that having a mental health diagnosis can convey.

- While chasing a false diagnosis, you might ignore another, more accurate diagnosis. False positives can provide a bogus sense of security, when you should be busily pondering the next move in your investigation.

- False positives can have two sorts of effect upon treatment: to promote treatment that is unnecessary, and to delay treatment that is needed. The resulting dollar costs (insurance expenditures, time lost from work) go almost without saying.

False-positive diagnoses are especially likely when we use criteria that rest exclusively on symptoms. (Counting symptoms is easy; understanding context can be difficult indeed.) To a degree, diagnostic manuals may promote overdiagnosis by encouraging multiple diagnoses.

Patients who have been given a false-positive diagnosis provide convincing evidence of the need for careful follow-up and reconsideration of the evidence. In 2005 Opal Petty died, after having spent 51 years in a Texas state mental hospital. Probably of borderline intelligence, she had begun behaving strangely as a teenager. For one thing, she wanted to go dancing, of which her fundamentalist parents disapproved. When a church exorcism failed to correct the situation, they had her committed. Diagnosed with schizophrenia, she languished in confinement until she was 67. Clinicians testifying on her behalf concluded that although she may have had a psychotic depression when first admitted, she had recovered soon afterward. A distant relative finally requested her release, and she lived the last 20 years of her life in her own home, apparently free of psychosis—and demonic possession.

PART II

The Building Blocks of Diagnosis

8 Understanding the Whole Patient

If someone comes to you with symptoms of mania and a history of bipolar I disorder, the most likely diagnosis is pretty much a slam dunk. But in regard to Carson (see Chapter 1) and his depression, does it make a difference that he was in the middle of a move when he contacted me that last time? Of course, the answer is an obvious "yes," and Carson's case shows the importance of environmental and historical information to our understanding of emotions and behaviors. My point is underscored by a 2005 editorial in the *American Journal of Psychiatry*, which noted that good clinical practice goes beyond (way beyond, I'd put it) the usual diagnostic checklists of symptoms to include full social and past mental health histories.

Another reason to mine every possible scrap of information is to reassure occasional patients who have no diagnosable mental illness, but are afraid that they do. Take, for example, Tom, whose marriage is falling apart and whose boss says that if he doesn't put in more overtime, the company will fold. Tom's stress and discomfort may make him worry that he has something more fundamentally wrong—perhaps that a mental breakdown is imminent. Here a complete history does double duty, pointing out both what he lacks (a mental disorder) and what he has (multiple problems of living). Because treatment for problems like Tom's is often less specific and perhaps less urgent than for a diagnosable illness, we want to be sure that we make context-dependent diagnoses such as job stress or marital discord only after we've ruled out other, more specific causes of emotional upheaval.

Of course, even mentally ill patients often have additional, unrelated problems that we must address.

Now age 37, Dorothy has been treated for schizophrenia for the past 15 years. Although she graduated from college with a major in English literature, she lives on a small disability income and what she can earn part-time bagging groceries and retrieving carts at her local supermarket. She shares rooms in an assisted-living apartment complex, does her own shopping, and keeps her own checkbook. Thanks to antipsychotic drugs, it has been a decade since she was last hospitalized, but nonetheless she feels deeply troubled. Her roommate, Janette, neither works nor keeps house, but spends her money (and some of Dorothy's) on bowling, video games, and pizzas that she orders in. Dorothy's social life is nonexistent: Janette yells and bullies her, and is such a slob that having friends over is not an option. Dorothy must do any cleaning herself. Although she feels used and manipulated by Janette, she also feels powerless to do anything about it. She knows that there is a long list of people waiting for an apartment; she fears that if she complains, she'll be asked to leave in favor of someone who is more compliant.

Apart from practical aspects of management, it is interesting and rewarding to know all about another person. Greater interest builds rapport, leading in turn to augmented sympathy (in both directions) and facilitation of our ability to work together. For all of these reasons, I consider it absolutely vital to consider the wide range of information often described under the heading of "personal and social history," along with details of the patient's family of origin. In this chapter we'll explore many items of this great building block of mental health history: the background information that can shape our understanding of symptoms and influence the diagnoses we give our patients. I've outlined this material in Table 8.1 for quick reference.

Childhood

Roland was an accountant in his early 40s. Throughout his adult life, his sour attitude had prevented him from forming close relationships. Shortly after I first met him, I learned some of his early history. Roland's mother had died when he was 2, and he was taken in by his aunt, who had two small children of her own. Roland was adequately fed and housed, but he never had a sense of belonging. At Christmas, his cousins would get elaborate gifts, while Roland received the barest tokens. One year, the other boys got Erector sets that would build a motorized parachute jump, whereas Roland's would only build a tiny truck you had to push.

TABLE 8.1. Outline of Personal and Social History

Childhood

Where was the patient born, reared?

Reared by both parents?

Number of siblings and sibship
  position.

Did patient feel wanted as child?

If adopted, what circumstances?
  Extrafamilial or intrafamilial?

Relationship with parents, siblings.

Were there other adults, children in
  home?

How was health as child?

Education: Last grade completed.
  Scholastic, behavioral, disciplinary
  problems.

Number and quality of friendships.

Age dating began.

Sexual or physical abuse. Details.

Sexual development.

Hobbies, interests.

Religion as child.

Losses through divorce, bereavement.

Family history

Mental disorders in close relatives.

Current relationship with parents,
  siblings.

Adult life

Currently lives with whom?

Type/source of financial support.

Ever homeless?

Current support network: family,
  agencies.

Number of marriages.

Marital difficulties, divorces,
  separations.

Number, age, and gender of children.

Stepchildren.

Occupation. Number of jobs lifetime?
  Reasons for job change.

Military service: branch, rank,
  disciplinary problems.

Combat experience.

Legal problems: civil, arrests,
  violence.

Current religion, attendance.

Leisure activities: organizations,
  hobbies.

Sexual preference and adjustment.

Age at first sexual experience. Details.

Suicide attempts: methods, association
  with substance use, consequences.

Personality traits and evidence of
  lifelong behavior patterns.

Current sexual practices.

Sexually transmitted diseases?

Substance use: type, quantity,
  duration, consequences.

Although a 2005 research report noted that half of all mental illnesses begin by age 14, much of the information about your patient's childhood years will go less toward diagnosis and more toward your general appreciation of what are sometimes referred to as "character-forming experiences." That in itself is of course valuable to know. But sometimes you will gain information about childhood years that may help you interpret the symptoms you encounter—perhaps the fact that a person imitates a parent

or other relative when responding to positive conditions of love and success or to stress from frustration or failure. Roland's second-class childhood (his relatives could have been a model for Harry Potter's horrific aunt
and uncle) had set him up for a lifetime of perceived rejection and isolation.

Early Relationships

What sort of child was the patient? Outgoing? Introverted? Quiet? Serious?
A show-off? A history of being a loner is often associated with later chronic
psychosis and personality disorder. Someone who has always been uncomfortable with others may be at risk for alcoholism. Older children sometimes
must shoulder responsibility for younger siblings, affecting their own experience of childhood and opportunities to form relationships as adolescents.

> Being "junior mom" to six younger siblings had certainly marked Jolie's
> life. As an adult, she persuaded her husband to take in foster children—up
> to seven at a time—until their marriage foundered on the shoals of their
> child-rearing responsibilities.

Information about how the person interacted with parents (was there
overinvolvement? distancing?), siblings, and others both in and out of the
household may be especially relevant to people like Jolie, who have no actual mental disorder.

The early social development of a patient with Asperger's disorder will
be marked by poor eye contact, lack of age-appropriate peer relationships,
and failure to bond with peers and family. The inability to understand and em-
pathize with the feelings and experiences of others extends into adult life.

> Despite her Asperger's, Audrey had recently formed a romantic relation-
> ship with Bert, a developmentally disabled young man. That Thanks-
> giving, when the two of them were celebrating separately with their re-
> spective families, Audrey telephoned Bert to say she loved him. Then she
> called again, and again—a total of 11 times, though Bert and his parents
> each repeatedly asked her to desist.

Losses

The dissolution of a relationship can be especially hard in childhood.

> When his father, a teetotaling preacher, left the family, Tyler was only 12,
> and he spent the next 20 years deeply resenting him. "I've always thought

it was a big reason I started using drugs," he said during one therapy session. "I was just so pissed off at the old man. I think that all along I've been trying to punish him."

Though the mechanisms of such associations are hard to understand, when a child suffers the death of a parent, it can sometimes be reflected in adult-onset depression. Studies have also linked major depression and GAD with parental divorce or separation. Loss of a father before age 14 may signal increased risk for personality disorder.

Education

Various disciplinary and scholastic problems are correlated with later behavioral difficulties.

> When 21-year-old Dudley was caught intoxicated on alcohol and burgling an apartment near where he lived with his mother, it was his third offense within the past year. "First probation, then 3 months inside haven't taught him a thing," said the assistant district attorney who was prosecuting his case. "He's clearly sociopathic." The clinician brought in by defense counsel noted that Dudley had been a model student, graduating from high school with high honors, and had had no legal difficulties at all until he started drinking a year earlier. After pointing out that the very definition of antisocial personality disorder includes early conduct disorder, which Dudley had not had, the consultant offered instead a diagnosis of alcohol dependence. The judge accepted the proposal that Dudley enter rehab.

Although it's possible that a person with budding antisocial personality disorder might have gotten through school without disciplinary problems, I've never encountered such a case. You can also use a patient's education history to help differentiate dementia from mental retardation, or a learning disorder from ADHD.

Sexuality and Abuse

Toward the end of childhood comes the time of the awakening and exploration of our sexual selves. Many adult patients will have memorable experiences to relate of that embarkation.

> At 15, Josephine's physical development had far outstripped her judgment: She and her long-time boyfriend found themselves becoming par-

ents when they were still children themselves. The resulting humiliation and lost educational opportunity followed them into young adulthood, culminating in drinking, depression, and divorce.

The sexual life of many a child is a far darker story, commencing with aggression and betrayal. Childhood sexual abuse is painful but vital to pursue, because it is a flag for many adult mental disorders—including bulimia nervosa, depression, alcoholism, and schizophrenia, as well as dissociative, somatization, personality (especially borderline), panic, and conduct disorders. Such a diversity across the diagnostic spectrum makes one wonder whether childhood sexual abuse, rather than having some specific effect, instead facilitates the development of pathology of many types. Regardless of possible causes and effects, I use the correlation in two ways. When I encounter someone who was abused as a child, I look for one of the disorders mentioned just above. And whenever I think a patient may have one of those disorders, I take extra care when checking for hints of abuse.

Although the data are somewhat less certain, the implications of childhood physical abuse are probably similar.

Adult Life and Living Situation

You can find many pointers to diagnosis from the basic facts of an adult's current life. Here are some of the issues I consider when I evaluate a new patient.

Age and Gender

These two basic patient characteristics have extremely important implications for diagnosis. Somatization disorder, for example, is found almost exclusively in women (especially young ones), which is why I consider this diagnosis strongly if my patient's name is Frances, but much less so if it is Francis. On the other hand, you'll encounter antisocial personality disorder mostly in young men, especially those living in prison. Although a few major conditions *don't* discriminate between the sexes (schizophrenia, bipolar disorder, and OCD pretty much complete the list), most mental disorders do play favorites. Table 8.2 comprises a partial listing.

TABLE 8.2. Gender Predominance for Select Disorders

Men predominate	Women predominate
Alcoholism	Anorexia nervosa
Antisocial personality disorder	Anxiety disorders (except for OCD)
Drug use	Bulimia nervosa
Factitious disorder	Dissociative disorders
Paraphilias	Kleptomania
Pathological gambling	Major depression
Pyromania	Somatization disorder

Sexual and Marital Life and Difficulties

Change in sex interest (up or down) are common flags for the different phases of mood disorders, and sexual behavior inappropriate for the circumstances is sometimes associated with disorders as diverse as dementia and substance use. Low sex interest is especially typical of somatization disorder.

With changing mores, multiple partners before marriage and sex outside marriage have become so commonplace that they no longer carry the whiff of scandal they once did. Nonetheless, when I encounter someone with more than one failed marriage, it raises my suspicions about the possibility of personality disorder. Absent clear evidence of mania, I would be especially careful to evaluate for personality disorder a patient who is inappropriately seductive, especially if the behavior targets the clinician.

Most people with schizophrenia once tended to remain single, but this may be less true today for two reasons: improved treatment, and a steep decline in the practice of institutionalization. However, someone with schizoid personality disorder is by definition likely to show little interest in sex with another person.

Current Environment

People survive in a wide variety of living situations. I've known many who thrive living by themselves, sometimes in circumstances that we would consider appalling. (To a question about where he lived, one man responded, "Well, the previous tenant was a Frigidaire.") Most people, however, do better with the safety and love that close friends and neighbors can bring. That's why the mental health evaluation doesn't consist solely in disease diagnosis; you must also judge whether the patient's support system is sufficient to maintain alertness for the symptoms of mania or depression, to watch for evidence of renewed drinking or other substance use, and to notify the clinician if the patient stops taking medicine that is vital to stabilize behavior and emotions.

I recently interviewed a young man recovering from substance use who lived alone in an apartment. When I asked about his support network, the sad truth was that he could name only his mental healthcare providers and his therapy group. The outlook for such a person must be less optimistic than for one who feels the constant support of friends and family. And changes in support can prove disastrous. For example, a person with agoraphobia may suddenly become housebound when a spouse or companion dies or moves away. Of course, the quality of the relationships can be as critical as their number. It is well known that patients with schizophrenia are especially likely to relapse if they have highly emotional relatives who freely shout and cast blame. I don't know of any solid data, but it stands to reason that any one of us who was rearing children alone, struggling in financial straits, or teetering on the brink of a divorce would feel more vulnerable in surroundings fraught with tension.

Where your patient lives could be especially relevant to the evaluation. The classic example occurs when a person with evolving dementia must move from familiar surroundings and becomes overwhelmed by the added disorientation. A lifelong city dweller who fears snakes may never have symptoms before moving to the country. Even such environmental factors as time of year can have a bearing on diagnosis. As noted in Chapter 1, Carson regularly became symptomatic with depression in the fall or winter and recovered in the spring.

Working and Financial Support

Apart from the financial support it provides, work is a cornerstone of self-esteem because it enables us to see ourselves as productive members of society. The type of work and the worker's perspective on it can suggest several diagnostic possibilities. Ilsa—who trained as a librarian, then spent years doing janitorial work at a large department store as she battled hallucinations and delusions—provides one example of how people with schizophrenia often drift downward on the occupational scale.

In the course of an interstate move, I asked Nick, an intelligent man with a ready wit, how he happened to fall into his current line of work carrying furniture. He said that he had formerly been pretty good at computer repair, but that his fondness for beer had led to repeated suspensions of his driver's license. When it was eventually revoked, he could no longer travel to a regular job. "What I like about humping furniture," he told me, "is that they pick me up each day and drop me off at the end. And it doesn't get between me and my 12-pack of Bud every night after work."

A long history of unemployment signals that something has been seriously wrong for many months or years; often that something is psychosis, substance use, or bipolar disorder. (Although a disability income suggests a serious, chronic illness such as schizophrenia, I've also known patients with somatization disorder or substance use disorders who managed to collect disability.) Another tell-tale pattern is the checkered job history of repeated firing and sudden quitting that is classic for antisocial personality disorder. But even a well-heeled celebrity may not be immune to the consequences of job-related behavior. At a New York Jets team reunion, former championship quarterback Joe Namath twice on camera told a reporter that he wanted to kiss her. That was his wake-up call to enter alcohol rehab.

My own long service in VA hospitals and clinics has taught me to be especially vigilant with people whose work history includes time served in the military or as firefighters or police officers. The dangers inherent in these professions warn that any symptoms of anxiety could be due to PTSD, and such symptoms should therefore prompt a careful search for evidence of psychological trauma. Those who do have PTSD are also highly likely to have depression and substance use disorders.

Legal Involvement

When you encounter a patient who has had arrests or convictions, you are likely to think first of antisocial personality disorder, conduct disorder, or substance use, because legal issues are included in these criteria sets. However, law enforcement officials often take an interest in patients with paraphilias (especially pedophilia and voyeurism) and with most of the impulse-control disorders (intermittent explosive disorder, kleptomania, pyromania, and pathological gambling—thus far, anyway, hair-pulling isn't illegal). In the throes of mania, a patient's judgment may be sufficiently er-

ratic to create conflicts with the law. Patients with schizophrenia occasionally have a history of violence, even to the point of homicide.

Family History

Although standard diagnostic systems don't use family history as a criterion,
most mental disorders run in families. Indeed, thousands of studies have
demonstrated that nearly the entire spectrum of mental disorders can be
transmitted from one generation to the next, at least partly through genetic
inheritance. That's why the existence of a biological relative with a mental
disorder can serve as a flag that your patient might have the same illness.

> A 34-year-old priest, Father Mark had spent 2 years working in the ar-
> chives at the Vatican. One afternoon, in a centuries-old Latin document,
> he came across a mention of the Apostle Mark. "Suddenly," he said later,
> "it became crystal-clear that this reference really meant *me*." Over the
> next several days, he became more and more agitated as he realized the
> implication: that he was himself the second coming of Christ. When he re-
> ported this revelation to other priests, it caused quite a stir. Before long,
> loaded with sedatives and accompanied by two burly novitiates, he was
> hustled back to the United States for treatment.
>
> When first evaluated, Father Mark still had grandiose delusions and
> heard voices telling him that he was destined to save the world. Partly be-
> cause his younger brother had for several years been treated for classical
> bipolar disorder, he was started on lithium. His symptoms rapidly re-
> solved, and, fully insightful that he had been ill, he resumed work. How-
> ever, he was never again posted to the Vatican.

Apart from mood disorders, family patterns similar to Father Mark's
can be found for a wide range of mental disorders. These include schizophrenia; many anxiety disorders (especially panic disorder, phobias, and
GAD); alcoholism and the use of other drugs; somatization disorder; Alzheimer's dementia; anorexia and bulimia nervosa; and personality disorders, most notably antisocial. Even narcolepsy, a sleep disorder in which
patients suddenly fall asleep at inopportune times (even while driving), is
strongly hereditary.

I do want to sound three notes of caution about using family history to
evaluate a patient. The first is that it is so easy for one family member's diagnosis to influence another's. It has happened to me, so I know that I
must take great care not to let my knowledge of the patient tilt my judg-

ment as to what a relative's symptoms signify. Researchers are well aware of this problem, which is why they developed the "blind evaluation": One clinician evaluates the patient while another, unaware of the patient's diagnosis, obtains and interprets the information about the relatives. Of course, you'll hardly ever have that luxury when making your own diagnoses, so you'll have to practice what I try to do: Be especially careful that prejudice doesn't affect clinical judgment.

The second cautionary note is that the diagnoses of relatives related by many patients and their families will be misleading or just plain wrong. The source may be a patient who has misunderstood—or, frankly, a clinician who has erred.

> My depressed patient Julia told me that her grandfather had been hospitalized for schizophrenia. Additional history from Julia's mother revealed that in fact there were three periods during which Grandpa had become convinced that he had special "cerebral powers"; he believed that he had altered the course of human history by the force of his thought waves. After each such episode, he had gradually returned to normal and resumed work driving a city bus. Despite Grandpa's alleged diagnosis, from the history I obtained, his psychosis was not chronic but episodic—and therefore highly suspicious for bipolar disorder. This suggested to me that Julia should be offered treatment to prevent mania.

The point is that whenever possible, you should obtain all the information possible to allow an independent evaluation of a relative's diagnosis. This suggests that we need to modify our diagnostic principle about family history from its previously stated version in Chapter 4 (see page 29).

Here is the third warning: The *absence* of a family history usually tells us nothing at all about a given patient. There are at least

> *Diagnostic Principle:* **Family history can help guide diagnosis, but because you often cannot trust reports, clinicians should attempt to rediagnose each family member.**

two reasons. The history may be faulty (informants may forget or conceal information; a patient may have been adopted and not know it). Even with good information, however, only about 10% of the parents, siblings, and children of patients with a major mental illness will have that same illness. That's why many patients will have no known close relatives who are affected. So regard a positive family history as a straw in the wind—but realize that even in the absence of a straw, the wind may be blowing anyway.

9 Physical Illness and Mental Diagnosis

Physical illness can play a vital role in creating or extending mental health symptoms. If we forget this fact, we imperil our diagnosis and our patients' health—indeed, their very lives.

James

As one of the forward party for our infantry battalion, I thought I was doing pretty well the morning I landed in Vietnam. The terror of nighttime mortar attacks, the horror of mutilated bodies, lay days in the future. For the first few hours of that first day, I kept my head down and spirits up as I went about the dull routine of setting up aid stations and inspecting field kitchens for cleanliness. But as evening drew near, I became first restless, then downright jittery. I had developed the most alarming collection of symptoms, starting with, well, alarm—anxiety too intense to be ignored, coupled with fatigue so great I could barely stir myself into action. I noticed that my heart was beating too fast, too hard, and too irregularly. I had trouble drawing a breath, and the sweat rolled off my forehead, though I was standing in the shade—sitting, rather, for my legs suddenly seemed too weak to support a soldier wearing a flak jacket and a steel pot helmet, and toting a medical bag and an M-16 rifle.

Was I going mad, caving in to pressure? Or was there something else? I was the only medical authority around, so I shakily reviewed the day's activity for clues to the reason for my acute unease. Suddenly I had it: I had forgotten (declined, actually, with the arrogance of youth) to take the salt tablets we had all been issued prior to landing. As retribution, I had developed an acute electrolyte deficiency. With a canteen of water, I washed down a couple of salt tablets and vowed to sin no more; within minutes, my panic attack had begun to abate.

My Vietnam experience illustrates the importance of physical health and its opposite, physical illness, to the mental health diagnostic enterprise. Indeed, if we don't seize upon these concepts as building blocks, they become roadblocks to understanding our patients' illnesses. Because physical symptoms in mental disorders can be hard to get our minds around, mental health professionals who are neither physicians nor nurses sometimes feel daunted by this material. However, it is extremely important for the patients—so every clinician, regardless of discipline, should read carefully about this element of mental health diagnosis. It is important enough that I've already awarded it diagnostic principle status.

How Physical and Mental Disorders Are Related

The effects of physical and mental disorders on one another can be complicated, but, taken in small steps, the relationships are easily understood.

Physical Disorders Can Produce Mental Symptoms

When Derek has one of his epileptic seizures, electrical impulses discharge throughout his brain. This makes him feel elated and causes him to have a visual hallucination—a jar of candy sitting on his desk. People with epilepsy can experience hallucinations in any of the other senses; some will feel depressed; still others may have trouble thinking or speaking. *Déjà vu* experiences can also occur. Like Derek, patients with brain pathology as varied as tumors or multiple sclerosis may experience mood changes. In fact, many physical diseases produce symptoms that closely mimic mental disorders.

> In *Saturday*, novelist Ian McEwan describes a street thug in the early stages of Huntington's disease. Within a few moments, Baxter's mood can swing from boiling anger to depression to bubbling euphoria, much like that of a patient in the throes of bipolar disorder. In the page-turning dénouement, the neurosurgeon protagonist operates to remove hematomas from Baxter's brain, thus saving a life he might have preferred to lose.

> The stuff of medical legend are patients mistakenly diagnosed as having schizophrenia or depression—and sometimes treated for those disorders for years—when the real problem is a thyroid or adrenal abnormality.

A 1978 study gives substance to these tales. Of 658 consecutive patients, 9% had medical disorders that produced mental symptoms. Depression, confusion, anxiety, and memory loss were the most frequent presenting problems. Most often the cause was an infection; pulmonary or thyroid disease; diabetes; or a disease of the blood, liver, or central nervous system. Nearly half the time, neither the patients nor their physicians had previously recognized these medical illnesses.

More than a generation later, we still don't adequately diagnose physical disease that causes mental symptoms. A study in 2002 reported that of 289 patients, 3 had previously undetected hypothyroidism, which in 1 case caused and in 2 others worsened a patient's mental symptoms. The investigators also found that previously known physical illness caused the mental symptoms of 6 patients and made worse those of 8. Their illnesses were as varied as drug withdrawal, alcoholic dementia, epileptic psychosis, postconcussional disorder, and myocardial infarction.

Physical Disease Can Worsen Existing Mental Symptoms

Even if it isn't the original cause, it's easy to see how the burden of heart disease, substance use, or AIDS could intensify the symptoms of someone who already has serious mental illness.

> Just as Gloria was recovering from her latest bipolar depressive episode, she learned that she had Addison's disease—adrenal insufficiency. "It shouldn't take Sigmund Freud to figure out that the news would drop me right back into depression," she lamented. Her family doctor agreed but pointed out, "Don't forget that the physiological effects of a metabolic or infectious disease can directly produce mental symptoms, such as depression, psychosis, and anxiety. That means your mood could improve a lot, once we get your endocrine system back under control."

Treatment for Medical Disorders Can Cause Mental Symptoms

Most medications have side effects, some of which can include mental symptoms. For example, psychosis is occasionally brought on by taking adrenal steroids, which are prescribed for illnesses as diverse as arthritis, infections, adrenal gland insufficiency, lupus, and asthma. In fact, probably the majority of all medications currently in use, including those that treat mental disorders, can produce mental symptoms of one sort or another.

Physical and Mental Disorders Can Be Independent Conditions

Even when medical illness doesn't cause or worsen mental symptoms, we must recognize and address physical illness in psychiatric patients. It is incredibly easy—it has happened to me—to become so focused on a patient's mental disorder that symptoms of an independent medical illness must knock loudly and persistently before we answer the door. Hence, the diagnostic principle that every new symptom should generate this thought first: Could a physical condition be causing this?

Uncharted Waters

There are some physical findings whose meaning we don't yet understand. For instance, for decades we've known that patients with schizophrenia often have enlarged brain ventricles. The degree of enlargement isn't great, and it doesn't always occur, so the finding isn't robust enough to enable diagnosis in an individual patient. We don't know what it means, but it's real. Here's another example: Recently researchers have reported reduced numbers of receptors for the neurotransmitter serotonin in the brains of patients with panic disorder. What does this mean? Once again, knowledge has preceded understanding.

The great healer, it is alleged, is time, which can also be a pretty darn good diagnostician. What we don't understand today often becomes clear as passing time reveals new symptoms or clarifies the meaning of older ones. Even without waiting, there are a couple of ways time helps us resolve relationships between medical illness and mental symptoms: (1) if the mental symptom and the medical disorder begin at about the same time, and (2) if the patient's mental or emotional symptoms remit after the medical disorder improves.

> When Sylvia's lupus worsened and she developed kidney failure, she became depressed; her appetite fell and she became weak and lethargic. After she started on dialysis, these symptoms of depression remitted. During a brief vacation trip to California, she missed two dialysis appointments in a row; once again, her mood headed south.

If neither of these time-related guideposts obtains, you might suspect a mental symptom if it is commonly associated with a medical condition. To that end, I've listed in Table 9.1 the mental symptoms of 60 medical disor-

TABLE 9.1. Some Medical Disorders That Can Cause Mental Symptoms

	Relative frequency[a]	Emotional/behavioral symptoms																	
		Depression	Mania	Anxiety	Panic	OCD-like behaviors	Labile emotions	Withdrawal	Catatonia	Insomnia	Hypersomnia	Hallucinations	Delusions	Depersonalization/ derealization	Déjà vu	Poor judgment	Suicidal ideas	PTSD symptoms	Flushing	Kluver–Bucy
Adrenal insufficiency	U	X		X				X				X	X				X			
AIDS	F	X	X	X				X				X	X				X			
Altitude sickness	U				X					X		X	X							
Amyotrophic lateral sclerosis	U	X																		
Antidiuretic excess	F												X			X				
Brain abscess	U											X								
Brain tumor	F	X	X				X					X	X	X	X					
Cancer	C	X		X	X												X	X		
Carcinoid	F																		X	
Cardiac arrhythmia	C			X																
Cerebrovascular disease	C	X	X	X			X			X		X	X			X	X			
Chronic obstructive lung disease	C	X		X	X					X		X				X	X			
Congestive heart failure	C	X		X	X					X		X								
Cryptococcosis	F		X									X	X							
Cushing's	F	X	X	X						X		X	X				X			
Deafness	C	X		X								X	X							
Diabetes mellitus	C	X	X	X	X															
Epilepsy	C	X	X	X					X			X	X				X			
Fibromyalgia	C	X		X	X															
Head trauma	C	X	X	X						X		X								
Herpes encephalitis	U	X		X					X			X								X
Homocystinuria	U								X											
Huntington's	U	X	X					X				X	X				X			
Hyperparathyroidism	F	X		X			X		X			X	X				X			
Hypertensive encephalopathy	F												X							
Hyperthyroidism	C	X		X	X		X			X		X	X							

Disorder	Freq[a]																						
Hypoparathyroidism	U	X					X	X	X						X	X					X	X
Hypothyroidism	C	X					X	X							X	X			X	X	X	X
Kidney failure	F	X										X				X			X	X
Kleinfelter's	F	X													X			X
Liver failure	C	X			X		X												X
Lyme disease	F	X	X		X			X		X					X	X			X	X
Ménière's	F	X	X		X										X						X
Menopause	N	X			X					X					X						X
Migraine	C	X																	
Mitral valve prolapse	C	X	X												X						X
Multiple sclerosis	F	X	X			X	X			X					X			X
Myasthenia gravis	F	X			X										X						X
Neurocutaneous diseases	F	X			X										X						X
Normal-pressure hydrocephalus	F	X							X											
Parkinson's	F	X			X					X					X						X
Pellagra	R	X			X										X						X
Pernicious anemia	C	X	X																X	X
Pheochromocytoma	U				X													X				X
Pneumonia	C	X			X															
Porphyria	U	X	X		X					X					X			X	X
Postoperative states	F	X			X			X		X					X			X	X
Premenstrual syndrome	C	X			X			X		X	X				X						X
Prion disease	R	X			X			X							X						X
Progressive supranuclear palsy	U	X			X			X							X						X
Protein energy malnutrition	C	X			X										X						X
Pulmonary thromboembolism	F				X										X						X
Rheumatoid arthritis	C	X								X					X						X
Sickle cell disease	F	X																	
Sleep apnea	C	X			X					X					X		X			X	X
Syphilis	U	X			X					X					X		X			X	X
Systemic infection	C	X	X	X	X										X						X
Systemic lupus erythematosus	F	X			X										X						X
Thiamine deficiency	F	X			X										X						X
Wilson's	U	X			X					X					X		X		X	X	X

Note. Adapted from *When Psychological Problems Mask Medical Disorders* by James Morrison, 1997, New York: Guilford Press. Copyright 1997 by The Guilford Press. Adapted by permission.

[a] For relative frequency: C, common; F, frequent; U, uncommon; R, rare; N, normal. See text for clarifications of the first four terms.

(*cont.*)

TABLE 9.1. Some Medical Disorders That Can Cause Mental Symptoms (cont.)

	Relative frequency[a]	Cognitive symptoms								Personality symptoms							
		Memory impairment	Disorientation	Minor cognitive impairment	Delirium	Dementia	Inattention	Slow thinking	Mental retardation	Irritability	Apathy	Disinhibition	Jocularity	Impulsiveness	Tenaciousness	Aggression	Criminality
Adrenal insufficiency	U	×	×	×	×					×	×						
AIDS	F	×	×	×	×	×	×	×		×	×						
Altitude sickness	U	×	×		×					×							
Amyotrophic lateral sclerosis	U					×											
Antidiuretic excess	F				×					×							
Brain abscess	U		×				×										
Brain tumor	F	×				×		×				×		×			
Cancer	C																
Carcinoid	F				×												
Cardiac arrhythmia	C				×												
Cerebrovascular disease	C						×				×	×	×	×			
Chronic obstructive lung disease	C	×			×	×	×	×			×						
Congestive heart failure	C			×	×	×											
Cryptococcosis	F	×	×		×	×											
Cushing's	F	×	×		×	×	×			×							
Deafness	C									×	×						
Diabetes mellitus	C				×												
Epilepsy	C								×						×		
Fibromyalgia	C	×		×			×	×									
Head trauma	C	×	×		×	×	×	×		×		×		×		×	
Herpes encephalitis	U	×															
Homocystinuria	U					×			×								
Huntington's	U	×				×				×	×	×				×	
Hyperparathyroidism	F	×					×	×		×	×	×					
Hypertensive encephalopathy	F	×	×		×			×		×							
Hyperthyroidism	C				×					×							

104

Disorder	Relative frequency[a]
Hypoparathyroidism	U
Hypothyroidism	C
Kidney failure	F
Kleinfelter's	F
Liver failure	C
Lyme disease	F
Ménière's	F
Menopause	N
Migraine	C
Mitral valve prolapse	C
Multiple sclerosis	F
Myasthenia gravis	F
Neurocutaneous diseases	F
Normal-pressure hydrocephalus	F
Parkinson's	F
Pellagra	R
Pernicious anemia	C
Pheochromocytoma	U
Pneumonia	C
Porphyria	U
Postoperative states	F
Premenstrual syndrome	C
Prion disease	R
Progressive supranuclear palsy	U
Protein energy malnutrition	C
Pulmonary thromboembolism	F
Rheumatoid arthritis	C
Sickle cell disease	F
Sleep apnea	C
Syphilis	U
Systemic infection	C
Systemic lupus erythematosus	F
Thiamine deficiency	F
Wilson's	U

Note. Adapted from *When Psychological Problems Mask Medical Disorders* by James Morrison, 1997, New York: Guilford Press. Copyright 1997 by The Guilford Press. Adapted by permission.

[a]For relative frequency: C, common; F, frequent; U, uncommon; R, rare; N, normal. See text for clarifications of the first four terms.

ders. I've adapted Table 9.1 from my book *When Psychological Problems Mask Medical Disorders*, which describes in greater detail these diseases that can cause mental symptoms. The table's purpose is to alert clinicians to the great variety of medical illnesses that can lead to such symptoms. In the second column, you'll find the relative frequency with which each disease is found in the general population:

> *Common*—Most adults have at least one friend or acquaintance who has, or who will have, this condition. (Prevalence ranges to 1 in 200.)
>
> *Frequent*—A town or small city will be home to one or more of these people. (Prevalence ranges to 1 in 10,000.)
>
> *Uncommon* —At least one such person in a large city or small state has the condition. Prevalence ranges to 1 in 500,000.
>
> *Rare*—Prevalence is less than 1 in a million.

Note that these frequencies do *not* indicate how often a disease produces mental symptoms; such data are simply not available. The good news here is that we don't often encounter such diseases. The bad news is that relative rarity lulls us into a sense of security. Unless we remain alert, we run the risk that we'll misinterpret the symptoms when they come calling.

Conversely, it is also important to know what physical symptoms are often associated with mental disorders. The sidebar "Physical Symptoms Commonly Linked with Mental Disorders" discusses some of these.

Clues to a Physical Cause for Mental Symptoms

Signs, symptoms, and items of historical information can suggest underlying physical illness. If you encounter any of these patient characteristics, which I've loosely adapted from a 1989 article in the *British Journal of Psychiatry* and from other sources, further investigation (physical exam, laboratory data, imaging studies) may be warranted. A physical cause for mental symptoms may be especially likely if your patient:

- Is having a first episode of the mental illness. Physical causes are less likely in recurring diseases.
- Is 40 or over. Advancing age increases the likelihood that someone is developing a major medical disease.

Physical Symptoms Commonly Linked
with Mental Disorders

Some physical symptoms are actually used as criteria for mental disorders; others serve as flags that a mental disorder may exist. Here I discuss some physical symptoms likely to turn up in patients who have mental disorders.

Sleep

Because it cuts across so many diagnoses, disturbed sleep is probably the most common physical problem you'll encounter. The diagnostic manuals list a number of specific problems with sleep as mental disorders, though in some cases you may choose to disagree. I know, because I do: Narcolepsy is as much a neurological disorder as is epilepsy, and surely mental health's claim on insomnia is no stronger than family medicine's. However, many of our patients do complain of difficulty sleeping, and we must carefully consider its possible diagnostic importance whenever we find it.

As was true with Carson, trouble sleeping will most often indicate a mood disorder. Insomnia, or sometimes hypersomnia (excessive sleep), is frequently encountered in major depression and dysthymia, and serves as a criterion for each. Patients with mania, who typically experience insomnia as reduced sleep requirement, may deny that it is a problem ("Why waste time sleeping when so much needs doing?").

Trouble sleeping is also a criterion for GAD, in which patients may complain of either insomnia or unrefreshing sleep. Poor sleep is one of the hyperarousal criteria for PTSD and its cousin, acute stress disorder. Inability to sleep or excessive drowsiness is also often symptomatic of drug or alcohol intoxication or withdrawal. An early hint of schizophrenia may be that the patient stays up until all hours pacing about the bedroom.

Appetite

A change in appetite is probably the next most frequent physical complaint of mental health patients. Decreased and increased food intake, often attended by weight loss or gain, serve as criteria for depression. Patients with anorexia nervosa will eat less and less, until weight loss becomes acutely life-threatening; however, such a patient may not admit to a lack appetite, only to a fear of being fat. Bulimia nervosa, on the other hand, involves gorging on huge amounts of food, such as an entire pan of brownies or box of candy at a sitting.

(cont.)

(cont.)

Panic Symptoms

The physical symptoms of panic include chest pain, chills, a choking sensation, dizziness, heart palpitations, nausea, numbness or tingling (which physicians call *paresthesias*), sweating, shortness of breath, and trembling. They may be experienced by a person who has any of several anxiety disorders, including agoraphobia, specific phobia and social phobia. Someone with GAD might complain of excessive fatigue, muscle tension, or trouble sleeping. Some of the same anxiety symptoms are often encountered during the use of illicit substances, and during withdrawal from use.

Other

Fatigue and either reduced or increased psychomotor activity are also typical of people with depression, whereas patients with mania become overly active. Manic patients may become inordinately interested in sex, whereas a depressed patient may lose all such interest. Whole chapters in diagnostic manuals are devoted to such problems as sexual arousal, pain with intercourse, and erectile dysfunctioning.

- Has recently given birth. Postpartum hormonal changes can create mental symptoms.
- Currently has a major medical illness. For example, in diabetes, episodes of low blood sugar can cause anxiety attacks.
- Takes medicine, either prescribed or over-the-counter. This clue will be stronger if symptoms began about the time medicine was begun.
- Has experienced neurological symptoms. These can include weakness on one side, numbness or tingling, clumsiness, trouble walking, tremor, involuntary movements, worsening headaches, dizziness, blurred or double vision, blindness in part of the visual field, trouble with speech or memory, loss of consciousness, slowed thinking, and trouble recognizing familiar objects or following commands.
- Has had a large weight loss (10% or more); eats an unusual diet (especially one that is very limited in variety, such as tea and toast or pasta and beer); or exhibits self-neglect. Any of these can cause symptoms from vitamin deficiency.
- Has a past history of serious medical illness, including those of the

endocrine system, heart, kidney, liver, lungs, or neurological system.

- Has had a recent head injury (with loss of consciousness) or falls. Even mild head injury can be associated with postconcussional disorder and other mental disorders.
- Has a recent history of alcohol or drug misuse, with the obvious implications for falls, malnutrition, and other physical problems.
- Has a family history of a heritable disorder, such as diabetes, Huntington's disease, or other metabolic or degenerative disease.
- Has changing levels of consciousness, any impairment in thinking, hallucinations other than auditory ones, or mental symptoms interspersed with periods of lucidity.
- Has certain alarming physical symptoms, such as fever, blurred vision, swelling of abdomen or ankles, jaundice, or chest pain.
- Has mental or behavioral symptoms that don't resolve, despite treatment that should be effective.
- Shows any evidence of worsening medical health that hasn't yet been evaluated by a physician.

Somatization Disorder: A Special Case

Each of the diagnostic building blocks is important; some loom larger than others. Somatization disorder is a mental condition that, as currently described, comprises exclusively physical (somatic) symptoms. Although it is common, affecting perhaps 1% of the general population, it is often overlooked by clinicians in the process of making diagnoses. Chapters 11 and 12 contain case histories, but for now we'll only address those aspects that pertain to physical symptoms.

In somatization disorder, the problem isn't so much the exact symptoms the patient has at any one time as the twin facts that there are so many of them and that they are so varied—and varying. They cause the patient to seek treatment or interfere with social, work, or personal functioning, and they include the following:

- Multiple pain symptoms in such locations as head, back, abdomen, joints, limbs, chest, or rectum; or pain related to body functions, including intercourse, menstruation, and urination.
- Gastrointestinal symptoms such as nausea, abdominal bloating, vomiting, diarrhea, and food intolerances.

- Sexual symptoms that include indifference to sex, difficulties with erection or ejaculation, irregular or excessive menses, and vomiting throughout pregnancy.
- *Pseudoneurological* symptoms (that is, symptoms with no anatomical or physiological basis) that include poor balance or coordination, weak or paralyzed muscles, lump in throat, loss of voice, retention of urine, hallucinations, numbness, double vision, blindness, deafness, seizures, amnesia (or other symptoms of dissociation), and loss of consciousness.

It is especially important to note that these patients aren't faking their symptoms; they think that they are really ill. In the typical pattern, first one symptom and later another becomes prominent as a patient visits doctor after doctor. The pattern suggests that what's important to the patient is the process of being sick, rather than the type of sickness itself. Somatization disorder is so important to many differential diagnoses and is so often forgotten that I've dedicated a diagnostic principle to it.

For the initial diagnostic evaluation, be aware of the following: (1) Patients with somatization disorder typically complain of a variety of somatic symptoms; (2) they often have mood and anxiety symptoms as well; (3) their symptoms respond poorly to treatment that usually works for most patients; and (4) if their symptoms do improve, new ones crop up to take their place. All of these factors explain why general health care providers often lose patience with these people and refer them elsewhere. By the time they come to the attention of mental health professionals, these patients may have seen many other doctors and therapists and received much medical care—usually to their clinicians' frustration and their own detriment.

> *Diagnostic Principle:* Consider somatization disorder whenever symptoms don't jibe or treatments don't work.

Using Physical Symptoms to Make a Diagnosis

Physical diseases won't often be the cause of your patient's mental symptoms, but when they do play a role, it is vital to find out right away. Anxiety symptoms, for example, can stem from a great variety of medical illnesses.

After several months of couple therapy, Milt and Marjorie's therapist noted that Marjorie had become increasingly irritable. Her hands shook visibly, and she often arose from her chair to walk back and forth. She complained that the temperature was too warm in the office, even in January, when the others were bundled up. It was during a discussion of her weight loss that the therapist suggested that she should be evaluated by her family doctor. Testing revealed moderately increased thyroid activity.

Physical disorders like Marjorie's can often be treated effectively; if ignored, they can wreak havoc. Here's how I think about them:

1. Make sure that information about general medical health is a part of every evaluation. This should include material obtained from the patient, as well as summaries from hospitalizations and medical workups.

2. Check to see that each patient has had a recent general medical evaluation; if your patient doesn't have a general physician, recommend one and ensure that a complete evaluation is performed. This is especially important if you note any of the indicators of medical disease suggested above in the section "Clues to a Physical Cause for Mental Symptoms."

3. Become familiar with somatization disorder. It is a truism that if you don't suspect a condition, you'll never diagnose it. Somatization disorder is too prevalent and has implications too important to risk passing by.

4. List physical disorders at the top of every patient's differential diagnosis. Even if you consider this possibility only momentarily before moving on, keep reminding yourself that it exists for the next patient, and the next. Eventually your vigilance will pay off.

Substance Use and Mental Disorders

The use of chemical substances—alcohol, street drugs, prescription drugs, or over-the-counter medications—can produce mental symptoms. The cause–effect relationship will be especially strong if the symptoms develop after use of a substance, and if the symptoms diminish once use stops. The association will be even stronger if the patient develops symptoms with each use, if each time they are the *same* symptoms, and if the patient has never had such symptoms prior to using that substance. I've already awarded diagnostic principle status to the important relationship between substance use and mental disorder.

That principle isn't limited to street drugs. For example, the use of anabolic steroids by athletes, from the professional level down at least through high school sports, has recently received a great deal of publicity.

> Beginning in high school, 19-year-old Efrain Marrero had injected synthetic body-building steroids to bulk up for football. When his parents learned what he was doing, they begged him to quit. He did, but rapidly sank into depression so deep that, as *The New York Times* reported in 2005, he shot himself to death in a bedroom at home.

You will need to make a list of all substances (legal and otherwise) taken by the patient, noting when symptoms began and when each substance was first used. Compare it to Table 9.2, which lists some of the types of medications that can produce mental symptoms, and to Table 9.3, which lists the mental and behavioral effects of alcohol and other substances of misuse.

Once again, let's revisit Carson (see Chapter 1) to assess our use of the diagnostic building blocks reviewed so far in Part II. We've used the history of his present illness; his family history (his grandmother reportedly was chronically depressed); and, from his personal and social history, the fact of his impending long-distance move. Each of these areas of information is necessary to fully understand the background to his misery. The sources of information we've used include Carson and his wife; we would also look at his previous medical records to shore up our memory that his previous episodes of depression occurred in the winter and spring. We've done all these things, yet there is still one important block to discuss—his present mental status. We'll take it up in the next chapter.

TABLE 9.2. Classes (or Names) of Medications That Can Cause Mental Disorders

	Anxiety	Mood	Psychosis	Delirium
Analgesics	×	×	×	×
Anesthetics	×	×	×	×
Antabuse		×	×	
Antianxiety agents		×		
Anticholinergics	×	×	×	
Anticonvulsants	×	×	×	×
Antidepressants	×	×	×	×
Antihistamines	×		×	×
Antihypertensives/cardiovascular agents	×	×	×	×
Antimicrobials		×	×	×
Antiparkinsonian agents	×	×	×	×
Antipsychotics	×	×		×
Antiulcer agents		×		
Bronchodilators	×			×
Chemotherapies			×	
Corticosteroids	×	×	×	×
Gastrointestinal agents			×	×
Histamine antagonists				×
Immunosuppressants				×
Insulin	×			
Interferon	×	×	×	
Lithium	×			
Muscle relaxants		×	×	×
NSAIDs[a]			×	
Oral contraceptives	×	×		
Thyroid replacements	×			

[a]NSAIDs, nonsteroidal anti-inflammatory drugs.

TABLE 9.3. Symptoms of Substance Use

	Alcohol/sedatives	Cannabis	Cocaine/amphetamine	Caffeine	Hallucinogens	Inhalants	Nicotine	Opioids	PCP (phencyclidine)
				Intoxication					
Use	Recent	Recent	Recent	Recent (250 mg)	Recent	Recent use or exposure		Recent	Recent
Behavioral changes	Inappropriate sexuality; aggression; labile mood; impaired judgment; impaired job or social functioning	Impaired motor performance; anxiety; euphoria; impaired judgment; social withdrawal; sensation that time has slowed down	Euphoria; blunted affect; hypervigilance; interpersonal sensitivity; anger, anxiety, or tension; changes in sociability; stereotyped behaviors; impaired judgment; impaired job or social functioning	Clinically important distress or impaired job, school, social, or other functioning	Depression or anxiety; ideas of reference; fears of insanity; persecutory ideas; impaired judgment; impaired job or social functioning	Apathy; assaultiveness; belligerence; impaired judgment; impaired job or social functioning		Euphoria → apathy; depression or anxiety; activity; impaired judgment; impaired job or social functioning	Assaultiveness; belligerence; impulsiveness; agitation; unpredictability; impaired judgment; impaired job or social functioning
Symptoms	Shortly after drinking: slurred speech; incoordination; unsteady walking; nystagmus; reduced attention or memory; stupor or coma	Within 2 hours: red eyes; increased appetite; dry mouth; rapid heart rate	Within hours to a few days: increased or decreased heart rate; dilated pupils; increased or decreased blood pressure; chills or sweating; nausea or vomiting; weight loss; agitation or retardation; muscle weakness; depressed breathing; chest pain; irregular heartbeat	Shortly after ingestion: restlessness, nervousness, excitement; sleeplessness; red face; increased urination; gastrointestinal upset; muscle twitching; rambling speech; rapid or irregular pulse; tireless periods; increased activity	Shortly after use: perceptual changes; dilated pupils; rapid pulse; sweating; irregular heartbeat; blurred vision tremors; poor concentration	During or shortly after use, 2+ of the following: dizziness; nystagmus; poor concentration; slurred speech; unsteady walking; lethargy; impaired reflexes; decreased psychomotor activity; tremors; muscle weakness; blurred or double vision; stupor or coma; euphoria		During or shortly after use, pupils constricted (or dilated, if severe overdose) and 1+ of the following: sleepiness or coma; slurred speech; impaired memory or concentration Specifier: With Perceptual Disturbances	Within 1 hour, 2+ of the following: nystagmus; numbness or decreased pain response; trouble walking; trouble speaking; rigid muscles; coma or seizures; abnormally acute hearing

Withdrawal

	Heavy, prolonged		Heavy, prolonged		Daily for several weeks	Cessation after several weeks heavy use, or use of antagonist
Use						
Symptoms	Within hours to a few days: sweating or rapid heartbeat; tremor; sleeplessness; nausea or vomiting; brief hallucinations or illusions; increased activity; grand mal seizures; anxiety		Within hours to a few days: dysphoric mood; fatigue; vivid bad dreams, increased or decreased sleep; increased appetite; increased or decreased activity		Within 24 hours of abruptly reduced use, 4+ of the following: dysphoria or depression; insomnia; anger, frustration, or irritability; anxiety; trouble concentrating; restlessness; decreased heart rate; increased appetite or weight	Within minutes to several days, 3+ of the following: dysphoria; nausea or vomiting; aching muscles; tearing or runny nose; dilated pupils, erect hairs, or sweating; diarrhea; yawning; fever; sleeplessness

10 Diagnosis and the Mental Status Examination

And here's the final piece of the diagnostic puzzle. In general, the MSE is simply a statement of how a person looks, feels, and behaves at the moment of examination. Nearly as important are the characteristics a person *doesn't* show. For example, although Carson's MSE (see Chapter 1) specifically reflected depression, feelings of panic, tearfulness, trouble concentrating, worries, and feelings of abandonment, he *didn't* have hallucinations or delusions. Findings such as these, which help rule out a diagnosis that seems otherwise a real possibility, are called *pertinent negatives*. They should not only be inquired after, but faithfully reported in the clinician's write-up.

In addition to noting pertinent negatives, we clinicians must keep in mind that though the MSE is important, it is really only a snapshot of a patient at a single point in time. It can be tempting to overemphasize particular symptoms observed during the MSE at the expense of other building blocks of diagnosis, and clinicians sometimes yield to this temptation (see the sidebar "Is the MSE Overrated?").

Appearance

Much of the MSE requires no questioning at all, only observation of the patient during an ordinary conversation. Nearly all the material in this section and the next two ("Mood/Affect" and "Flow of Speech") falls into that category.

Is the MSE Overrated?

Although the MSE is an important part of diagnosis and the database, can it ever be overrated? I'm afraid that it sometimes is. Traditionally coming at the very end of a diagnostic examination, the MSE is nonetheless where too many clinicians begin. Scientific studies of diagnosis have shown that we clinicians may too quickly jump to conclusions based on a single, arresting symptom. That's because we wrongly assume that really dramatic symptoms can mean only one thing; in the case of hallucinations and delusions, for example, this would be schizophrenia.

We forget that there is probably no mental symptom that can have only one interpretation. Even a symptom as seemingly specialized as the belief that one is pregnant (when one is not) can be found in diagnoses as diverse as mania, depression, dementia, and substance use. Consider the writer Virginia Woolf: On at least five occasions throughout her life, she became acutely and severely ill with delusional ideas about her supposed guilt and the worthlessness of her work. She hallucinated voices so terrifying that she could never bring herself to describe them. Yet within weeks or months she recovered completely—each time except the last, when she weighted her fur coat with a stone in the pocket and drowned herself in the icy March waters of the river Ouse. The lesson: Mental status symptoms should never put us into a box, but onto a decision tree.

Far from being the only important factor in diagnosis, the MSE often isn't even the *most* important. MSE information doesn't usually make or break a diagnosis; much of the time, the longitudinal evaluation has greater diagnostic value than does the cross-sectional appearance. What the MSE should do is set flags that warn you of the possibilities, which you must evaluate in the context of all you have learned from the patient's own history and from the information provided by relatives, old charts, and previous clinicians.

General Appearance

Information concerning general appearance should be evident even to an unpracticed eye. You probably won't be able to diagnose your patient based on appearance alone, though it can signal some possibilities. As Mark Twain almost said, clothes make the individual. For example, if you see an adult who wears tattered, bizarre, or dirty clothing (or is otherwise generally untidy), schizophrenia and other psychoses, dementia, and the more extreme effects of substance use come to mind. If the patient is a teenager or child, the options will be broader still. And of course, excessive thinness can signal anorexia nervosa, especially if the person is a young woman.

> An office patient I once evaluated turned out to be one of the most anxious individuals I have ever known. My first clue was upon shaking hands with Douglas, when I felt a bulge of enlarged muscle at the base of his right palm. He said that he was a draftsman, and he habitually clutched his pen as if it was trying to escape. Over the years, that muscle had grown huge from the tension of his grip.

Level of Attention

How alert is your patient? If the patient is drowsy or inattentive, delirium, possibly coupled to a medical disorder or a substance use problem, may be responsible. On the other end of the attention spectrum is hypervigilance, in which the patient glances frequently around the room, as though trying to locate the source of voices or a threat. Hypervigilance suggests PTSD, but it is also often associated with paranoia and other psychoses. Perhaps more frequently encountered is someone like Lester, who accompanied his wife to counseling, though evidently not in spirit. His wandering gaze, refusal to give eye contact to anyone in the room, and frequent responses of "Huh? Oh, sorry!" clearly proclaimed his lack of investment in the proceedings. He reminded me of our high school civics course, conducted—I wouldn't say taught—every spring by the baseball coach. Even when he lectured, he mostly gazed out the window that overlooked the diamond. It was crystal clear that he wished himself elsewhere (a sentiment fervently endorsed by his students).

Of course, ability to sustain attention is famously associated with ADHD—a condition typically of children and adolescents, but increasingly found to affect adults too. More than once, ADHD has been finally diagnosed in a parent whose child has just been evaluated for inattention and motor restlessness.

Amount of Activity

Your patient's activity level can be an important indicator of diagnosis. The most common observation is increased motor activity, such as the jiggling leg or frequent hand wringing that indicates simple anxiety, or perhaps the desire to decamp. Abnormal body movements can indicate that the person has been using a medication, perhaps one of the older, now less popular antipsychotic drugs such as Prolixin or Haldol; then you might suspect a psychotic disorder. The classic back-and-forth "pill-rolling" tremor, which may indicate naturally occurring Parkinson's disease, can also result from these medications. An involuntary movement of lips, mouth, and upper limbs referred to as *tardive dyskinesia*, and the restless inability to sit still referred to as *akathisia* (such a patient feels the need to keep quite literally on the move), are two additional movement disorders related to these drugs. Table 9.3 describes motor behaviors related to substance misuse.

Although excessive motion is probably the more common finding in mental health patients, a facial expression that shows little mobility—sometimes seeming nearly frozen—can be found in patients suffering from dementia or severe depression. The classic, nearly complete immobility of catatonia is now rare.

Mood/Affect

Let's briefly discuss three qualities of mood: its type, *lability* (the degree to which it changes in a given time frame), and appropriateness.

We think of mood as being diagnostic: We tend to equate euphoria with mania, and sadness with major depression or dysthymia. But who among us hasn't experienced these feelings at one time or another, without other indicators of illness? Indeed, much of the time, a person's emotional state doesn't really tell us much about diagnosis. Anger (and its cousin, hostility), anxiety, shame, joy, fear, guilt, surprise, disgust, and irritation are emotions that can occur in mental disorders, though most of the time they are perfectly normal. Patients who worry about normal moods will often benefit from simple reassurance.

Excessive lability of mood may yield more accurate diagnostic inferences. For example, a person whose mood often shifts between extremes (from laughter to weeping and rapidly back, or into sudden fury without apparent cause) should be considered for the diagnoses of somatization disorder, mania, and the dementias. Unheralded outbursts of temper occasionally indicate medical conditions such as brain infections or tumors. A mood that hardly budges (decreased lability) can suggest schizophrenia, severe depression, Parkinson's disease, or dementia.

The third quality of mood is its appropriateness to the person's content of thought. When I interviewed Joan, she giggled as she talked about the recent death of her mother. That sort of inappropriateness of affect to content brings to mind two possibilities: mania and schizophrenia of the disorganized type. Joan's history was one of episodes of psychosis, followed by depression, then long stretches when she was completely normal—clearly suggesting bipolar mood disorder. You'll also encounter inappropriate mood when someone with somatization disorder discusses a current physical problem such as paralysis or blindness with none of the apprehension you'd expect for such a serious condition.

Depression is the mood symptom most often noted during the MSE. Because of its ubiquity, potential for harm, and response to treatment, I look for depression in every new patient—and a lot of old ones. This is important enough to rate its own diagnostic principle. Of course, *always* is always a bit over the top, but depression is so common, so important, and so often missed that I've left in the intensifier.

> **Diagnostic Principle:** Because of their ubiquity, potential for harm, and ready response to treatment, *always* consider mood disorders.

Flow of Speech

Although flow of speech can reveal several possible clues to diagnosis, let's first acknowledge that most of us have speech quirks that aren't usually pathological at all. Examples include verbal tics (such as "you know," "whatever," "awesome," and "like, no way"), *circumstantial speech* (where the person relates several life histories before coming to the point), and speech so distractible that it nearly drives you nuts trying to communicate.

Probably the best-known type of actual speech pathology is known as *loose associations*, or sometimes *derailment*. Loose associations occur when thought coherence breaks down, so that one idea skids into another that isn't clearly related. Although you can understand the sequence of words, the direction they take is nowhere on the compass. The result is illogical speech or writing that may mean something to the patient, but that doesn't communicate this meaning to others. Here is an extreme example:

> "I found out that the English tea which the British drink. And that clam chowder isn't different, like Indian corn is American food. But England has a king, queen, and a prince. Princess Anne is married to an Englishman. Now medication is for help of accidents, sickness, burned people, and blackouts and dizzy spells like me. The truth of Europe, in fact Japan has tea, too. And America. Thanks."

Loose associations and other, less common speech patterns (such as *incoherence*, *neologisms*, *perseveration*, and *echolalia*) are usually said to be characteristic of schizophrenia, though they can also occur in mania and dementia.

How rapidly someone responds to questions is called *latency of response*; marked deviations often point to a mood disorder. Very long latency is characteristic of severe depression, whereas reduced latency, in which the patient answers almost before you reach the question mark, is often found in mania. In *poverty of speech*, a patient will spontaneously speak little or not at all; it can suggest depression or schizophrenia.

Content of Thought

In the history of the present illness, you will have already encountered most of the material usually considered content of thought. The implications of this information are pretty straightforward.

No matter how you frame them, delusions and hallucinations almost always mean psychosis. However, the sort of delusion you encounter can help define the type of psychosis. Delusions of influence, persecution, passivity (a patient is being acted upon by some outside influence), reference (comments are being made about the patient), thought control, or thought broadcasting (patients feel their thoughts are being transmitted, as by radio waves) nearly always suggest schizophrenia, especially paranoid schizophrenia. Delusions of ill health (having a terrible disease) or even of being dead can indicate either schizophrenia or severe depression. Delusions of grandeur, in which patients believe they have great powers or are famous beings such as God or Madonna (either of them), are classic for mania but can also be encountered in schizophrenia. Delusional guilt suggests either depression or delusional disorder, whereas a delusion that one has become impoverished usually indicates depression.

Also note mood *congruence*, which refers to how well mood matches the content of the person's delusion. When I asked a woman I once treated for a postpartum manic psychosis why she seemed so happy and contented, she said it was because she knew she had "the little baby Jesus at home in his crib." Such mood-congruent delusions usually indicate a mood disorder. On the other hand, the delusions of schizophrenia are often mood-incongruent, as with the young man who believed that he was the illegitimate son of Jay Leno and that he could change the weather. Despite these grandiose delusions, he knew that his mental condition had prevented him from maintaining a job and having a normal social life, and he felt severely depressed as a result.

You might encounter hallucinations of any of the senses in a psychosis caused by a medical or substance use disorder such as delirium tremens, dementia, brain tumor, toxicity, or seizures. In schizophrenia, whereas most hallucinations are auditory, some are visual, and infrequently you will encounter hallucinations of the other senses. The vivid, dream-like states that we have when awakening or falling asleep are respectively called *hypnopompic* and *hypnagogic* hallucinations, but they are completely normal. Also normal are illusions, *déjà vu*, overvalued ideas (such as a belief in the superiority of one's religion or ethnic background), and depersonalization that is neither protracted nor extreme.

Although phobias or obsessions and compulsions often signal a specific anxiety disorder, keep in mind two general issues. One is that, as with anxiety in general, a minor degree of these symptoms is common and not at all abnormal. The second, which we'll discuss further in Chapter 12, is the clinical tendency to focus on dramatic phobias and compulsions while ignoring the quiet little depression that may be lurking underneath.

Finally, we must mention thoughts about suicide, homicide, and other forms of violence. Suicidal ideas most often point to depression, though they can also indicate a personality disorder (especially borderline), substance use, or schizophrenia. If ideas concerning violence indicate any mental disorder at all, it will usually be one of the three conditions just named. But violence and homicide are more typical of plain old criminal activity. Remember the Godfather.

Cognition and Intellectual Resources

The abilities to reason, do math, and think abstractly (such as recognizing similarities and differences) largely depend on the person's education and native intelligence; they will therefore be prominently deficient in mental retardation and developmental disorders such as autism. They can also be clouded by serious mental illnesses such as dementia, schizophrenia, and mood disorder. Problems with comprehension, fluency, naming, repetition, reading, and writing, other than those you might expect from non-native speakers, suggest the need for neurological evaluation.

Orientation is only occasionally deficient, and then almost always it indicates a cognitive disorder—either delirium or dementia. Occasionally a psychotic patient may claim to be Zog from Mars who lives in the Fifth Dimension, but we would say that such a person is delusional, not disoriented. Impairment of short-term memory can point to dementia, delirium, a psychosis, a mood disorder, or just plain anxiety.

Insight and Judgment

The amount of specific diagnostic information you can gather from the patient's insight may be less than overwhelming. Poor insight into the fact of having a mental disorder often indicates psychosis, but it is also common in patients with dementia and delirium, and can even occur in alcoholism. You'll also encounter deficient insight in diagnoses we don't automatically associate with psychosis, such as severe mood disorders, dissociative identity disorder, anorexia nervosa, body dysmorphic disorder, and instances of OCD so severe that the individual may not recognize that the compulsive behaviors are irrational.

Both insight and judgment also heavily depend on factors that no one would consider abnormal. The person's age is one: Up to the early teen years, children lack perspective on their own behavior or emotions, and even later on they still do not have a fully developed ability to comprehend the consequences of their own actions. Hence the 2005 U.S. Supreme Court ruling against capital punishment for minors. To a degree, the insight and judgment of adults are also affected by native education, intelligence, and cultural issues such as superstition and prejudice.

Like insight, judgment may be affected by psychosis and delirium. Any personality disorder can also affect insight (who among us readily admits to having character flaws?), but judgment is especially vulnerable to the more severe forms of personality disorder, such as borderline and antisocial.

With the conclusion of Part II, you now have insight into the full range of information you'll need to make accurate diagnoses in your patients. This is the raw material we use during the diagnostic levels already described in Part I. Always keep mentally prepared, however, for new information that could necessitate a reassessment of the facts—as you thought you knew them.

PART III

Applying the Diagnostic Techniques

11 Diagnosing Depression and Mania

For several reasons, I've chosen to begin Part III with the mood disorders. Perhaps most important, mood disorders (they are still sometimes called *affective disorders*) are among the major ills that affect mental health patients. They also rank near the top of the safety hierarchy (Table 3.1), and they present the most complicated challenges to every diagnostician, regardless of discipline or level of experience. Whenever I lecture on diagnosis, I explain that once you understand the mood disorders, the rest of diagnosis is a relative breeze.

Mood disorders present a variety of challenges:

1. Clinicians must consider numerous depressive syndromes, including major depressive disorder (with its various subtypes and specifiers, such as atypical, melancholic, and seasonal), dysthymia, and the depressive episodes of bipolar disorders.
2. The opposites of depressed mood are mania and its variants (hypomania, mixed states, and the high phases of cyclothymic disorder).
3. Once we make a diagnosis, we have to consider the question of comorbidity of mood disorders with other conditions and with one another.
4. Depression shares borderlands with bereavement and other losses, problems of living, and adjustment disorders. There is also the question of suicide as rational behavior versus treatable illness (see the sidebar "Can Suicide Ever Be Rational?" at the end of this chapter).

Syndromes of Depression

Mental disorders have often been compared to onions: you peel away layer after layer until you arrive at the core. Syndromes of clinical depression are like onions in a different sense: There are many different kinds of onions—red, yellow, white, pearl, Bermuda, Walla Walla (which are popular here in the Northwest), scallions, and many others. Each type may be used somewhat differently, depending on its unique characteristics, which you must first identify. So it is with types of depression. Table 11.1 lists the forms we'll consider in the chapter, along with some brief definitions. In addition to the examples given here, you'll find others involving depression in later chapters. By the time you've finished reading, you'll really know your onions.

Kent

Let's start with this relatively uncomplicated example of a man who seems classically depressed.

> Kent was referred for evaluation by his family doctor, who noted that, though physically healthy, he was "sagging in the mental department." By education and training an electronics engineer, Kent had worked in California's Silicon Valley for 7 successful years. To poise himself for further moves up the corporate ladder, he had enrolled in an MBA program at a local university, and was just one class short of graduation when the bursting dot-com bubble downsized him out of a job. With thousands of his colleagues also looking for work, he spent a dispiriting 8 months pounding the pavement before he finally found another job—selling cars for a brother-in-law who "had never even finished college," as he told the interviewer.
>
> Kent complained of months of depression, which he blamed on his loss of status and struggle to meet the mortgage payments on his expensive house in San Jose. However, during the first interview, his wife pointed out that he had been having problems with both insomnia and a diminished appetite for weeks before he'd been laid off. ("He didn't even show much enthusiasm for the fly fishing outfit I got him for his birthday.") Now he expressed guilt that he couldn't provide adequately for his family, and distress at the low energy and concentration that hampered his efforts at work. He denied having suicidal ideas, but his wife said that the previous week, he had told her that he didn't much care whether he lived or died.
>
> Kent had had no psychotic symptoms or prior episodes of mental illness, and his family history was negative for mental disorder. Although he

**TABLE 11.1. Differential Diagnosis with Brief Definitions
for Depression**

- *Depression due to a medical condition.* Physical illness can cause depression, which need not meet criteria for a major depressive episode.
- *Depression due to use of a substance.* Alcohol, street drugs, or medications cause depressive symptoms, which also need not conform to the definition of major depression.
- *Major depressive disorder, either single episode or recurrent.* For weeks or longer, the patient feels depressed or cannot enjoy life and may have problems with eating and sleeping, guilt feelings, loss of energy, trouble concentrating, and thoughts about death. There can be no episodes of mania or hypomania.
- *Bipolar depression* (bipolar I or II disorder, most recent episode depressed). Currently depressed, the patient has a history of mania or hypomania.
- *Melancholic depression.* This is a special type of major depression characterized by early morning awakening, appetite and weight loss, guilt feelings, and failure to feel better when something happens that would ordinarily be enjoyable.
- *Atypical depression.* Certain symptoms are the opposite of those usually experienced in major depression—increased appetite, weight gain, and excessive sleeping.
- *Seasonal affective disorder.* In this condition, also known as *seasonal mood disorder,* patients regularly become depressed at a certain time of the year, especially fall or winter.
- *Postpartum depression.* A woman develops major depression within a month of having a baby.
- *Dysthymia.* These patients typically remain ill for years with symptoms less severe than those of major depressive disorder; they don't have psychosis or suicidal ideas.
- *Bereavement.* For weeks or months, a person whose relative or friend has died has symptoms of depression that may or may not qualify as major depression.
- *Adjustment disorder with depressed mood.* Some people respond to life stresses by developing depressive symptoms.
- *Somatization disorder with mood disorder.* Patients who have an extensive history of many bodily complaints for which no physical explanation can be found often also have depression, and sometimes even symptoms of mania.

drank alcohol when he was in college a decade earlier, he hadn't touched it since.

Analysis

Using the numbered steps in our decision tree for a patient experiencing depression (Figure 11.1), here's how I would think about Kent's history. He had no history of mania or hypomania that would suggest a bipolar dis-

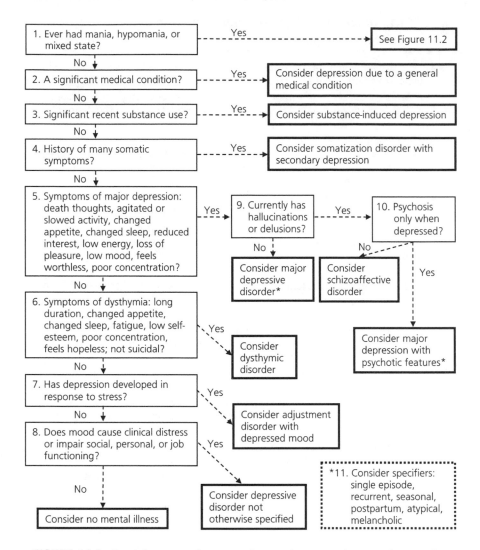

FIGURE 11.1. Decision tree for a patient who experiences depression or loss of pleasure.

order (step 1). Although his mood was terrible, his family practitioner had given him a clean bill of physical health (step 2). He didn't drink or use drugs (step 3) and had no history of multiple somatic symptoms (step 4). We therefore quickly arrive at step 5, where we note that he had quite a few of the typical major depression symptoms. Lack of psychotic symptoms at step 9 should lead us first to consider major depressive disorder.

The asterisk directs us to step 11, which reminds us of the variety of sub-types we can diagnose. Kent had symptoms of neither the melancholic nor the atypical form (see Table 11.1), and he obviously did not have postpar-tum depression, so we would say he had a single episode of major depres-sive disorder—the term most often used now for *clinical depression.*

Let's also mention a few of the diagnostic principles that, by either their presence or their absence, have helped us arrive at this conclusion. We have relied heavily on the collateral history from Kent's wife, which proved more accurate than Kent's own history of when the depression be-gan. His ancient history of drinking was trumped by 10 recent years of so-ber living. The social setting of an intact marriage has helped to assure us that personality disorder would be unlikely to play much of a role in his di-agnosis, and anyway, we would want to avoid that diagnosis if there was a significant possibility of a major Axis I mental disorder. There are no un-usual symptoms that would draw us away from a diagnosis of major depres-sion, which is a common diagnosis (a horse, not a zebra).

Comment

In my opinion, the diagnosis of major depression has a major shortcoming: Although it offers the illusion of precision, it obscures the fact that in real-ity, depression has many causes. Because they are encompassed by one name, we are tempted to view very different patients as having the same illness, and *that* encourages us to prescribe similar treatments (often anti-depressant medications) for all. Of course, many patients respond well to the standard regimens, but throughout this book you'll find patients with major depressions occurring in contexts that should suggest treatments other than antidepressant medications.

Marilyn

Once you have in mind the appropriate differential diagnosis and decision tree, the process of diagnosis is relatively straightforward, as in the case below.

A 23-year-old graduate student in cultural anthropology, Marilyn had signed up to spend 4 months in Guinea observing and recording the pronunciation of native forest dwellers' fast-vanishing language. Three weeks before she and two other students, led by an instructor, were scheduled to leave for western Africa, she requested an appointment with the dean of her professional school. "I thought that the thrill and activity of this trip would help me ditch the depression I've had for several years," she confessed. She still had trouble with loss of sleep and appetite, and her mood was low "most of the time." Later, consulting with a clinician friend, the dean repeated this information and asked for an opinion. The answer was unexpected. "Right now, I just can't say," replied the clinician. "We don't have nearly enough information." Here's what an interview later revealed.

Marilyn's depression had first come to light when she was just 15. Although she was pretty and intelligent, competitive in volleyball, and earned nearly all A's, she hadn't adjusted well to high school. By her sophomore year, she felt that she didn't have what it took to make it as either a scholar or an athlete. Though she had a few close friends, she often worried that she wasn't going to make the grade socially, either.

Born to a Korean woman who was not married to her biological father, Marilyn had been adopted when she was just a week old. Her parents were both college graduates; her mother wrote for a biweekly newspaper, and her father served for many years as a news anchor for a local television channel in a large East Coast city. Two older siblings, who were not adopted, had excelled in school and were now entering into professional careers.

Marilyn admitted that she felt sad and lonely "most of the time, even when I'm with other people." Although she readily agreed that she had little in the way of self-esteem, her interest and concentration in her studies were good; she had never had suicidal ideas. She absolutely denied any substance use (including prescribed or over-the-counter medications), and her mother, during a telephone conference call in which Marilyn participated, agreed. She volunteered that Marilyn had never had a significant medical disorder, "not even the flu."

Analysis

Based on Marilyn's history, we can quickly pass through steps 1 through 4 of the decision tree in Figure 11.1. Marilyn had just a few symptoms of major depression (step 5), not enough to justify that diagnosis. Her long duration of overall mild symptoms sounded much more like dysthymia (step 6), which is the main diagnosis we should consider.

It is important to recognize, as did the clinician consulted by Marilyn's dean, the need for a comprehensive evaluation; without longitudinal information, Marilyn's appearance wasn't really very specific for any diagnosis. Information about her biological parents might have helped, as suggested by the family history diagnostic principle, but family history is more useful in starting the train of diagnostic thought than in determining its final destination. Although her mother's belief that there had been no substance use is reassuring, of course it is not proof; when indicated, objective tests (urine or blood) should be considered. You might think that Marilyn's depression worsened in response to the anticipation of an extended assignment overseas, which would suggest an adjustment disorder with depressed mood. However, that conclusion would contradict the safety diagnostic principle: We should first consider more treatable, more specific diagnoses.

Although I have said that we could quickly eliminate substance use and medical disorders in discussing Marilyn's disorder, I do not mean—and I will *never* mean—that we can be cavalier about them. The trouble is that they aren't usually at the root of a given patient's problem, so you could blithely ignore them 50 times without incident and reap tragedy on the 51st. Throughout the rest of this book, if I say, "We can safely eliminate . . . ," I mean only that we'll accept it as proven for the purposes of discussion. Whenever evaluating a new patient, I always carefully consider physical and chemical causes.

Comment

Dysthymia, or dysthymic disorder, harks back at least to Emil Kraepelin in the early 1900s. Yet, for all we have learned from its long history, we still relive the old arguments about just where this mild yet prevalent type of depression fits into the family of mood disorders. Of course, the difference in symptoms between dysthymia and major depression is obvious, and other terms have been used over the years to describe types of depression similar to dysthymia. Clinicians have long noted that the chronic low mood and poor self-esteem of patients with dysthymia seem almost part of character. Recent editions of the DSM *still* retain depressive personality disorder in the "provided for further study" appendix. Today we seldom encounter *neurotic depression,* a term once frequently used to describe depressions that were supposedly reactive to an intense disappointment or some other external stimulus. In counterpoint to this older thinking, recently some studies have found family histories of bipolar disorders in patients with dysthymia.

Dysthymia is pretty common, affecting perhaps 6% of the general adult population, but you'll also find it in children and adolescents. Although people with dysthymia are less impaired overall than those with major depression, they and their families nonetheless bear a heavy burden; some writers note that these patients tend to channel whatever energy they possess into work, with little left over for personal relationships. The good news is that, like many other types of depression, dysthymia can be effectively addressed with standard antidepressant treatments—provided we diagnose it correctly.

Timothy

The disorders we've encountered so far entail more or less typical depressive symptoms of varying severity. However, it would endanger both the diagnostic process and the patient to rely wholly on symptoms. The following example shows how important it is to seek the diagnosis in the history, as well as in the cross-sectional symptoms.

> Timothy, a journalist now in his late 30s, had covered the war in Sudan for a major news organization. Shortly after receiving an emergency blood transfusion, he contracted hepatitis C and was started on interferon. "Within a few days I began to feel like I had the flu—achy muscles, tired all the time, stomach pain—and I couldn't sleep more than a couple of hours before I woke up exhausted." However, he denied problems with his appetite, and he had never felt suicidal; even his sex interest had remained good.
>
> Reassigned to the United States, he chafed at the relatively dull stories on his new beat. He complained of trouble focusing on his reporting, and began brooding about his health. Noting his insomnia and loss of concentration, his internist concluded that he was depressed and started him on Prozac. "For all the good it did, I might as well have taken Tic-Tacs," Timothy said. "Twelve weeks later, I wasn't any worse, but I sure wasn't any better, either." In answer to a question, he pointed out that he followed his religion, which forbade the use of alcohol or tobacco in any form.
>
> Noting that Timothy and his wife had previously seen a therapist to deal with the marital problems surrounding their infertility, his doctor next referred him for counseling. It was during "that fruitless 8 weeks" that Timothy, surfing the Internet one day when he should have been working, came upon a blog that described the mental effects of interferon treatment. He learned that about a third of patients treated with interferon develop serious depression. "I felt outraged and relieved at the same time," he later said. "I was seriously ticked off that I hadn't been warned about side effects of the drug, but delighted to find a treatable cause."

Since his hepatitis was in remission, he stopped the interferon. Within days, his depressive symptoms remitted completely.

Analysis

The absence of a history of mania or hypomania gets us past step 1 of Figure 11.1, but we need to consider whether the hepatitis itself could have caused Timothy's depression (step 2). Typically, patients with hepatitis C complain of poor appetite, weight loss, and fatigue, but not depression. The fact that his depression started with the interferon helps move us along to step 3, which is where we stop. The important diagnostic principle that we should always consider a substance use etiology is about all we need: Timothy was taking a medication known to produce depression. Here we see a benefit of the decision tree approach, which leads us straightaway to the safest—and correct—diagnosis. A less wary clinician might have settled for an adjustment disorder or for the "wastebasket" diagnosis of depressive disorder NOS.

Comment

It is easy to assume that "significant recent substance use" refers exclusively to *misuse* of alcohol or street drugs. Timothy's experience demonstrates otherwise: Medications, both prescription and over-the-counter, can also cause mental symptoms. The fact that his depression responded within days of his discontinuing interferon is powerful evidence, though not conclusive; only a resumption of interferon would confirm his diagnosis, and Timothy was understandably cool to the idea of taking the interferon challenge. Nonetheless, we can feel pretty confident that we've found the cause of his depression. A medication used for conditions as varied and serious as multiple sclerosis, leukemia, lymphoma, and melanoma, interferon can also produce symptoms of anxiety, delirium, and psychosis. Of course, it is only one of the many types of drugs mentioned in Table 9.2 that can produce mood disorders.

Why does it take interferon and other medications so long to produce emotional symptoms? To arrive at the final common path of depression requires that a drug first reach an effective blood level, which then must cause enzymatic or physiological changes in the brain. Similarly, it may take days or weeks of using a corticosteroid to produce psychotic symptoms. The bottom line is this: Just because a patient on medication for weeks has only recently developed symptoms, don't shrug off this possible cause of mental disorder.

Annette

The following vignette underscores the value of examining a wide-ranging differential diagnosis before accepting the facile explanation for a set of symptoms.

> During 19 years with her airline, Annette had always maintained her weight at 117, svelte for her height of 5 feet 5 inches. Now she was in distress as she spoke to her family physician.
>
> "I've gained nearly 15 pounds in just 6 months—15! I'm huge! I'm so depressed, I feel like crying all the time." As if to prove her point, Annette wiped her eyes. "And my face, it's all puffy."
>
> Her family practitioner learned that she had been having trouble getting to sleep, and that her interest in her hobbies (she played the piano and collected dolls) had dwindled to "nearly nothing." So far, she had had no death wishes.
>
> Though she'd never had "the opposite sort of mood, like a mania," Annette had been depressed once before, a few years after she started flying for a living. She thought that her symptoms then were, if anything, a little worse. She was working short hours during one of the cyclical downturns in air travel, and she had just been dumped by the man she had lived with for nearly 4 years. Her doctor then had diagnosed a "situational depression" and had given her an antidepressant (she couldn't remember which one); within a couple of months, she'd improved.
>
> Annette had no relatives with mental disorder, and she had never drunk alcohol to excess or used drugs. Her doctor noticed that she had a moustache that seemed heavy for a woman and a few wispy hairs on her chin. "Those have started just recently, too," Annette volunteered. "As if I needed anything else wrong with me. I've tried to pluck them out, but mostly I just don't care."
>
> After the analysis of a 24-hour urine specimen revealed an elevated corticosteroid content, her doctor told her she had Cushing's syndrome, probably caused by a benign tumor on her adrenal gland.

Analysis

The path to Annette's diagnosis is straightforward and short. Racing through step 1 of Figure 11.1 with her denial that she'd ever had highs of mood, we come to the question of a significant medical condition (step 2), and immediately we are rewarded. Her physician suspected Cushing's syndrome from the physical examination, which typically includes weight gain (especially of the body, but not the limbs), a rounded "moon" face, physical weakness, and an increase in body hair. Then testing revealed that Annette's adrenal glands were overproducing steroids. Steroid medications prescribed for diseases such as asthma or rheumatoid arthritis can also cause Cushing's, but it is usually associated with tumors of the adrenal glands or of the pituitary gland—the so-called master gland located in the brain. Depression (sometimes of serious proportions) often results, as can anxiety, delirium, and even psychosis. Of course, once we reach this step in our decision tree, the search for other causes of Annette's depression would be put on hold until the underlying medical condition had been treated.

Using the diagnostic principles is a bit tricky, because some of them collide. Annette's earlier history of depression that resolved with treatment might have led us down the garden path to a current diagnosis of major depressive disorder; happily, recent history trumps past history to put us right. Tame horses (not zebras) might also have dragged us to the common illness of a recurrent mood disorder, but the principle of looking first for a physical disorder keeps us on course as we navigate the decision tree.

Comment

Table 9.1 presents a long list of physical illnesses that can cause depression. Of course, some of these are quite rare, but overall you could reasonably expect to encounter a good double handful of them at some time during a professional career. It will repay learning these, if only to reassure yourself that you're on the lookout for something another clinician could have missed.

Robert

Of course, we prefer to make do with a single diagnosis, but that isn't always possible. Some depressed patients require at least two.

> As a teenager, Robert was intensely interested in math. When he was a freshman in high school, he used his babysitting money to purchase one of the first electronic calculators. It could only do basic arithmetic, but he used it to work out his own method for figuring square roots. Forever after, the kids at school called him "Square Root."
>
> Square Root Robert was quiet, but not a loner. He had friends in the science club and on the newspaper, for which he wrote a science column.

Based on his science fair participation, he won a scholarship to what he called a "second class" university. After sailing through college with high marks and earning a degree in math in just 3 years, he worked as an actuary for an insurance company. He used to smile ruefully and say, "I dreamed of being an accountant, but I didn't have the personality."

As long as Robert could remember, he had felt "mostly a little sad, and always a little hurt." His sleep and appetite were about average, and he could focus well enough on his work; however, he frequently complained of low energy, and he said that he never expected much from the future. He brought doughnuts to work every Friday, but the gesture never seemed to win him any real friendships. He believed that his chronic low self-esteem and lack of drive had led him to remain single. He'd had only fleeting relationships with women, though when he did have a girlfriend (each of his relationships was pretty short-term), his sex interest and ability were "adequate."

Now 56, Robert was successful in his career, but his personal life had become so miserable that he sought care. As he told the mental health clinician who interviewed him, "I can scrape together the oomph to get me through the day at work, but once I get home, I collapse. I don't fix dinner; I don't really care if I eat. Living or dying isn't that important any more. I just want to go to sleep. I can't even do that very well, just lie awake half the night. For weeks now, I just wish it would all end—or that I would."

The clinician noted that Robert had never misused alcohol or street drugs; he had recently been given a clean bill of health from his family practitioner. Robert denied the suggestion that he had ever had a mood swing in the opposite direction. "Don't I wish!" he scoffed.

Analysis

To diagnose Robert's condition requires two trips through the decision tree. After paying obeisance at the shrines of steps 1, 2, 3, and 4, we note that his long-standing history of low mood and self-criticism did not include symptoms severe or numerous enough (extra credit: identify the diagnostic principle here) to answer "yes" at step 5. However, throughout his adult life he would seem to qualify for a diagnosis of dysthymia (step 6).

Now let's heat up our leftovers. Robert's recent, more acute episode added some yet unexplained symptoms that force us to start over on the decision tree. This time, the introduction of insomnia, death wishes, and reduced interest would earn a step 5 "yes" answer. With no psychotic symptoms (step 9), we arrive at our second diagnosis: major depressive disorder.

Which diagnosis do we list first? The alphabetical approach offers simplicity, but a diagnostic principle places us on firmer ground: It encourages us to list first the disorder that most requires treatment. In Robert's case, that would be his major depression. We'll list his dysthymia second, even though it started first.

Comment

Clinicians sometimes term the combination of these two depressive disorders *double depression*. Despite the fact that it can go undiagnosed, this combination occurs more often than you might imagine; no principle says that having one mental disorder will protect a person from others. Once the major depression is treated, the patient may settle back into the symptoms of dysthymia.

Most patients with dual diagnoses have two disorders from different chapters of the diagnostic manual—schizophrenia and alcoholism, for example. The symptoms of double depression, however, can look like one big illness, and maybe that's the way we should view it. A recent study found few differences among patients with several types of long-standing depression: chronic major depression, double depression, recurring major depression without full interepisode recovery, and chronic major depression grafted onto an existing dysthymia. Perhaps each of these terms is just a proxy for severity, and chronic depression is really only one disorder—a spectrum disease that sometimes worsens, sometimes improves, without ever completely resolving.

Regardless of what we call it, what we really want to know is this: How should we treat double depression, and what is the prognosis? A number of studies suggest that patients with double depression (for convenience, we'll continue to use the term) may be less likely to recover, as well as more likely to have continuing symptoms, impaired social lives, greater comorbidity with still other disorders, and hypomanic episodes. Double depression may also be more likely to require cognitive-behavioral therapy in addition to antidepressant medication.

Carson (Again)

One last time, let's revisit Carson, our graduate student whose depressions regularly occurred each fall or winter and remitted each spring. I had interviewed him at the point when he was again acutely distressed, apparently due to the prospect of moving his family across the country to a strange town, away from family and friends. We have met him at the beginning of Chapter 1 and discussed his differential diagnosis in Chapter 3.

Analysis

Let us consider first his very recent distress around the issue of moving. Carson's lack of mania or hypomania, current substance use, or physical disorders earns a pass at steps 1–4; the fact that he currently had relatively few symptoms leads us past step 5, whereas the brevity of his low mood earns a "no" for dysthymia (step 6). The obvious stress-related nature of his condition (step 7) brings us to adjustment disorder with depressed mood. We'd have to go through the decision tree again, with a step 11 side trip, to arrive at his other diagnosis of a seasonal mood variant of major depressive disorder. Because it was currently summer, only the adjustment disorder required immediate attention, so we'll list it first.

Comment

I would guess that people have been blaming events for their moods ever since they first learned to observe cause and effect. That said, in the wake of the DSMs the type of depression formerly known as *reactive* has sunk nearly out of sight, a victim of our inability to agree on what constitutes a legitimate stressor. One clinician's precipitating stress might be another's unrelated anecdote. When I was in training, we marveled at the published report of a patient who had become depressed upon learning that his dog had fleas. The concept of reactive depression lives on officially only in the conditions of bereavement and postpartum depression—and in the form of adjustment disorder that afflicted Carson.

You'll notice that I've put adjustment disorder way down on the differential diagnosis for depression (see Table 11.1). There are two reasons: It is much less well defined than most of the other diagnoses, and it is supported with far fewer scientific follow-up data. Nonetheless, 10% of adults in some mental health populations are diagnosed with adjustment disorder. Is this in error? The relevant data simply don't exist. I can tell you that adjustment disorder is meant to be a category of exclusion, for use only if no other possible diagnosis is appropriate. If someone's symptoms qualify for major depressive disorder, you shouldn't call it an adjustment disorder. A diagnosis of bereavement is generally preferred if the person has recently suffered the loss of a loved one.

An adjustment disorder diagnosis might be appropriate for acutely developing responses to a severe stressor, such as a threatening physical illness, parental breakup, or upheaval in the workplace. Even when the diagnosis is warranted, it comes with some risk: Although the label carries relatively less stigma for the patient, it may be associated with suicidal behaviors and even with completed suicide. And, perhaps the greatest risk of all, it implies that the situation must be left to work itself out. There isn't much practical you can do, after all, to address the root causes of, say, a heart attack or a fire that just burned the patient's house down.

Carson did not currently qualify for major depressive disorder, and his former treating clinician and I therefore agreed that this newest episode was most likely only a reaction to multiple stresses: a new program of study, impending fatherhood, and a new and unfamiliar home in some far-off and unknown part of the world. We communicated this to Carson, and the next day he had recovered his spirits as he and his wife drove off to meet their new life adventure. The episode underscores the diagnostic principle that we should be chary of symptoms that develop in response to a crisis; they may well turn out to be transient and not indicative of the patient's overall condition.

Andrea

You will probably remember Andrea Yates, the Texas mother who, one June morning after her husband left for work, fed breakfast to her five children—and then drowned them, one by one, in a tub of bathwater. Andrea herself provided information for Suzanne O'Malley's book *"Are You There Alone?"*, which carefully relates the details of her illness and its aftermath. All of the information I've given here, then, is in the public record.

> By the time she was pregnant with her fifth child (her only daughter), several clinicians had already identified Andrea as one of the sickest patients in their experience. Her symptoms read like a textbook summary of grave psychopathology: markedly reduced speech (sometimes called *poverty of thought*), poor attention span, low mood, and delusional guilt about being a bad mother. At one time or another, she cried and had constricted range of affect, feelings of worthlessness, and hopelessness. During her second psychiatric hospitalization, four months after the birth of her fourth child, she became nearly mute; a month after release, she tried to cut her own throat.
>
> During her fifth and final pregnancy, Andrea improved, but after childbirth—coping with a new baby and still trying to home-school her other children—she once again became severely ill. She stopped eating

and speaking, and her insomnia worsened; for long periods, she would just stare into space. She developed the belief that the "mark of the beast" (the number 666) had been written on the top of her head, and she rubbed her scalp raw attempting to remove it.

Andrea's upbringing had been conventional and unremarkable; she had never misused alcohol or drugs, and her physical health was good. An older brother carried the diagnosis of a bipolar disorder.

After her arrest, she told a jail psychiatrist, "I am Satan," and she explained that a camera had been installed in her home to monitor her performance as a mother. She believed that her children were "not righteous, because I am evil." She could hear a variety of hallucinated sounds: the voice of Satan coming to her over the jail intercom; the voice of a character from the movie *O Brother, Where Art Thou?*; and the sounds of ducks, teddy bears, and a man on horseback, all pouring forth from the cinder blocks of her cell.

Under Texas law, and with conflicting psychiatric testimony, Andrea was judged able to tell right from wrong (never mind that she didn't know which was which) and found guilty of murder. She barely escaped a sentence of death.

Analysis

Which of our two mood disorder decision trees to use (Figure 11.1 or Figure 11.2, to be presented later) presents a bit of a problem, for it isn't exactly clear now (it certainly wasn't then) whether Andrea ever had a bipolar disorder. At least one clinician who saw her in jail believed that she did, and this judgment was partly supported by her brother's diagnosis of a bipolar disorder (the family history diagnostic principle). However, at the time of her trial, there was no clear evidence of previous mania or hypomania, so we'll use the tree in Figure 11.1. Our information brings us quickly to step 5, where all of us will agree that she had many, many symptoms of severe depression. At step 9, we can say a loud "yes" to current hallucinations and delusions. Nowhere do we find information that she had symptoms of psychosis other than when depressed (step 10), so we have a diagnosis: major depression with psychotic features. Now step 11 asks about any additional specifiers, one of which is postpartum. The final diagnosis is a postpartum psychotic depression. (This is also where we'd arrive if we had used Figure 11.2.)

Focusing on her psychosis, several psychiatrists diagnosed Andrea as having some form of schizophrenia or schizoaffective disorder. They'd have done better using the psychosis decision tree provided in Chapter 13: Figure 13.1 leads us to severe depression with psychosis. In other words, if those clinicians had used a systematic approach, she might at least have had the benefit of a correct diagnosis at trial.

Andrea's depression was foreshadowed by her previous history of postpartum depression and by a superabundance of symptoms that are absolutely typical for depression—three diagnostic principles in one sentence. The quality of Andrea's delusions also helps guide us: (1) They were not bizarre (each was something that was possible—cameras could have been planted in her house, she could have had a mark written somewhere on her); and (2) they were mood-congruent (in keeping with someone who had a severe depression). Each feature is both typical of mood disorder and less consistent with schizophrenia. In a differential list, I'd put schizophrenia dead last as the least safe diagnosis, which would force us to ignore it until the possibilities of the mood disorders diagnosis had been adequately explored.

In the story of Andrea Yates, we can discern another common diagnostic dilemma. Prior to the ultimate tragedy, she had been treated successfully with an antipsychotic medication (Haldol). The fact that she appeared to respond well to this treatment may have persuaded some of her clinicians that her main diagnosis should have been schizophrenia, not a mood disorder. However, this conclusion conflicts with her history and the symptoms she presented. Once again, this case illustrates the importance of the decision tree and of safety-oriented differential diagnosis.

Comment

The postpartum period is one of those special circumstances that can modify the diagnosis of major depression. Various studies suggest that many postpartum women, up to perhaps 15%, will have enough symptoms to warrant a diagnosis of major depressive disorder. This is quite different from the so-called baby blues, a far milder syndrome that many (possibly most) women experience and shrug off by the 10th day after delivering a baby. Still not clear is whether women in the postpartum period are at any greater risk for depression than during other periods of their lives.

No one knows just why these emotional states occur, or why they sometimes progress to an actual mental disorder. The many hormonal changes that take place in a woman's body following childbirth must play a major role, but no specific mechanism has yet been identified. We do know that mental difficulties in the postpartum period are by no means limited to depression. Postpartum events can trigger bipolar disorders that in about 1 in 1,000 patients reach psychotic proportions—as was Andrea's tragic experience. The occurrence rate for those who have experienced such a psychosis (about 25% of subsequent pregnancies) is daunting, or should be. The entire tragedy could have been averted if Andrea's clinicians had only recognized and forcefully pointed out that those who have once experienced postpartum depression are highly likely to have it again. (Charles Dickens's wife reportedly experienced it 12 times!) The good news is that this devastating experience can be prevented. But first it must be recognized and correctly diagnosed.

Increasingly, other mental diagnoses are recognized to occur subsequent to childbirth, including OCD (in which the content of the obsessions is harming the infant) and PTSD (sometimes to the point that a woman will refuse to bear more children). Some women develop panic disorder, though others actually experience reduced anxiety following childbirth.

Mania and Its Variants

A patient once said, "Mania is worse than depression. At least for depression, there's a floor, and you know it can't get any worse. But with mania, the sky's *no* limit; you just keep going up and up—until you lose propulsion and crash."

A pathological upswing of mood signals a whole new spectrum of diagnoses, requiring a new decision tree and several changes in the differential diagnosis. The implications of these diagnoses for treatment and prognosis are huge. When considering any of them, we must look for hints not just in the patient's recent history, but in the past and in family histories as well. Although a type of psychosis called schizoaffective disorder can form a part of the differential for the mood disorders, we'll defer that discussion until Chapter 13. Table 11.2 presents the differential diagnosis for mania and its variants.

Herbert

The typical symptoms of mania are as classic as they are well known, and the typical bipolar pattern of illness followed by complete recovery can practically hit you in the face. Yet clinicians continue to miss the diagnosis with appalling frequency—at times treating patients for unipolar major depression, at others for schizophrenia or some other psychotic disorder.

TABLE 11.2. Differential Diagnosis with Brief Definitions for Mania and Its Variants

- *Manic symptoms due to a medical condition.* Physical illness can cause mania or hypomania.

- *Manic symptoms due to use of a substance.* Alcohol, street drugs, or medications can cause symptoms of mania or hypomania.

- *Mania.* For a week or longer, the patient feels elation or irritability; is grandiose; and is unusually talkative, hyperactive, and distractible. Poor judgment leads to problems with social life and work, and often results in hospitalization. Patients with an episode of mania are said to have bipolar I disorder; most of them will also have episodes of major depression.

- *Hypomania.* A patient has symptoms much like mania, but less severe. Patients who also have an episode of major depression and no full-blown mania are said to have bipolar II disorder.

- *Mixed states.* Some patients have mixed episodes, in which they fulfill criteria for both mania and major depression.

- *Cyclothymia.* Patients experience repeated mood swings that are not severe enough to qualify as mania or major depression.

After 6 years working as a pharmacist, Herbert had had an affair with a woman he'd met when he sold her a bottle of lotion. His wife had never learned of his infidelity, but the memory stuck with him, and he always felt guilty. For one thing, it reminded him of his own father, who had suffered from what would now be called bipolar I disorder. When manic, he would drink heavily, then physically abuse both his wife and little Herbert.

Just when Herbert turned 30, that guilt boiled over. At the party his wife gave him, he burst into tears when she gave him his present—an antique mortar and pestle he had admired for months but felt they could not afford. Days later, he called in sick to work. He spent nearly all of his time in bed, much of it sleeping; when awake, he ruminated about the "trick" he had played on his wife. He worried that he had infected her with herpes. Though his physician explained that the chances were negligible, still he couldn't shake his concern. He worried about the size of his penis: several times a day he would measure it with a carpenter's folding rule, and more than once he clicked on e-mail spam that offered to "Grow your p*nis." Additional symptoms piled up—anorexia, weight loss (10 pounds in just 3 weeks), frequent tearfulness, and finally thoughts of shooting himself with his service weapon. At last, he agreed to start taking medication. Within a week he had improved, and in a month he was back at work.

Although from time to time he still worried about herpes, Herbert remained well for the next 2 years. Then, once again on his birthday, he began to think about sex. He began talking rapidly; within days he developed grandiose thoughts. He became convinced that he was the reincarnation of William Faulkner, and he began several "first chapters" dealing with the further doings of the people in Yoknapatawpha County. He even worked late several nights writing a Pulitzer Prize acceptance speech. However, the two policemen who came to remove him forcibly to the hospital turned out to be buddies from his high school graduating class. They all had a wonderful time reminiscing and catching up on their recent lives. His friends departed, still chuckling and exchanging witticisms, leaving Herbert behind. When his wife finally kicked him out, he moved into his camper.

Analysis

Note that *any* history (not just current symptoms) of mania or hypomania starts us off in bipolar territory, even if the patient's current mood is depressed. The lack of any history of medical problems or substance misuse gets us past steps 1, 2, and 3 of the decision tree for a patient with elevated, expansive, or irritable mood (Figure 11.2). Then step 4 leads us through steps 9 ("yes") and 11 ("yes") to step 12 and the diagnosis of bipolar I disorder.

Had we evaluated Herbert when he was 30, rather than years later, we would have found no history of mania, and his diagnosis could well have been major depression, rather than bipolar disorder—applause for the diagnostic principle that recent history beats ancient history! However, the depressive episodes of patients with bipolar disorders differ in some respects from those of patients who will never have mania or hypomania. Patients with bipolar depression are more likely to have hypersomnia, mood lability, and psychomotor retardation. Bipolar depression also may begin quite suddenly and at a relatively early age. An earlier clinician should have been alerted to the bipolar possibility by the history of mania in Herbert's father. However, an individual patient with a first episode of depression may show none of these features, so we must forever remain alert for evidence of ensuing symptoms of mania or hypomania.

Comment

In the years after lithium proved effective in treating and preventing mania, the tendency of American clinicians to diagnose what is now called bi-

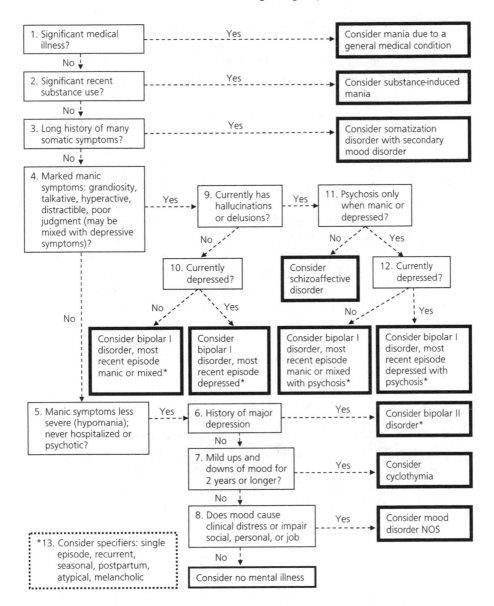

FIGURE 11.2. **Decision tree for a patient who has had elevated, expansive, or irritable mood.**

polar I disorder soared. Yet even in 1980 a study reported that 56% of patients with this disorder had at one time been diagnosed with schizophrenia. A study in 2000 reported that 69% of patients with bipolar disorder had been misdiagnosed, usually as unipolar. Even today, we *still* often don't get it right, or when we do we don't get it early—on average, it takes several years from the onset of first symptoms to make the correct diagnosis of bipolar disorder.

More difficult to redress is the misdiagnosis of *unipolar* major depression in a patient who really has bipolar disorder. That was the fate of 40% of the patients in a 1999 study. Although this mistake can sometimes be avoided by strictly applying current diagnostic criteria, the first episode of many patients with bipolar disorder is one of depression. Then the ultimate correct diagnosis can be suspected initially in patients who have a bipolar family history, or who respond to antidepressant drugs or bright light therapy by becoming manic. Other hints at an eventual bipolar diagnosis include a rapid onset of depressive symptoms, onset in the teens or early 20s, and unstable mood before or after the depression. Because patients don't always recognize that their own symptoms imply illness, it's important to ask relatives or friends about prior manic or hypomanic episodes, and to report mood lability if it occurs down the road.

Erma

So much of mental health diagnosis depends on degree—consider the importance of how much a person drinks, gambles, or eats. The symptoms of mania or hypomania are no exception. When intense, as in the case of Herbert, they can lead to hospitalization, disrupted relationships, or even financial ruin. When milder, if they are noticed at all, they can imply a couple of different diagnoses.

> A news reader for a local radio station, Erma complained that her listeners could tell what kind of a mood she was in. "Every once in a while I get e-mails from people who say, 'What's wrong? Your voice doesn't have its usual sparkle.' "
>
> Erma used to believe that she was responding to pressures at home; now she realized that her moods were causing her on-air vocal changes. "Once I got divorced, I went right on having ups and downs of mood. Only now, I fight with the people at work."
>
> Quizzed closely about her moods, she described them this way: "They last a few weeks at a time, never longer. When I'm down, I feel as

though I'm running on about half-power. I'm still me; I just don't scintillate." During these down phases, she was grumpy and sometimes rude, but her sleep and appetite were about as usual. "And I know what you're going to ask—I *never* have suicidal ideas. I've worked too hard to get where I am to throw it away." When she was up, on the other hand, "I'm a 50-megawatt powerhouse. I feel like talking and dancing, both at once."

Erma spoke clearly and distinctly, her inflections reflecting years of training and experience behind a microphone. She said she didn't think her mood swings followed the seasons, and they definitely didn't react to her environment. "I was up for several weeks after my husband left me for our babysitter, and down the month after I got a raise."

At a recent checkup, Erma's family practitioner had pronounced her physically healthy. A Chinese American, she flushed easily whenever she drank alcohol, and she therefore avoided it almost completely. She had never used street drugs and took no medications.

Analysis

Erma's up periods would earn her a ride on Figure 11.2. The history makes it clear that Erma had no known step 1 (or 3) medical complaints that could explain her symptoms. The fact that, like many people of Asian descent, she became acutely uncomfortable with even modest amounts of alcohol would rule out a step 2 alcohol-related illness; we'll take her word that she didn't use street drugs, either. When feeling up, she didn't present the far-out picture of mega-grandiosity that characterizes step 4 "true mania." This would move us on through step 5 to step 6, where her relatively minor depressive symptoms spoke against bipolar II disorder. Her ups and downs had persisted for several years (a step 7 "yes"), leading to cyclo-thymic disorder as our final diagnosis.

The lilt (or its absence) in Erma's voice is an excellent example of a sign, which, as the diagnostic principle says, often beats symptoms in identifying a mental disorder. Her listeners didn't have to know her personally—didn't even have to *see* her—to know when something was amiss. She herself identified another principle that can lead patients and clinicians astray: For years she had thought her moodiness was due to marital problems, but after her divorce she discovered that she was still moody. The mere fact that one event follows another doesn't mean there is a causal connection; it's a terrific example of the fallacy of *post hoc ergo propter hoc,* a Latin maxim that translates to "after the fact, therefore because of it." Remember, it's a fallacy.

Comment

Had Erma experienced even one episode of major depression, we would say that she suffered from bipolar II disorder. With only minor degrees of depression, however, cyclothymia would be the warranted diagnosis. The diagnoses of bipolar I, bipolar II, and cyclothymic disorders are closely related, in that they have similar symptoms and treatment.

Indeed, there may be yet other bipolar conditions that have still not been adequately described. Some clinicians use the labels *bipolar III* for those situations where treatment for major depressive disorder causes the patient to switch briefly into hypomania, and *bipolar IV* for major depressive disorder without a discrete hypomanic episode (just a sunny temperament that is sometimes called *hyperthymic*). However, neither of these two has as yet been given any official stamp of approval. It may be only custom that has averted the use of something on the order of *bipolar V* for cyclothymia—which was, after all, regarded as a personality disorder as recently as the 1970s. And who knows where it will stop? The Romans have lots more numerals.

Rosa

I've mentioned several times before that you should always take a complete history, no matter how obvious the symptoms appear. I'll repeat this yet again here, and Rosa's history demonstrates why.

> When she was 46, Rosa noticed that she stumbled when she walked. It happened inconsistently—maybe it was worse when she was tired—and at first she tried not to pay much attention. She was too excitable anyway, her husband had always said, and for once she didn't want to seem alarmist.
>
> "It's not like I lurch from side to side or anything," she finally told her family doctor. "It's more of a limp, like I just can't quite get my legs to play nicely together." The doctor couldn't find much that was wrong, diagnosed conversion disorder, and remanded her to a therapist—for her mood.
>
> Rosa felt fatigued and rather depressed. She had been a homemaker for 25 years; now her two children were off to college, and she hadn't enough to do. With the encouragement of her counselor, she became active in her church women's fellowship. Her limp nearly disappeared; perhaps the therapy was working, she thought. Over the next couple of months her mood first brightened, then moved steadily through sunny to outright ecstatic.

Rosa became agitated. She would grip the coat sleeves of strangers on the street to tell them how faith had cured her. She sold her living room furniture and donated the proceeds to a television evangelist. When her husband objected, she called 911 to report that he had struck her; a policeman escorted him from the house.

Meanwhile, her limp had returned, and a peculiar, rapid-fire stuttering made her speech increasingly hard to understand. Recognizing that something was amiss, her therapist persuaded her to return to her family practitioner. Another physical exam led to a neurological consultation, and to the eventual diagnosis of multiple sclerosis. Treatment with glatiramer acetate, specific for her disease, reduced her physical symptoms, and her mood gradually returned to normal.

Analysis

Climbing through the decision tree in Figure 11.2 is pretty quick in Rosa's case, with a hit at step 1. This apparent success shouldn't allow us to rest on our laurels with the feeling that our job is done. Although we try to follow the Occam's razor principle and simplify diagnosis whenever we can, it was still possible that Rosa's manic symptoms were unrelated to her physical disease; as we've learned, chronology doesn't always equal causation. However, the remission of her mood disorder once the physical symptoms were under control pretty well eliminated any likelihood that she had two independent conditions.

Comment

By now, the symptoms of mania (and hypomania) have pretty much become common knowledge, even to laypeople. That which we know well tends to be uppermost in our minds, so it comes as no surprise that every once in a while, someone with a physical condition that is associated with euphoria and the other symptoms of mania/hypomania goes misdiagnosed. It's a shame that Rosa's first diagnosis wasn't based on the differential diagnosis/decision tree model; doing so might have saved a lot of anguish.

The number of physical disorders that can cause manic or hypomanic symptoms is modest (you'll find some in Table 9.1). However, from time to time I read reports of such symptoms newly associated with a medical condition. These conditions include low blood sodium, uremia (kidney failure), blood vessel malformations in the head, and open heart surgery. Without a doubt, some of these represent true cause-and-effect situations; just as surely, others are pure coincidence. The trick is to know which is which (see the sidebar "Recognizing Physical Causes of Mania or Hypomania"). As I've noted (well, harped on) previously, the only safe approach is initially to suspect an organic cause for *every* patient.

Comorbidity

The patients we've met so far in this chapter have had only mood disorders. However, depressive or bipolar disorders commonly occur with other disorders; in fact, a lot of research suggests that this is the rule. Sometimes this co-occurrence is referred to as dual diagnosis, but some clinicians reserve this term for a substance use problem combined with a non-substance-related disorder. For the sake of clarity, I'll try to avoid using it.

You will encounter mood disorders combined with nearly every other mental health diagnosis in several possible relationships, which aren't mutually exclusive:

Recognizing Physical Causes of Mania or Hypomania

Some useful indicators can actually help differentiate physically caused mania or hypomania from bipolar disorders. (A sidebar on page 159 informs us that we aren't so lucky with physically caused depression.) Suspicion of physical causes should increase for patients who have some of the following characteristics:

- Late onset of first manic or hypomanic episode (35 or older)
- Clear history of potential physical cause, such as AIDS or recent closed head injury
- Lack of depressive episodes
- No prior mental hospitalizations
- No family history of bipolar disorders
- Irritability or dysphoric mood
- Threatening or assaultive while manic
- Grandiose delusions of worth, power, or special relationships (as with a deity)
- Cognitive dysfunctions, such as defects of orientation and concentration
- Poor response to standard treatment for mania or hypomania
- Rapid resolution of symptoms once a physical cause has been ameliorated

---

- Two disorders can begin together, or one (primary) precedes the other (secondary).
- Two disorders are present at the same time, or they alternate.
- One disorder induces the other, or they are completely independent. (The former isn't technically comorbidity, but it happens often enough to rate mentioning.)
- The symptoms of one disorder conceal another, such as when a person's heavy drinking masks the fact of depression.

The case histories that follow draw our attention to another issue: Which diagnosis in any pair should you list first, and which later? This issue has more than academic interest. A vast body of research has shown that, for example, secondary depressions respond differently to somatic treatments such as electroconvulsive therapy and antidepressant medication.

Arnold

Arnold had become depressed when he was just 15. His father had recently died of alcoholism; he himself was foundering in several classes in his sophomore year of high school; and he saw "no future in life" and had begun to lose weight. He also couldn't sleep without a couple of pulls at the port wine his mother for years had generously employed as an antidepressant and painkiller. After his grades sank even further, he left school and "just hung out," he told his clinician a decade later—"doing about as much as I wanted to, which was nothing at all." After several months, his depression lifted without any intervention at all. Then he lied about his age and enlisted in the Army.

Arnold was posted to Vietnam, where he served nearly 2 years of his 3-year enlistment. During this time, because he was bright and competent, he was promoted three times; because he had a talent for getting into trouble with his staff sergeant, he was busted twice. He returned to civilian life as a former private first class with a heroin addiction. "There was a lot of it available over there," he told the VA clinician who interviewed him after he was discharged.

Maintained on methadone for the next 15 years, Arnold did reasonably well, using heroin only occasionally and maintaining steady employment as a printer. As he gained experience, he moved into desktop publishing and was ultimately offered a partnership in his small firm. After several years, he married a woman who had been divorced once. Her first husband had periodically misused alcohol, so she knew the drill. "Use just once," Beth told Arnold, "and I'm out of here. No, *you're* out of here!" The methadone and that promise kept him clean and sober for the next decade.

But in the late 1990s, Arnold's methadone maintenance program fell victim to VA cost cutting. As he tapered off the drug, his mood darkened, and he grew more irritable than he had felt in many years. Although he went to work faithfully, his interest flagged. In his Narcotics Anonymous support group, which he still attended regularly, he heard similar stories from others. One Friday evening, a speaker described the emotional symptoms of methadone withdrawal—depression, irritability, and sometimes a sense of expansiveness—and said that they sometimes lasted for months.

Although this description prepared Arnold for discomfort, it seemed that his friends were weathering withdrawal better than he was. As the weeks wore on and he remained completely off methadone, the muscle aches and restlessness diminished, but his mood dipped lower. He barked at Beth, he growled at his boss; and his work output gradually slowed to a crawl. For the first time in years, he had begun to think about scoring some heroin—and taking a massive, lethal overdose.

Analysis

With substance use and depression, we have the ingredients for a classic example of comorbidity. A degree of depression can be expected when a person is withdrawing from heavy use of any opioid; methadone is no exception (see Table 9.3). But if Arnold's diagnosis were a simple coast through Figure 11.1 to step 3, we would expect that the longer he went without the drug, the more his depression would improve. In fact, quite the opposite occurred: As time passed, both the number and intensity of his symptoms increased (there's a diagnostic principle here concerning the likelihood of major depression), and we end up at step 9 with major depressive disorder. Arnold's history shows how important it is to consider the time course of symptoms, not just the symptoms themselves.

As to arranging these two diagnoses, I like to list diagnoses chronologically. But, because we believe that Arnold's mood disorder was of major proportions and independent of the substance use, it would require our immediate attention. Safety first. Besides, his substance use was currently in check.

Comment

In Chapter 4 (page 30) we've met Jakob, whose drinking produced both psychosis and depression. As I've already noted, we wouldn't refer to that relationship, where one illness directly causes another, as *comorbidity*. Patients like Arnold, however, have two (or sometimes more) mental disorders that have no obvious causal relationship. It can take some detective work to sort out the symptoms of each independent disorder to arrive at a diagnosis of true comorbidity.

The work of that detection can be distressingly difficult. It is so easy to encounter evidence of one diagnosis and misconstrue it as support for another. Just think about the symptoms of major depression you can find during the course of intoxication or withdrawal from various substances—they include sleeplessness, social withdrawal, apathy, low mood, and weight loss (see Table 9.3). You can also find symptoms reminiscent of mania—such as rambling speech, periods of tirelessness, heightened psychomotor activity, poor judgment, euphoria, belligerence, and impulsiveness. Alcohol and other drugs can also release inhibitions and induce anxiety states or psychosis, sometimes leading to the morbid thinking that results in suicidal behavior. Table 6.1 lists mental disorders you might encounter in a substance-using patient.

Another deterrent to easy detection is the fact that shame can render patients secretive about abusing substances. Fortunately, most people will tell the truth if you question them directly about how much they drink or whether they use drugs. All in all, is it any wonder that a study of inpatients found that nearly 20% of patients with mood disorders also had substance use disorders, of which under one in four had been diagnosed by the physician in charge?

Connie

The depressions we have read about up to now have all been of the sort that respond to standard treatment with antidepressant medications or structured psychotherapy. However, the effective treatment of many other depressed patients depends heavily on an exact diagnosis that may be quite different from the ever-popular major depression.

> During 2 years of severe depression, Connie had been treated with psychotherapy and 12 different medications for depression and anxiety, and then a long series of electroconvulsive treatments—none with lasting

benefit. Her physician had mentioned the possibility of psychosurgery, but suggested that first she consult another clinician, to see whether there was any other possibility before taking such a drastic step.

There could be no questioning the gravity of Connie's depressive symptoms. At their worst, which was most of the time, she complained of loss of appetite and weight, trouble sleeping, poor concentration, fatigue, and death wishes. She had made three suicide attempts of increasing severity, and thought about suicide daily. Because she couldn't cope with her three children, she had lost custody of them to her former husband. (She had lost *him* to chronic pain with intercourse and lack of interest in sex.) Her job had disappeared in the morass of six lengthy hospitalizations. "I'm totally desperate," she said. "I wish they'd just go ahead and cut."

Something about the way Connie brightened after talking for a while made the consultant reach back for some additional history. With Connie's permission, her mother was contacted by telephone. She recalled some difficulties that Connie hadn't mentioned previously. Connie had been chronically ill from the time she was 13. Besides severe headaches, she had had a number of strange complaints, including fainting spells, an attack of paralysis, and even a brief episode of blindness for which no cause could ever be determined. In fact, each of the doctors they had consulted during her adolescence and early adult years had pronounced her remarkably fit. She revealed that Connie had consulted doctors or taken medication for difficulty breathing, heart palpitations, chest pain, dizziness, nausea, abdominal bloating, menstrual irregularity, and pain in her back and extremities.

Connie admitted that she had been a sickly child and "always ailing" as an adult, right up to the time that she began having the depression. Recently, the physical disorders had bothered her less. Although she had experimented with marijuana when she was in high school, it had only made her feel sick. "More sickness, I didn't need at all," she remarked with a wry smile. She had avoided drugs and alcohol since.

Analysis

The differential diagnosis we would construct for Connie is very similar to Table 11.1, though we'd need more information to determine whether we should diagnose some form of anxiety disorder. Let's analyze Connie's depressive symptoms with Figure 11.1. For the sake of simplicity, we'll assume that Connie hadn't had symptoms of mania or hypomania in the past (step 1). At step 2, she had certainly had numerous medical complaints that could suggest a medical disorder underlying her mental symptoms. However, through the years she had been seen by several specialist physicians as well as her family practitioner, and each of them had ultimately pronounced her physically sound. That bounces the ball squarely back into our court. No recent step 3 substance use moves us along to step 4, where we agree that she had had many somatic symptoms in the past. Note that its placement early in our various decision trees calls our attention to somatization disorder, regardless of how severe the depressive, manic, or other symptoms may have been.

Here's a problem: How do we list the two disorders? If we slavishly (uh-oh, the word's a dead giveaway, isn't it?) follow the same rules we used for Arnold, we'd mention the depression first. But from all that is written about somatization disorder, we know that directly addressing a co-occurring mood disorder (which occurs in about 80% of the cases) is fraught with hazard: Depressed patients with somatization often don't respond to standard treatments that help most other depressed patients. Listing somatization disorder first puts the disorders into chronological order, which suggests in turn that the depression might need special handling. Similar calculations would apply to other disorders that occur with somatization disorder, including anxiety disorders, anorexia nervosa, and bulimia nervosa.

Incidentally, the tip-off to Connie's diagnosis was the observation that in the face of a very severe depression, she brightened up after conversing for a while—another example of the diagnostic principle that signs beat symptoms. It may not be invoked very often, but it carries power. Keep it in mind.

Comment

Without a doubt, differentiating primary clinical depression from secondary depression that occurs with somatization disorder is one of the most difficult problems mental health clinicians face. (Of course, diagnosing secondary depression that accompanies *any* primary disorder is a challenge; see the sidebar "Recognizing Secondary Depression" on page 159.) To understand why this problem exists, we'll need to explore a little history.

Somatization disorder has been recognized for more than 150 years. Known for millennia by the ancient term *hysteria*, it was well described in 1859 by the French clinician Paul Briquet. In the 1960s, Robins, Guze, and other American clinicians formalized Briquet's findings and used his name for the syndrome they identified. They included more symptoms than are used in today's diagnostic criteria. Of course, there were such physical complaints as various body pains, sexual dysfunctioning, chest and abdominal complaints, and complaints like an attack of paralysis (see Chapter 9, page 109). They also found that these patients typically had symptoms of depression, anxiety, or even psychosis. In the intervening years, follow-up studies repeatedly demonstrated the predictive value of their work. However, when DSM-III was adopted in 1980, all of the emotional symptoms of Briquet's syndrome were removed from the description, leaving only the physical symptoms. This left clinicians free to diagnose any additional mood, anxiety, or psychotic condition for which a patient happened to meet criteria.

One outcome is, I believe, that many clinicians today haven't learned a basic principle of somatization disorder—namely, the almost uncanny ability of patients to sense and conform to the interests of their caregivers. The first example is still the best. On the neurology ward operated by Jean-Martin Charcot in the Salpêtrière hospital in late-19th-century Paris, patients with hysteria (as it was then known) imitated patients with epilepsy. The interest shown by clinicians from all over Europe encouraged these women to elaborate a ritualized form of pseudoseizure that became known as *grand hysteria*. Thus commenced a worldwide pandemic, which collapsed when Charcot died in 1893.

I don't mean to imply that such people ever aim to deceive their clinicians, either in Charcot's time or in our own. Often their symptoms evolve in an unconscious collaboration between clinician and patient. You can understand why a gastroenterologist who encounters abdominal pain and vomiting, or a mental health clinician who finds depression and anxiety, might well diagnose conditions common in their respective fields. When following up positive responses, the clinician asks about other symptoms typical of the diagnosis. The patient notices the clinician's interest and supplies any number of other symptoms, and the syndrome seems to be confirmed.

Today's patients with somatization disorder discern and mirror their clinicians' interests in mood, anxiety, and even psychotic disorders. That's why I call somatization disorder an *iatroplastic* condition: Clinicians don't cause it, but by their interests they certainly do mold its form. Whereas physical and laboratory examinations yield a lack of demonstrable pathology in the case of physical complaints, we still have no such tests for emotional symptoms. Although someone could have two independent disorders—say, somatization disorder and major depression—Occam's razor suggests that just one is far more likely. The bottom line: A direct assault on such a mood disorder seldom provides the relief these patients seek.

Recognizing Secondary Depression

Would that it were simple. About the only easy aspect of secondary depression is its definition: a depression in someone who has a previous serious (that is, it threatens life or the capacity for self-care) medical illness or non-mood-related mental disorder. By some estimations, about 40% of depressions are secondary.

The problem with the diagnosis is this: After years of careful investigations, researchers can only tell us that most secondary depressions are relatively mild (patients like Connie notwithstanding). The symptoms tend to be pretty garden-variety, and there simply aren't any symptoms that clearly differentiate secondary from primary depression. That leaves us with precious few generalizations to make:

- As a group, these patients are more likely to be younger males with a family history of alcoholism.

- Of depressed men with alcoholism, about 95% will have a secondary depression; the figure for women is about 75%. (Yes, this means that among people with alcoholism, primary depression is about five times more common in women than in men. Go to the head of the class.)

- A patient who is psychotically depressed or who has symptoms of melancholy (awakens in early morning, feels worse in the morning, has marked loss of appetite, has unwarranted guilt feelings, loses pleasure in nearly everything, feels no better when something good happens) is unlikely to have a secondary depression.

- Depression in patients with somatization disorder is almost certain to be of the secondary kind. In all my years of experience, I've known only one such patient who I was sure also had a primary depression.

- Depression secondary to medical illness is likely to develop later in life and less likely to include the symptoms of suicidal ideas, guilt, or delusions.

- You may not be able to decide definitively whether depression is "real" or is the expected reaction to medical illness, but don't automatically pass it off as the latter. Rather, look for such telltale indicators as previous episodes, history of mania or hypomania, family history of mood disorder, and duration (longer duration is more likely to be found in major depressive disorder).

Borderlands

The boundaries of the mood disorders have been sharpened up considerably, but a number of fuzzy lines still snake between various forms of pathology or between the normal and the pathological. In this section, we'll explore a few of them.

Bereavement and Loss

Long ago, depressions were commonly divided into two types: those that occurred in reaction to some external event (such as loss of a job or a death in the family), and those that, without external cause, sprang from within the individual. The first type was called *endogenous* (coming from within); the second type was termed *exogenous* or *reactive*. Once the DSMs began to spell out diagnostic criteria, the term *reactive depression* fell out of favor; it was too hard to define what constituted an adequate precipitant for depression. The principal remnant of this simple, logical, but ultimately flawed division of depression into two parts is bereavement—a diagnosis that serves to exclude from consideration for major depressive disorder those who have very recently (within 2 months) suffered the loss of a loved one.

Of course, when someone you deeply care for dies, you naturally feel grief-stricken. What we as clinicians (and we as bereaved persons) struggle with is to etch the boundary between a clinical depression that requires treatment and the natural grieving process that must be soothed and endured. The diagnostic manuals define the difference only as a matter of time: If mood symptoms last longer than 2 months, they no longer qualify as the natural reaction to loss. But so simplistic a distinction contradicts the experience of many patients and clinicians; increasingly, it no longer makes scientific sense either.

Solid research suggests that bereavement is different from depression. Besides its brevity, it is usually less severe than melancholia and unresponsive to antidepressant medication. A bereaved person's low mood is triggered by memories of the departed individual, whereas those with non-bereavement-related depression feel bad regardless. And it is unusual for bereaved people to have severe feelings of guilt, worthlessness, suicidal ideas, or the slowing of speech and action called *psychomotor retardation*. Bereavement, then, tends to seem rather normal, unaccompanied by seriously impaired activities of living.

Over the past few years has arisen the concept of *complicated bereavement* or *traumatic grief*, which is associated with impaired functioning and relatively poor outcomes. Somewhat similar to PTSD, it is meant to comprise some of the following symptoms: preoccupation with the dead person; longing or yearning; disbelief and inability to accept the death; anger or resentment over the death; and avoidance of reminders of this loss.

As a disqualifier for major depressive disorder, bereavement is currently unique—other losses, such as that of a career or a marriage, don't count. However, researchers have recently found that a person who feels devalued by a humiliating event (such as a public put-down by a boss, a divorce brought about by the infidelity of a spouse, or rape) can develop depression similar to grief. And that, of course, lands us right back at the concept of reactive depression. Confusing, isn't it?

For me, here is the bottom line. We expect feelings of grief and sadness after a major loss, and we should be careful not to join the stampede to diagnose mental disorder. However, we should also recognize that for a sizeable minority, bereavement eventually morphs into major depression. Accordingly, any depression that hangs on and on demands careful reevaluation. And at any point in the grieving process, the presence of any severe symptom such as suicidal ideas, psychosis, or psychomotor retardation requires immediate treatment for major depression.

Minor Degrees of Depression

If there are major depressions, there must be minor ones, right? That thought seems to have struck many researchers, because numerous studies have recently described forms of minor depression that may bear different names, unique criteria, or both. What's resulted so far is a microcosm of the diagnostic chaos that existed before the DSM started getting its act together back in 1980. One writer even proposes a form in which the patient doesn't actually experience any depression or anhedonia! Most definitions boil down to a relatively brief (2 weeks or more) episode of relatively few depressive symptoms, in much the same way that dysthymia has fewer symptoms than major depression.

Minor depression, however defined, actually nets some pretty interesting findings. Some studies report anatomical changes in the brains of such people, and the diagnosis predicts early death in old men (but not old women). Just like people with major depression, people with the minor variety tend to have difficulty functioning in their everyday lives, and they respond to standard treatments such as the SSRIs and maprotiline. Minor depression can also be found as a secondary diagnosis in conditions as varied as Alzheimer's dementia and alcoholism, and it has been identified in patients with bipolar disorders.

Moreover, like patients with major depression, patients with minor depression can have both emotional and cognitive symptoms, though vegetative symptoms such as sleep and appetite changes aren't often reported. And though minor depression may be relatively mild, it isn't necessarily brief; just as in the major variety, symptoms tend to persist for weeks or months. Family histories are about the same as for major depression, suggesting that the two forms may spring from the same ground. One problem with the concept is this: Because prevalence data variously put the number of such patients as high as 20% of the general population, it dangerously blurs the line between normal and abnormal. And that—the delimitation from normal—is one area where any worthwhile diagnosis ought to excel.

At least one authority has suggested that the greatest value of minor depression may be in helping to predict major depression later on. However, others who look at the various lines of evidence suggest that differing degrees of depression overlap: A person who develops a mild depression may progress in stages through moderate to severe symptoms later on. In effect, depression may best be viewed as existing on a continuum.

Can Suicide Ever Be Rational?

The existence of rational suicide has been hotly debated for many years. Favoring the concept are moral philosophers who regard humans as free agents whose choices can include how and when they will die. Arguing against it are those who cite numerous scientific studies reporting that an overwhelming number of people who committed suicide had some form of a mental disorder. (Overwhelming, perhaps, but not unanimous—nearly every such study includes a few individuals for whom no mental disorder could be demonstrated.)

Western medicine traditionally regards suicide as an irrational response to over-whelming stress. One consequence of this view is a logical lapse on our part: Because suicide is a symptom of mental illness, we reason that only mentally ill persons commit suicide. We therefore reject the possibility that occasionally a mentally healthy individual, perhaps threatened by the physical pain or disability of a terminal illness, may desire to stop living. An apparent example was the professor and mystery fiction author Carolyn Heilbrun, who killed herself in 2003 after saying for years that she would one day do just that.

In Oregon, where I live, terminally ill patients may obtain from their physicians lethal medication to help them avoid wrenching pain and incapacity at life's end. In any given year, whereas several score of patients request such medications, only about 30 have actually used it. A number of careful studies have found no evidence of coercion or ulterior motives, such as on the part of relatives.

In 1995, James Werth surveyed 400 other psychologists in an attempt to define rational suicide. The group's definition boiled down to the following:

1. The individual's condition should show little hope of remission.

2. There must be no coercion.

3. The decision making should be sound, as shown by these characteristics relevant to the decision maker: mental competence; rejection of other options only after due consideration; values consistent with this decision; consideration of the impact of the suicide on others; and consultation with other professionals, such as therapists, hospice personnel, and spiritual advisors.

I'm as concerned as the next responsible clinician to maximize the value of anyone's life, but I believe that this must be done with due consideration for its value to the individual who has to live it. There is no easy answer here.

12 Diagnosing Anxiety and Fear

First, let's define some terms. *Fear* is emotional discomfort caused by a sense of approaching danger. A *phobia* is an unreasonable and intense fear that is associated with some situation or object. What distinguishes the commonplace fear of, say, spiders from the delusional fear of persecution? It is that spiders usually pose no real threat, and the phobic person knows this, whereas the delusional person doesn't have the benefit of insight. *Anxiety* is also fear, but it isn't caused by something specific the person can identify. *Worry* is mental distress relating to concern for something that might happen. Usually, anxious or worried people have unpleasant physical sensations, such as tense muscles, fatigue, insomnia, and restlessness. A *panic attack* is a discrete episode of intense anxiety accompanied by acute physical symptoms, such as chest pain, choking, dizziness, pounding heart, numbness, sweating, shortness of breath, and trembling.

To a degree, fear, anxiety, worry, and even panic in the form of an acute fright are sensations that normal people experience, and we must therefore discriminate them from ordinary uneasiness. Of course, we clinicians aren't usually consulted for ordinary uneasiness, but even so we need to make sure (by asking) that the anxiety a patient presents has caused *marked* distress or has in some way interfered with social, work, or interpersonal functioning. Table 12.1 presents the differential diagnosis for anxiety states.

Panic Disorder and Phobias

Many normal people experience the highly unpleasant sensations of panic attack. In fact, perhaps a third of adults in the general population have had at least one such attack. It's when they recur often enough to interfere with normal life that they require treatment.

TABLE 12.1. Differential Diagnosis with Brief Definitions
for Anxiety States

- *Anxiety due to a medical condition.* Physical illness can cause panic or other anxiety symptoms.
- *Anxiety due to use of a substance.* Alcohol, street drugs of misuse, and prescribed medications can all cause anxiety symptoms.
- *Panic disorder.* Repeated panic attacks (brief, sudden episodes of intense dread, accompanied by a variety of physical and other symptoms) with worry about having additional attacks can occur by themselves, but are often accompanied by agoraphobia.
- *Agoraphobia.* Patients fear situations or places (entering a store, being away from home) where they might have trouble obtaining help if they should become anxious.
- *Specific phobia.* Particular objects or situations—such as animals, storms, heights, flying, being closed in, or blood or needles—cause anxiety and avoidance.
- *Social phobia.* The prospect of embarrassment when speaking, writing, performing, or eating in public causes anxiety and avoidance.
- *Obsessive–compulsive disorder (OCD).* Patients have thoughts or behaviors that appear senseless, but the patients feel nonetheless compelled to repeat them.
- *Posttraumatic stress disorder (PTSD).* Patients repeatedly relive a traumatic event, experiencing hyperarousal and avoidance or numbing along the way.
- *Generalized anxiety disorder (GAD).* Without experiencing actual panic attacks, patients feel anxious or tense about a variety of different problems.

Ruth

Sitting alone in the waiting room, Ruth breathed heavily into a paper bag. With mounting dread, she had felt the old symptoms: Her heart was pounding, and her breathing was strangled as though her throat would close forever. She had hoped she could get through at least 1 week without the feelings, and now, on day 5, just as she was at last about to tell someone about them, they were on her again. As she sat there, she again feared that she was on the verge of going crazy and tearing off her clothes. As she had that thought, she noticed that she was sweating and shaky.

At age 29, Ruth was a saleswoman at an appliance store. She had been married briefly, and now lived with her boyfriend, Sammy, the assistant store manager. When not in school, her 7-year-old daughter stayed with Grandma.

A few weeks earlier, the episodes of anxiety had driven Ruth to one of her rare visits to her family practitioner. The electrocardiogram she'd demanded was, she was told, "completely normal, just like the rest of your exam." Because she seemed nervous, she was given a prescription for Valium. But Ruth, who had tried marijuana in college, didn't like the "spacey, unrooted" feeling it gave her, and she'd avoided drugs since.

She told the doctor that she tried to stay near a doorway when indoors. Because she lived in earthquake country, she always worried how she'd escape in the event of the "big one." Recently this concern had grown; now, if she had to go into the stockroom, she'd ask Sammy to accompany her. That made *him* nervous, since the store's antinepotism policy was strictly enforced. Ruth tried to shop only when Sammy could accompany her. If ever she had to go alone, she would dash in for her gallon of milk, pay at the self-check, and practically run back out before the panic could take hold.

The attacks seemed to come at odd times. Once, when she was driving home, she had to stop the car because she couldn't focus on the road. Another time it caught them both off guard, when she and Sammy were beginning foreplay while watching a sexy movie on cable. However, the present attack in the waiting room aborted itself and faded away, almost as suddenly as it began. By the time the clinician called her name, Ruth was applying fresh lipstick.

Analysis

In the absence of health problems and of any history of substance use for Ruth, we can quickly move through the first three steps of the decision tree for a patient with symptoms of fear, anxiety, panic, or continuing worry (Figure 12.1). Then, moving unrewarded through the tree, we eventually hit pay dirt: Ruth was afraid of being in a place where escape would be difficult (step 14), such as her local supermarket or the storeroom at work. She also (step 15) had unexpected attacks during which she experienced panic accompanied by a number of physical symptoms. In short, we should strongly consider a diagnosis of panic disorder with agoraphobia. Had we focused on the panic attacks and initially overlooked her symptoms of agoraphobia, we would have arrived at the same conclusion. Along the way, we would have considered both somatization disorder and a mood disorder, both commonly associated with anxiety symptoms. In fact, because depression so often accompanies panic attacks, asterisked step 17 even reminds us to check for it.

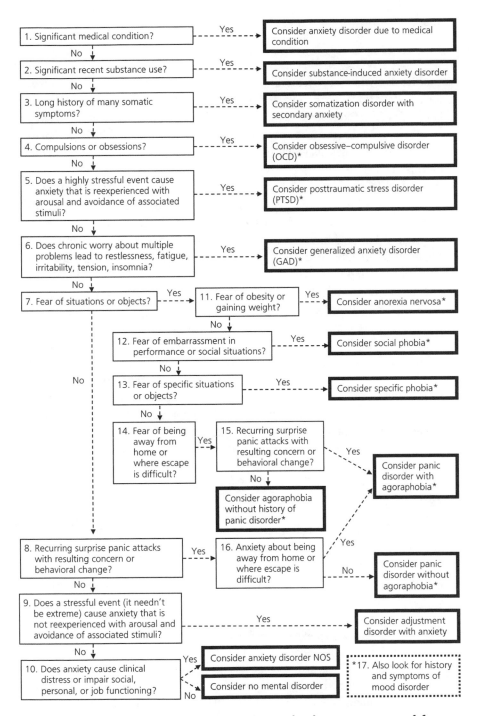

FIGURE 12.1. Decision tree for a patient who has symptoms of fear, anxiety, panic, or continuing worry.

Comment

Charles Darwin had repeated attacks of shortness of breath, lightheadedness, palpitations, trembling, and feelings of faintness, which would probably qualify him today for a diagnosis of panic disorder. Various authors have suggested that because he was famously reclusive, he also had agoraphobia. Others feel that his symptoms may have been related to physical conditions such as Ménière's syndrome or Chagas disease (a parasitic infestation found in rural areas of South and Central America). Anyway, fitness prevailed, and he survived. More recently, an adolescent girl has been reported to have panic disorder with agoraphobia as the result of a seizure disorder. Additional physical causes of panic and other anxiety symptoms are included in Table 9.1; substance-related anxiety symptoms are covered in Tables 9.2 and 9.3.

Agoraphobia only infrequently occurs by itself; in fact, it may not even be a separate disorder. When panic disorder and agoraphobia occur together, they are currently considered to be a single disorder, not comorbid. I say "currently," because there doesn't yet seem to be consensus on the point. For diagnostic purposes, it doesn't really make much difference: We care less about code numbers than about what's wrong and how to combat it. For that, it suffices to recognize whether the patient has panic attacks, agoraphobia, or both. Although one study reported 64% cumulative sustained remission at 10 years after exposure treatment, there is some evidence that agoraphobia symptoms may reduce the likelihood of improvement at follow-up for patients with panic disorder.

Zena

Fear is one of the most common words we have to describe negative feelings about the world and our relation to it. When we encounter something we fear—whether it is a specific object, circumstance, or social situation—we immediately imagine that we will be harmed, be embarrassed, or suffer other untoward consequences.

> Though she was an experienced teacher in her mid-30s, Zena had trouble writing on the blackboard in front of her seventh-grade class. A couple of times she has felt panicky, but usually she only experienced trembling, dizziness, and a sinking feeling of dread. When she thought she heard the kids laughing behind her back, she also felt hot and flustered, and she shook even harder. When no one was watching, she could write just fine, so she came to school early every day and posted as much of the lesson as

she could before the bell rang. Last year, she had requested two extra blackboards, so she could write everything in advance. But it was hard to do so completely, because she had a number of different subjects to teach, and she needed to post assignments and other material as she went along. "Besides the shakes," she told the clinician, "it always makes me feel that I have to use the toilet, even if I've just gone. I can't be charging out to the loo several times a day."

Analysis

Zena's clinician would first have to rule out medical and substance use causes for her symptoms (steps 1 and 2 of Figure 12.1). Once that was done, it would be on to a "no" at steps 4 and 5—she had no obsessions or compulsions, and she hadn't suffered from a serious trauma. Neither did she worry about multiple problems (step 6); just one was plenty for her. Rather, Zena's distress took place in a performance situation ("yes" at step 7 and at step 12)—specifically, writing in public—and her diagnosis would therefore be social phobia. Her clinician should next review the symptoms with her to ensure that they weren't overlooking additional diagnoses, notably mood and other anxiety disorders.

Comment

When diagnosing phobias, clinicians face two problems. The first is not realizing that a fear exists; although patients are usually very clear about *what* they fear, they often don't complain of it. It may turn up only when they seek help for another mental health problem, such as depression or a different anxiety disorder. The second problem is separating abnormal fears from what is normal. After all, most of us cringe from something—whether it is heights, thunderstorms, or visiting the dentist—yet we aren't about to diagnose the majority of the general population with an anxiety disorder. We only make a diagnosis when symptoms cause enough difficulty to interfere with the person's life in some meaningful way. (Zena came to work early to write on the board, and she suffered distress whenever she had to write in front of the class.) Sometimes we forget to observe the boundary between illness and wellness.

Other social phobias that involve facing strangers include fears of speaking (which is especially common), eating, writing, or playing a musical instrument. Specific phobias include fears of animals, the environment (storms, heights, water), blood/injection/injuries, situations (flying, being closed in), and circumstances that could lead to illness, choking, or vomiting. In all types, the person may either avoid the phobic situation or endure it with severe stress or anxiety symptoms. As with other anxiety disorders, the anxiety experienced can take a variety of forms. Many persons experience symptoms that fall just short of a classic panic attack, including a sense of impending doom, intense uneasiness, or marked tension.

Rawson

Granted, physical conditions causing anxiety symptoms are a bit uncommon. But it is their very rarity that causes them not to stick uppermost in the diagnostic mind. Rawson fell victim to just such a lapse of vigilance.

> A British transplant to the United States, Rawson was 25 and worked on the rewrite desk of a daily newspaper. Twice he had become dizzy when eating lunch. The second time, his editor personally walked him down to see the company nurse; she found that his elevated blood pressure rapidly returned to normal as he rested in her office. She recommended that he consult a doctor, but he didn't have one—he'd never been ill, and he didn't smoke, drink, or use drugs.
>
> A few months later, he began to complain of anxiety attacks. At first, they only occurred every couple of weeks; later they came more often. At most, they lasted only 10 or 15 minutes, but they were scary: Rawson felt lightheaded, he had trouble catching his breath, and his heart seemed to beat wildly. Perhaps worst of all, they left him drenched in sweat and dreading the next attack, which always seemed to loom just over the horizon.
>
> On the day he finally sought medical advice, he felt fine, and his vital signs were all normal. "It's like getting your wireless repaired," he joked, "it always works fine in the shop." He did complain of occasional headache, feelings of weakness, and shaky hands. His energy was low, and he occasionally felt depressed. His appetite had drifted downward, so that he'd lost nearly a stone. "That's 14 pounds," he added helpfully.
>
> "Your physical health is terrific," the doctor told him, "but you certainly are anxious. I think you may have an underlying clinical depression." That's how Rawson was started on antidepressants and antianxiety drugs. When the attacks continued, he was switched from one antidepressant to another—a total of four in the course of 10 months. Yet his symptoms continued; the feeling of dread was marginally better, but the headaches were even worse, and he still had the drenching sweats. Finally, during another visit to his family practitioner, he had an attack right there

in the office. His blood pressure, normal when the nurse first checked few moments earlier, climbed to 180/125. A series of tests revealed that he had a pheochromocytoma on one adrenal gland. Surgical removal cured his panic attacks and depression—and his blood pressure problems.

Analysis

I'd like to believe that I wouldn't have made the same mistake as Rawson's family practitioner, but I couldn't swear to it. It is easy to overlook a decidedly uncommon possibility such as a pheochromocytoma, which accounts for only about 1 in 1,000 cases of hypertension. The differential diagnosis/ decision tree approach to diagnosis forces us to think every time about substances and physical disorders that can cause mental symptoms. However, the diagnostic principle about atypical symptoms also provides a clue: Headache isn't a symptom usually associated with panic disorder, and though sweating is, it is usually far less prominent than in Rawson's case.

Comment

Of course, you'll want to know how to tell when anxiety symptoms are medical, not mental. The answer is that you can't—at least, not on the basis of the anxiety attacks themselves. You have to rely on always being suspicious, looking for symptoms that are a little different from standard anxiety symptoms (such as Rawson's headaches and high blood pressure). The most difficult part is always to keep in mind something you infrequently encounter: mental symptoms with physical origins. Quite a few medical conditions can cause panic attacks; you'll find some of them listed in Table 9.1.

Wilson and Harold

Speaking of physical causes, there's another whole class of causes to keep alert for, especially when you're trying to get to the bottom of anxiety symptoms. The next two vignettes present a couple of them that are legal.

> When Wilson was younger, he loved coffee. Drinking a lot was fine, as long as he was in college; later, however, he drifted into the arcane world of musical instrument repair, which required patience and a steady hand.

Thus his habits clashed with his livelihood, until he turned to decaffeinated coffee, of which he now drank six cups or more each day.

All was well until a few months earlier, when by accident a trainee clerk at his favorite coffee store gave him regular beans. The result was several days of feeling excited but restless, upset stomach, heart palpitations, and sleeplessness that was "nearly total." Unable to reassemble the silver flute he'd been working on, he journeyed to his family doctor to try to figure out the cause.

The morning his father was diagnosed with lung cancer, Harold quit his 20-year cigarette habit cold turkey. By bedtime, he was pacing the floor and angry, though he hadn't a clue what he was angry at. Surely not his father? After a sleepless night, he felt "incredibly uptight," and he fried up and devoured a double helping of bacon and eggs, which for health reasons he usually avoided. By 10 A.M., he couldn't concentrate at work; he could think only of having a puff—just one deep drag—of a cigarette. Either that, or some more breakfast. At noon he called his wife and wondered aloud whether he'd be able to stay off tobacco. "Being dead would be better than this," he almost sobbed.

"I've already gotten you in to see our doctor, later today," she responded. "I knew this was going to be tough."

Analysis

Because the history sits out in plain sight, there should be no problem in diagnosing either Wilson or Harold, both of whom actually came only to the attention of their respective family practitioners. The use of Figure 12.1 seems trivial, but I would recommend as an exercise formulating a complete differential diagnosis. Typical symptoms of intoxication and withdrawal for all major classes of drugs, including caffeine and nicotine, are given in Table 9.3.

Comment

The problem with such examples is that beneath the obvious can lurk other syndromes that are independent of any substance use. I'm especially talking about a mood disorder here, though others are possible. When patients are either using substances or withdrawing from substance use, they can develop a variety of anxiety symptoms, including outright panic attacks, phobias, generalized anxiety, or even occasionally obsessions and compulsions. Because the anxiety disorders are so often comorbid with other anxiety disorders, you often have to make two (or more) trips through the decision tree. Does this mean that the person truly has more than one illness? Perhaps not—we just haven't yet advanced far enough that we can understand the nuances, as with PTSD and depression.

GAD, PTSD, OCD, and Comorbidity

In his freshman year with the Boston Red Sox, Jim Piersall was hospitalized for a severe mental problem and treated with electroconvulsive therapy. He published his story in 1955 in a hugely popular book called *Fear Strikes Out*, which included material from his childhood. The following is based on Jim's account.

Jim

From the age of 9, Jim worried constantly. He dated his worrying to the first time his mother entered a mental hospital for a serious but unnamed illness. Treated in an era before the advent of effective medication, she periodically improved enough to be released. However, young Jim never knew when she would have to be readmitted, and so, because she might be taken away again at any moment, he was afraid to go to school and afraid to come home again in the afternoon.

He commenced to "worry about everything"—about school, about whether his classmates would like him, about what mood his father would be in each evening. In the spring, he worried whether he'd be promoted; in the fall, he worried about who his new teacher would be. As he grew up, it got only worse. In the sixth grade, he worried that the weather would affect his ability to play ball; would he be any good when he was grown? Tense and unable to unwind, he had difficulty sleeping and felt that he always had to be on the go. Even when he was grown, physically healthy, and married, with a healthy child and a steady job, he worried about the future.

Analysis

Because young Jim was in good physical health and, at the age of 9, hardly a candidate for substance use, we can move right through steps 1, 2, and 3 of Figure 12.1. Nowhere in his narrative did Jim describe obsessions or compulsions (step 4). Did his mother's hospitalization act as a step 5 stressor? There's no evidence that he relived it, or that he had physiological symptoms such as marked startle response. These *pertinent negatives*, as clinicians call them, lead us on to step 6, where we can agree that even as a youngster, he chronically worried about many things. Our decision tree urges us to consider the diagnosis of GAD.

However, GAD cannot explain his severe breakdown as a young adult, which resulted in mental hospitalization and subsequent electroconvulsive treatment. The evidence concerning that illness is meager; Jim was always a bit circumspect about divulging details. Although he provided some information in his second book, *The Truth Hurts*, it wasn't the whole truth.

> In his freshman year with the Red Sox, Jim was restless, at times sleepless. He sometimes felt that the Red Sox were trying to get rid of him by making him a shortstop. His speech was sometimes logical, sometimes "completely haywire," and he was ejected from games for engaging in fistfights on the field. When admitted to the hospital as violent, he was noted to be talking fast. After his electroconvulsive treatment, he returned to the Red Sox. He subsequently played 17 seasons in the major leagues, and twice won the Golden Glove award.
>
> After 20 years of good health, when he was no longer playing baseball, Jim suffered an episode of depression, during which he had crying spells. Exhausted and suffering from a loss of self-confidence, he again entered a hospital. With medication, he apparently recovered as completely from his second episode as he did from the first.

Although such skimpy information doesn't allow a definitive diagnosis, it provides a pretty good example of how we'd use available information to make our best guess—the way we might evaluate, say, a word-of-mouth history provided by someone's relative. Here's how I'd reason: A history of psychosis (paranoid suspicions during his first episode) and of mood disorder (typical symptoms of depression during his second) suggests that Jim might have had a psychotic depression, perhaps in the course of a bipolar disorder. An episodic course would be highly unusual for schizophrenia (we'll use the diagnostic principle about atypical features). Jim's mother also had a serious mental illness that was episodic, providing yet another possible clue to the nature of her son's difficulty. Here I would assert my favorite diagnostic principle and say that he was still undiagnosed, though in my heart of hearts I suspect that a personal examination would confirm a bipolar disorder. Although Jim's GAD long predated his mood disorder, I would of course list the latter first, because that was the diagnosis in need of immediate attention.

Comment

The worries of GAD go far beyond ordinary "worry-wart" status, which raises the problem with any mental disorder: How do you differentiate it from the garden-variety troubles we all have? That's where the issue of impairment or clinically important distress steers us away from the temptation to hang a diagnosis on just about everyone we know. Of course, that criterion isn't perfect; as clinicians, we must still judge what level of distress or disability to certify. But as with so many other mental diagnoses, we can use it to ensure that only people whose lives are truly affected will be considered patients.

There is one more important consideration for GAD: The person must not be just worried about isolated specific issues, such as might occur in a different Axis I disorder. Here are some examples: Gaining weight would be a source of worry for someone with anorexia nervosa; contamination would worry a patient with OCD; and the prospect of having a panic attack would greatly trouble a person with panic disorder.

Although it affects as many as 5% of all adults, GAD is comparatively new, having made its bow only a generation or so ago. Before that, it was just one of many anxiety states covered by the old term *anxiety neurosis*. Women are more often affected than men, and it is more prevalent in midlife than in childhood or adolescence. Although it may fluctuate in intensity, it is a chronic condition that, like major depressive disorder, can be highly disabling. An important feature of GAD is that many patients (perhaps the majority) later develop a mood disorder. Indeed, on follow-up, nearly every patient with GAD has a comorbid diagnosis. No one is quite sure what this means in terms of causal relationships, but it is important to keep in mind for anyone who has GAD symptoms. It's what happened to Jim Piersall.

Wilbur

Fear can be focused on a single entity, as with specific phobia, or on a type of situation, as with a social phobia or agoraphobia. On the other hand, clinicians must sometimes link fear with other symptoms and historical features to make the correct diagnosis.

When Wilbur was only 19, the Army drafted him. Lacking any special skills, he trained as a cook and served honorably through two tours in Korea. Because of his job, he never expected to see much combat, so he remained in the Army as a career. "I always figured I could open a restaurant after I finished my 20 years."

That's how Wilbur came to be caught up in Lyndon Johnson's big Vietnam buildup in the middle 1960s. He found himself stationed in the Mekong River Delta, which he described as "the only place on earth you could stand chest-deep in water and have dust blow in your face." His battalion of the 9th Infantry Division participated in a sweep of the countryside from Saigon up through Tay Ninh province in 1966. When the armored personnel carrier a few feet ahead of his rolled over a 2,000-pound bomb buried in the road, men riding on top were thrown dozens of yards. Shrapnel struck Wilbur's neck and right arm, but it was when the head and spinal cord of his best friend landed on his vehicle that he threw up and passed out. He remembered little of the next 24 hours, though he was told that he had helped to collect body parts and that he richly deserved his Purple Heart and Bronze Star.

"After I got back, I was never the same," he told the clinician years later at the VA outpatient clinic. "I couldn't quite accept the fact that I was out of the war zone; I was always on the alert, always scanning the horizon for threats." Occasionally, as when awakening from a nap, he would think he was back "in country"; just for a moment, he might think he could see Viet Cong lurking behind his sofa. His wife had complained that many nights she would awaken to find him screaming in fright and kicking her—hard. Finally, she'd had enough and moved back in with her parents.

"I didn't blame her a bit," Wilbur said. "I was a nervous wreck, always jumping at the slightest sound. I wouldn't watch a movie on TV if there were soldiers, and I was always tired and grouchy. *I* wouldn't want to live with me!"

The clinician unearthed other problems. Ever since he returned from the war, Wilbur's appetite had been off, and his weight had dropped almost 20 pounds. "Everything tastes like C-ration boned chicken," he complained. Although he had found a job as a clerk at his county farm bureau, he was irritable with clients and repeatedly forgot to file the paperwork. He was eventually told, "Get some help, or we'll have to let you go."

The clinical review disclosed that Wilbur's tour of duty had ended before soldiers' heavy use of heroin had begun. "We drank some—you could get a fifth of Jim Beam for three bucks at the commissary—but I never caught the habit. I might've smoked a joint or two, but never since returning home. I'm not suicidal." While admitting to feeling "wired" or "uptight" much of the time, he denied having actual panic symptoms, such as pounding heart or shortness of breath.

Analysis

Mental trauma often goes hand in hand with brain injury, which is therefore all the more important to consider in evaluating a patient who may have PTSD. Wilbur had returned from Vietnam physically scarred though intact, but for less fortunate others, careful questioning might reveal neurological deficits that can help explain their symptoms (step 1). The fact that Wilbur did not use substances is hardly rare, but remarkable in that so many veterans do (step 2). The number of men with somatization disorder is vanishingly small (step 3), and there were no evident phobias or obsessions (step 4). Indeed, as presented, the diagnosis fairly explodes off the page. The dead giveaway is, of course, the severe step 5 emotional trauma that preceded the onset of Wilbur's anxiety and avoidance symptoms. Panic symptoms can accompany the PTSD experience, but they aren't required for diagnosis.

Comment

Wilbur is far from the most difficult type of patient with PTSD. At the VA, I've evaluated returning combat survivors so fearful and suspicious that for years they'd lived alone in the remote hills of California. Elaborate criteria aside, PTSD is determined by four basic concepts: (1) A seriously traumatic event produces a feeling of fear, helplessness, or horror; (2) the person attempts to avoid these feelings; but (3) through thoughts or images, they continue to occur anyway; and (4) they evoke symptoms of increased physiological arousal, such as insomnia, hypervigilance, and startle response. The symptoms must last a month or more. Besides its relationship to combat, PTSD can also develop when civilians experience natural trauma such as hurricanes, earthquakes, and tsunamis), as well as motor vehicle accidents, rapes, and other human-caused forms of violence.

Be alert for several confounds in the differential diagnosis of PTSD. Patients with OCD perceive their automatic thoughts as inappropriate, and they won't have experienced a specific traumatic event. Patients with PTSD sometimes behave automatically and later may not remember what they did, setting up a possible confusion with dissociative disorder. Had Wilbur's only stressor been that his wife left him, we might instead consider the residual category of adjustment disorder with anxiety (step 9). Unhappily, at the VA as in civilian courts, financial gain can provide a motive for malingering—which, because it is both pejorative and hard to treat, should be considered as a last resort in any differential diagnosis.

You'll need a careful review to ensure that you aren't missing yet another disorder that must be addressed in treating these patients, for whom anxiety may be only the tip of the mental distress iceberg. Carefully consider the asterisked step 17 at the bottom of Figure 12.1, since many patients with PTSD have associated depression. Nearly always in combat veterans, and often in civilians as well, anxiety and depressive symptoms are almost inextricably entwined. In my opinion, one of the many challenges of evaluating a patient with PTSD is to demonstrate that there *isn't* a history of concomitant major depression. Also frequently comorbid with PTSD is dependence on alcohol, illicit drugs, or prescription drugs, and sometimes on all three.

Peter

The drama of anxiety and its cousins can nearly eclipse signs of other problems. Histories like Peter's demonstrate the importance of doing a full evaluation, even when the chief complaint is a request for help with a specific problem.

A cousin brought Peter for mental health evaluation. Because he was so afraid of contamination, Peter had resisted leaving the house, where he lived with his younger sister and his mother, an evening shift supervisor at Wendy's. A biology major, Peter had recently dropped out of junior college. "I did well for the first semester, but then I just couldn't bear to touch those specimens any longer," he told the student clinician who gathered the initial history.

For the past 3 months, Peter had also refused to eat raw vegetables ("Can't tell what they've been grown in"). He had gradually developed rituals, such as frequent vigorous handwashing and grasping doorknobs with the cuff of his shirt. An "inner voice" reminded him to wash his hands, even if he'd just done so a few minutes earlier. If he didn't, he'd feel "terribly anxious, as though something truly catastrophic was about to happen." He became tearful as he said, "I feel totally washed up, quite literally. Who wants to spend his days scrubbing the skin off the backs of his hands?"

The student clinician agreed with Peter's own assessment of OCD, for which behavior therapy seemed an appropriate option. However, during a subsequent interview, the supervising clinician saw something else. Peter's gaze was almost continually downcast, and his eyes reddened when he mentioned his girlfriend, who had broken off their relationship "because I didn't even want to hold hands with her any more, let alone make love. I just didn't have the interest."

On close questioning, Peter admitted feeling sad most of the time, beginning even before the obsessions started. He had had no suicidal ideas, but he mentioned that he had dropped out of school after he found that his interest, even in his chosen field of plant physiology, had flagged to the point that he couldn't concentrate well enough to study for exams. Although he denied ever using street drugs, he admitted that about the only relief he got was when he drank beer; over the past month or two, he had gradually increased his consumption to a 6-pack nearly every evening. "At least it gets me to sleep at night," Peter commented.

Peter's immediate family was well, but his father's cousin had been treated with lithium for some sort of a mental breakdown, during which he had "gone off the deep end" and spent a great deal of money.

Analysis

In discussing Peter's differential diagnosis, we must consider the entirety of Tables 11.1 and 12.1. Although his history contains no evidence of a physical disorder that could explain either his depression or his obsessions and compulsions, for safety's sake he should have a careful medical examination. Alcohol use could not explain the anxiety or depression, both of which had begun weeks or months before he began drinking beer. That moves us on through the first steps of two decision trees.

You can easily step through the rest of Figure 11.1, arriving at major depression. Then, following Figure 12.1, you can work your way through to the (not unexpected) diagnosis of OCD. I'd list the depression first, emphasizing its importance as the primary problem. The compulsions I'd regard as a secondary phenomenon. Armed with that information, the recommendations for Peter's treatment change to antidepressant drugs or cognitive-behavioral therapy, which might very well resolve both sets of problems. The vignette also presents a good example of the very last level in our roadmap (Figure 1.1)—reevaluate as new material comes to light—and of the family history diagnostic principle (the cousin who probably had bipolar disorder).

Comment

The benefit of multiple diagnoses is clear: When clinicians learn that patients being treated for one condition actually have several, they often enlarge the treatment program. In contrast to double depression (see the case of Robert in Chapter 11, page 137), where it can be hard to separate the symptoms of two types of depression, you would think that the presence of symptoms and historical data from diagnostic groups as diverse as anxiety and mood disorders would make it hard *not* to notice comorbidity. Experience and scientific studies suggest otherwise: Clinicians commonly pass right over comorbid diagnoses.

One solution is more information; you can request previous medical records and talk with relatives and other informants. Another is to use more assiduously the mental health review of systems, which asks questions about emotional and behavioral issues other than the patient's chief complaint—hallucinations, delusions, phobias, obsessions, compulsions, panic attacks, depression, mania, problems with sleeping or eating, the use of drugs or alcohol, and forgetfulness. Such a plan has been formalized in structured interviews such as the Structured Clinical Interview for DSM-IV-TR (SCID), which forces a systematic inquiry about all aspects of a patient's mental health history. Although the value of the SCID and similar interviews has been demonstrated over and again, clinicians' willingness to use them remains to be shown. After all, a lengthy questionnaire requires more time than clinicians can typically devote to a single interview, and its somewhat lock-step format could conceivably interfere with other goals, such as forming rapport.

Linda

No matter how bitter the complaints of anxiety, we need to look beyond the obvious for evidence of other conditions. This requires a breadth of perspective that I feel is too often lacking in our contemporary approach to patients.

> At age 61, Linda was one of the older patients I have ever treated for anxiety. When we first met, her main complaint was "fear and heart palpitations" that for many months had plagued her and a whole string of clinicians, who had prescribed a variety of antidepressant and antianxiety medications. On our first visit, Linda told me that none of them had made much difference "except that they all made me more anxious—even the pills I took for anxiety!"
>
> No one had ever considered the diagnosis of somatization disorder, which fortunately I always include in my differentials for anxiety and mood disorders. I soon learned that Linda had felt sickly all her life, com-

plaining to her bevy of clinicians about trouble swallowing and walking, blurred vision, weakness, dizziness, nausea, abdominal bloating, food allergies, diarrhea, constipation, menstrual irregularity, and a variety of pains throughout her body. Chronically depressed since age 15, off and on she had felt hopeless, had complained of trouble with concentration and thinking, and had suffered loss of interest in her usual activities. Though she had had ideas about killing herself, she had never made a suicide attempt.

With this information, I was able to offer a treatment plan somewhat different from the one that had been pursued before (it emphasized behavior modification). Within a few months Linda was no longer having panic attacks, and her restless search for physical cures for her various maladies had come to an end. The importance of somatization disorder is signified by its place in Figure 12.1.

Analysis and Comment

Actually, there isn't a lot to say about somatization disorder that I haven't already written in Chapters 9 and 11. The search of the decision tree stops at step 3, which previous clinicians had ignored. Technically, you could make multiple diagnoses, including somatization, anxiety, and mood disorders. In my opinion, that really isn't necessary, because anxiety symptoms are so very common in patients with somatization disorder. Furthermore, with few exceptions, treating the somatization addresses all the problems, and why confuse things with unneeded verbiage?

Acute Stress Disorder

If you examine the diagnostic manuals, you'll find that I've omitted acute stress disorder (ASD)—the diagnosis DSM-IV created to fill the hole created by PTSD's time requirement of 1 month—from Table 12.1 and Figure 12.1. The problem with ASD is that it imparts pathological significance to reactions that we might often consider to be normal. Some researchers have reported a strong degree of overlap between PTSD and ASD; others have noted that the diagnosis isn't especially good at predicting who will recover quickly and who will need health care services down the road. All in all, you probably won't spend a lot of time thinking about ASD.

13 Diagnosing Psychosis

The psychoses aren't so terribly common. Historically, however, they were of signal importance in helping to establish the mental health healing professions. Many of the great names of 19th-century mental health—Kraepelin, Bleuler, Alzheimer—cut their diagnostic teeth on schizophrenia, bipolar psychoses, and cognitive psychoses. Today, the economic impact of schizophrenia alone is huge: For the United States in 2000, the total of direct and indirect costs was as high as $40 *billion*. And in nonmonetary terms, schizophrenia and its close relatives are responsible for a mountain of human effort, recrimination, and misery, preoccupying patients, relatives, and caregivers alike. For all these reasons, diagnosing schizophrenia is one of the more important skills of any mental health clinician, though it is exceeded by the ability to tell when a psychotic patient does *not* have schizophrenia.

Psychosis means being in some sense out of contact with reality. In a practical sense, this loss of touch can be manifested by having symptoms in one or more of the following five groups. By the way, whereas I don't ordinarily favor rote memorization of criteria (that's what we have books for), I do make an exception in the case of these basic criteria for schizophrenia, which clinicians often need in the pursuit of diagnostic clarity.

Psychosis requires at least one, schizophrenia two, of these five:

1. *Hallucinations.* In the absence of external stimulation, the person perceives sensory input. The result is a belief that the person hears voices when no one is speaking, or sees people, objects, even whole tableaus that are not really there. Although hallucinations of smell, touch, and taste can also occur, they are far less common than those of hearing or vision.

The film *A Beautiful Mind,* which portrays the psychosis of the real-life mathematician John Nash, brings home to the viewer just how real these hallucinated sensations can seem to the psychotic person.

2. *Delusions.* Believing something to be true that is not, the individual cannot be persuaded otherwise. These false ideas often involve persecution, such as by government agencies, but others may be grandiose. Delusions of guilt, poverty, ill health, infidelity by a spouse, and influence or thought control through information media (e.g., newspapers, television, radio) are also possible.

> Consider, for example, Daniel Paul Schreber, whose memoirs Sigmund Freud famously analyzed. Schreber, a judge in Dresden, developed the notion that he was being transformed into a woman so that, as God's wife, he could become pregnant and thus save humanity.

3. *Disorganized speech.* The person's mental associations are governed not by logic, but by puns, rhymes, or other rules that may not be clear to the outside observer. The resulting output is so badly impaired that communication is difficult or impossible. A passage from the first page of James Joyce's novel *Finnegans Wake* provides an unintended example:

> The great fall of the offwall entailed at such short notice the pftjschute of Finnegan, erse solid man, that the humptyhillhead of humself prumptly sends an unquiring one well to the west in quest of his tumptytumtoes: and their upturnpikepointandplace is at the knock out in the park where oranges have been laid to rust upon the green since devlinsfirst loved livvy.

It is noteworthy that though her diagnosis remains in doubt, Joyce's daughter, Lucia, lived in a madhouse for 47 years until her death.

4. *Disorganized behavior.* Actions that don't appear directed toward a goal may suggest psychosis. Examples include making signs (e.g., of the cross), assuming postures, maintaining unusual or uncomfortable positions for long periods, and removing one's clothes in public.

> I once helped treat a patient who had been admitted years before to a mental hospital. He had spent nearly a decade lying so rigid in bed that his wrists and ankles had become frozen, and he could neither walk nor feed himself.

5. *Negative symptoms.* Symptoms are called *negative* when they indicate the absence of something that most nonpsychotic people have. Examples of negative symptoms include low range of emotional involvement (of-

ten called *blunted affect* or *flattened affect*), poverty of speech, and loss of the will to accomplish things (termed *avolition*). By contrast, positive symptoms such as delusions and hallucinations are conditions that most of us lack. Frustrated relatives sometimes mistakenly interpret negative symptoms as indicating laziness or apathy.

> Medication had already abated the hallucinations and delusions of my patient Eric. Now age 34, he spent his days lounging around his apartment, which his mother subsidized. Although Eric hadn't worked in 6 years, he seemed totally unconcerned when we talked about it. "Oh, I guess I'll get a job later on," he'd say, often with a yawn. When he came to my office, he would slouch in the chair and look just about anywhere but at me. His voice was a little monotonous, and he always wore the same half-smile that never touched his eyes. As long as I knew him, he never changed much, never found work, and never really smiled.

Table 13.1 presents the differential diagnosis for psychosis, and Figure 13.1 presents the decision tree for a patient with psychotic symptoms. Note in Figure 13.1 that, against my usual practice, I've included no possibility of normality: Anyone who has even the briefest of psychoses is going to need some sort of mental disorder diagnosis.

Schizophrenia: Its Subtypes and Variants

Patients with chronic psychosis typically tend to develop symptoms when young—usually as teenagers or young adults. The early evidence of illness may be hard to differentiate from normal adolescent rebellion. I've included the following vignette not because it presents a difficult diagnostic challenge, but to illustrate the development and nature of a classic syndrome as a baseline for later examples of chronic psychosis.

Ronnie

> As a small child, Ronnie had always seemed different. Preferring to build intricate castles and raceways with his blocks, he'd never played much with other children. He had several imaginary friends whose company he kept right through eighth grade. He was often laughed at because of his odd expressions, such as referring to himself in the third person, and he liked to wear clothing that was old and unfashionable. Having no play-

TABLE 13.1. Differential Diagnosis with Brief Definitions for Psychosis

- *Psychosis due to a medical condition.* Physical illness can cause a psychosis that doesn't necessarily meet the criteria for schizophrenia.

- *Psychosis due to use of a substance.* Alcohol, street drugs of misuse, and prescribed medications can all cause psychotic symptoms.

- *Cognitive disorder with psychosis.* A patient with Alzheimer's disease or some other dementing illness develops psychotic symptoms, often persecutory delusions.

- *Somatization disorder with pseudopsychosis.* Some patients with somatization report hallucinations or delusions that can superficially resemble those of schizophrenia.

- *Mood disorder with psychosis.* A patient with an episode of severe mania, depression, or a mixed state has psychotic symptoms that last only during the active phase of the mood episode.

- *Schizophrenia.* These patients have been ill for many months and have at least two of the five types of psychotic symptoms listed in the text. Mood, disorders, substance use, medical conditions have been ruled out as causes.

- *Schizophreniform disorder.* These patients have all the other necessary conditions of schizophrenia, but have been ill less than 6 months.

- *Schizoaffective disorder.* During the same month-long episode of illness, a patient has had an episode of mood disorder (major depression, mania, or mixed) with psychosis (two or more types of psychotic symptoms). For a significant period, there has been psychosis without mood symptoms.

- *Delusional disorder.* For at least a month, a patient has delusions, but none of the other symptoms characteristic of psychosis.

- *Shared psychotic disorder.* Rarely, a patient develops delusions similar to those of a relative or other close associate.

---

mates, he could spend all his time studying, and every year he broke the grading curve. This only further estranged him from his classmates.

Just after Ronnie turned 17, his studies began to slide. His high school counselor mailed home a note that said he seemed lonely; he spent most of every lunch hour in the library reading. Ronnie had denied that he had any problems. He claimed that he was only interested in science and physics, and wanted to "do math" as an adult. The counselor had concluded that he was a sensitive youth who might have a mild depression; neither Ronnie nor his parents were much interested in medication, and he soon dropped out of counseling.

His first year in college started out well enough. Ronnie lived at home, in his old room whose walls were covered with the pictures of NFL

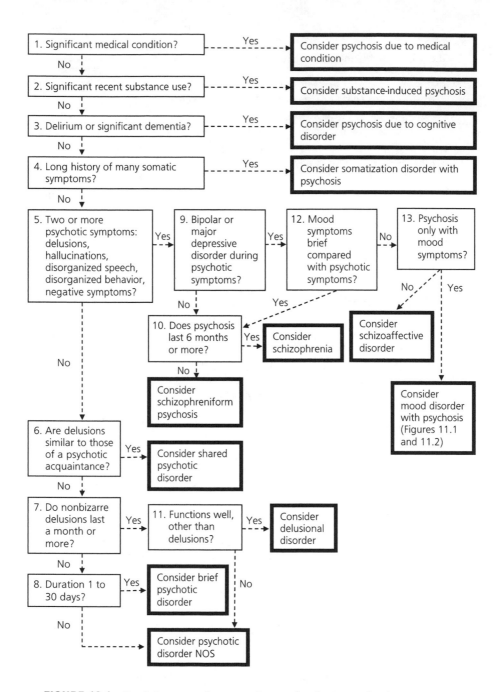

FIGURE 13.1. Decision tree for a patient who has psychotic symptoms such as delusions, hallucinations, disorganized speech, and/or disorganized behavior.

quarterbacks his father had put up years earlier; Ronnie had never cared enough to remove them. Ignoring the mandatory humanities course and focusing on science, he threw himself into his work. Nearly every day, he came home right after class, then stayed in his room. He didn't eat meals with his parents—he'd adopted a vegan diet—and his room soon began to smell of discarded crusts and long-opened cups of tofu spread. At first his mother tried to clean his room, but he added a dead-bolt lock to his bedroom door and wore the key around his neck on a fraying piece of string. He wouldn't even allow her to change the sheets, which gradually turned a greasy grey.

Ronnie's physics professor showed his midwinter exam to the dean. It consisted almost entirely of carefully executed drawings, pentagrams, and upside-down crosses, with text that seemed to combine classical mechanics with Biblical phrases. Before they could question him, Ronnie stopped attending class; he stayed in his room and spent his time creating and revising a website devoted to his study of infinity. His mother had taken quite a lot of higher math in college, but when she came across his website one day while surfing the net, what he had written there seemed a mishmash of geometric symbols and religious verses. It made no sense to her.

Whenever she managed a word with Ronnie, usually as he was on his way to the toilet, he would only mutter something she couldn't quite hear. He grew his hair long and started on a wispy beard. He had always been a gentle, quiet boy, but now he yelled at his mother when she asked him to shave and get a haircut. At night she would sometimes awaken when it sounded as if he was pacing the floor or talking to someone. Someone in his class had introduced him to nonfiltered cigarettes; now he went through a couple of packs a day. That bothered both of his parents, neither of whom smoked. Despite the time he spent at his work, his science and math grades were heading the same direction as his humanities grade. Just before spring break, his advisor finally telephoned him to say, "Either get some help, or we'll have to drop you."

In his second session with the clinician, Ronnie began to tell this story: Early in the fall, he had begun to notice that the professor addressed many of her remarks directly to him. At first he was pleased to be singled out in such a large lecture hall. He'd glance carefully around to see whether the other students noticed, but they all seemed intent on taking notes. Later he realized that the professor was actually talking *about* him, to the others—giving them messages about Ronnie's private life, even his sexual thoughts. One day while walking in the quad, he heard a voice just behind him that said, "He's a wanker, all right." He quickly turned around, but there was no one anywhere near him. Later that evening in his room, he heard the same voice, again criticizing his sexuality.

Ronnie told the clinician that he had always had plenty of friends, but during a later interview, his mother noted that he had always been "something of a lone wolf." She mentioned a great-uncle who by family tradition had been termed "senile," but his history was one of a deteriorating illness requiring chronic hospitalization from the age of 38.

Although he denied that he was doing it, several times during his initial interview Ronnie laughed, even though nothing obviously funny had happened. To the interviewer, he seemed to be responding to internal thoughts. When he wasn't laughing, he seemed to have no facial expression whatsoever. Twice Ronnie interrupted the interview to go outside and smoke, saying that he felt too nervous to continue.

Analysis

The absence of issues relating to health, substance use, and memory help move us quickly through the first several steps in Figure 13.1. (Any faint possibility of a cognitive disorder should be further assessed with a brief version of an MSE, such as the Mini-Mental State Exam [MMSE] developed by Folstein and colleagues. This issue is discussed further in Chapter 14.) We note that Ronnie had several step 5 symptoms, but there was no evidence of either depression or mania, bringing us to the step 10 question about duration of symptoms. His hallucinations and delusions had lasted for a relatively short period of time, but his deteriorating hygiene and negative symptom of loss of will to pursue his studies would persuade us that his illness had gone on longer than 6 months. So, whereas schizophrenia is typically my diagnosis of (almost) last resort, in Ronnie's case it would be the most likely diagnosis to consider.

Along the way, we've used several important diagnostic principles. The collateral history from his mother that he was a loner had more credibility than Ronnie's own, and his laughter during the interview was a sign trumping his denial that he was having unusual thoughts. The family lore about his uncle's diagnosis was at odds with the more probable impression of a chronic psychosis, possibly schizophrenia, which would help support Ronnie's own diagnosis. This shows the value of obtaining what details you can about family history, then forming your own impressions, rather than taking relatives' diagnoses at face value.

Two additional possible diagnoses deserve comment. Ronnie's childhood isolation and discomfort with social relationships might suggest a premorbid schizoid or schizotypal personality disorder. These two personality disorders often herald later schizophrenia, but I would follow my own diagnostic principle and decline to diagnose any of them without more information and the opportunity to talk with Ronnie after he had been treated. The other secondary diagnosis might be nicotine dependence. Although the vignette doesn't provide enough criteria for a formal diagnosis, can anyone doubt that he was hooked on cigarettes? That's the case in an astonishing 80% or more of patients with schizophrenia, who are about three times more likely to smoke than the general population of adults. The reasons aren't yet clear, though recent research suggests that nicotine may temporarily improve not only a patient's defective thinking, but also the person's sensation, such as the ability to smell.

Comment

In diagnosing schizophrenia, novice and expert clinicians must both struggle—the novices to get it right, the experts to avoid getting it wrong. The latter often happens when experts who come to "feel" the diagnosis of schizophrenia (what's the diagnostic principle lurking here?) forget to consider other possibilities. A couple of generations ago, experts on opposite shores of the Atlantic would have come to very different conclusions when diagnosing psychosis: By a wide margin over their European colleagues, American clinicians tended to use the term *schizophrenia* in questionable cases. The gulf between the two sides began to narrow in the early 1970s, as American clinicians gradually adopted scientifically validated, conservative criteria for schizophrenia. Even so, errors still occur. As a diagnostic aid, I have put together a list of characteristics that can be used to distinguish schizophrenia from other forms of psychosis (see the sidebar "Distinguishing Schizophrenia from Other Psychoses" on page 210).

Once we've agreed that a person does have schizophrenia, there is still the problem of determining the appropriate subtype. These are the familiar terms we've thrown around for years, and they're based on the five classes of psychotic symptoms listed at the start of this chapter. Quite frankly, this step in the diagnostic process isn't so terribly important; subtypes don't predict all that much, and some patients change from one subtype to another over the course of time. Nonetheless, we do it anyway— partly out of habit, partly because the terms have some value in describing the typical symptoms of patients.

• *Paranoid.* Whereas these patients have prominent delusions and auditory hallucinations, their speech and behavior remain well organized and their affect appropriate. Illness often begins later (when patients are in their 30s or older) than for other patients with schizophrenia.

> For many years Kevin had believed that he was being pursued by a secret U.S. government agency—he wouldn't say which one. "They'd find out, and I'd be even more of a marked man." Although he continued to hold down a responsible job and support his family, he spent much of his free time checking his phone and fax lines at home and office for bugs.

• *Catatonic.* Patients with this form of the illness, seldom encountered today, typically are markedly slowed down—sometimes to the point of immobility. They may show *negativism* by turning away from you or refusing to follow a command; *posturing* by spontaneously posing or assuming a bizarre posture; *stereotypies* (behaviors that are not goal-directed, such as repeatedly flashing an "OK" sign); *muteness*; and *echolalia* or *echopraxia*, the meaningless repetition of another person's words or actions.

> When I first met Bruno, who had been psychotic for many years, he was lying on his back in bed, rigid and mute. An attendant showed me that when the pillow was carefully removed, his head didn't budge: now it hovered in midair, an inch or two above the mattress. It seemed that he could remain that way for hours.

• *Disorganized.* These patients may have some disturbances of behavior (though less obvious than in catatonia), plus disorganized speech *and* flattened or inappropriate affect. The symptoms of patients with this subtype, which used to be called *hebephrenic*, begin quite early in life. As with all forms of schizophrenia, men develop symptoms somewhat younger than women.

> With a several-year history of well-diagnosed schizophrenia, Hilda knew all the hospital staff members by sight. However, on this admission, she couldn't communicate so much as her name. Her brother had brought her to the emergency department, because for weeks she had been hiding in her room, refusing even to come out for meals. When he finally got her to the emergency room, her hair was matted and her nails had grown long and ragged. She evidently hadn't bathed for many days; her clothes were

mismatched; and one of her shoes was missing its lace. As the interviewer entered, Hilda giggled and hid her face in her hands. Answering the question "Why are you here?" she replied, "I've got jolly sixpence." Then she started taking off her clothes.

• *Undifferentiated.* This final group, which is the subtype of schizophrenia most often diagnosed today, comprises all those patients who don't qualify for any of the previous three categories. Because his psychosis contained both paranoid and disorganized elements, this was the diagnosis Ronnie eventually received.

Although schizophrenia isn't rare, it occurs infrequently enough that early in the course of a young person's illness, we may fail to recognize that a serious process is afoot. Another issue to keep in mind is the need to keep revisiting a schizophrenia diagnosis—patients can change, and even the best diagnosticians make mistakes. The diagnosis of psychosis is a high-risk mental health area, where the stakes are people's lives and families' happiness.

Winona

The typical symptoms of schizophrenia are relatively easy to spot. A greater clinical challenge is to identify issues that are not typical and to recognize what they mean.

Winona had excelled during her first 2 years at an East Coast women's college. She had earned good grades in a demanding major (physical chemistry), and had served as underclass representative to the Student Senate. She'd had several boyfriends; one had proposed marriage. Over the summer, she had held down two jobs, one of them as lab assistant to her advisor.

In mid-October of the new school year, Winona's roommate dropped out of school. The official reason was "fatigue," but everyone knew that she was pregnant and, unwilling to have an abortion, had gone home. Winona's new roommate had just transferred in as a junior. Almost immediately, Winona noticed that Sherrie was watching her closely, apparently tracking her movements around their small dormitory room.

Within days, others on campus had joined the effort to keep tabs on her. By a system of hand waves and nods, one student "could pass me off to another, so the record would be complete," Winona told her clinician later. At first, these signals were barely perceptible, but over the next few weeks they became more and more blatant. Soon she detected mocking in the tone of her professors, which proved to her that the faculty had joined the plot.

Winona made a trip to her student health service. The faint ringing sounds in her left ear that had bothered her for the past couple of weeks had grown louder, and she demanded a hearing test. The audiologist was unoccupied at that very hour, so she had her test, which was completely normal. The doctor then asked whether she'd been using alcohol or drugs; a little offended, she replied that she had not. "And I haven't been depressed, either, if that's what you're thinking." All in all, the visit was a complete bust—her health seemed to be perfect.

A few days later yet, Winona understood about the ringing. It had been a way of warning her to be wary of Sherrie, who wanted to steal her boyfriend (never mind that she didn't have one currently). In fact, she had begun to hear tinkling laughter with the ringing, which, as she explained later, "gradually morphed into voices. It's embarrassing how simple it all seems now."

Uppermost in Winona's mind was her anger at Sherrie's persecution: "I don't see why I should suffer, just because she can't get a guy."

Analysis

Winona's health overall had been excellent, as attested by her student health visit. This fact gets us past steps 1, 2, and 4. A few minutes' additional interview would confirm that she had no significant cognitive symptoms (step 3). At step 5 we note that she had both delusions and hallucinations. Though for now we would accept her denial as regards depression, her clinician would need more questioning to rule out any hidden depression (step 9). Because she had been ill for only about 6 weeks, far less than the total of 6 months needed for schizophrenia, step 10 recommends that we consider the diagnosis of schizophreniform disorder.

Comment

Schizophrenia usually begins slowly—"insidious" is the word clinicians use to describe the glacial pace at which this disease announces itself. But in 1939 a Norwegian clinician named Gabriel Langfeldt described a psychotic illness that began more rapidly and often resolved entirely. From this concept, through many diagnostic twists and turns, has evolved our current usage of *schizophreniform psychosis* to mean a psychotic disorder that lasts at least a month but less than 6 months.

Within a generation, American clinicians have gone from being almost unbelievably permissive in how we diagnose psychosis to having the strictest criteria set in the world. Some now say that the current criteria may actually be too conservative—that they promote false negatives. A few patients who should receive the diagnosis of schizophrenia don't, or at least don't in a timely fashion. The time factor may be vital; although the definitive study has yet to be done, recent studies suggest that the longer we wait before beginning treatment, the poorer the outcome. As little as 7 days may make a difference, but the effects of delay may go out to 1 year or more. That's one of the virtues of schizophreniform disorder: It allows us to proceed with treatment while keeping our options open as regards final diagnosis.

Like schizophrenia, schizophreniform disorder is in all likelihood a group of disorders that we should (but probably won't) refer to in the plural as the *schizophreniform psychoses*. As a group, they are just a parking place for some patients until we can figure out something better to call them. After half a year or so, some patients will be rediagnosed as having a psychosis related to substance use or a physical disorder; others will turn out to have a mood disorder. And a substantial minority who continue to be ill with their original symptoms will be rediagnosed as having schizophrenia. A few, perhaps 20%, will experience complete remission within the 6-month time frame; they are the only ones who can retain the diagnosis of schizophreniform disorder (see the sidebar "Prognosis and Schizophreniform Psychosis"). Be discerning when you read about this condition; I've encountered writers who disregard the time requirements and continue to use the diagnosis for a patient who has been ill for years.

Organic Psychoses

Numerous physical illnesses can cause psychotic symptoms, which can sometimes look remarkably like those of schizophrenia. Table 9.1 lists some of these causes, four of which are illustrated in the following vignettes.

Edwina

Though she'd tell you she hated the word, Edwina was still spry. She had been a writer all her adult life, and from the retirement home where she'd lived for the past 5 years, she continued to pen a weekly column—about

---

Prognosis and Schizophreniform Psychosis

Schizophreniform disorder incorporates criteria for predicting which patients are likely to recover completely from their current episode of illness. The outlook is more likely to be favorable if we can identify some features that in follow-up studies have predicted a good prognosis. The patient who has two or more of the following is likely to recover:

- Confusion
- Psychotic symptoms that begin early (within the first month of the illness)
- Good premorbid social and work functioning
- Good preservation of affect

Winona had three of these factors—delusions from the first days she was ill; excellent functioning socially and in her job (school) before becoming ill; and the ability to show anger while ill (therefore, her affect was probably not blunted). However, even when most acutely ill, she did not seem confused. Her clinician told her and her parents that she would probably recover completely, which is in fact what happened.

---

retirement. She didn't smoke or use alcohol, and took no medications other than vitamin C. Because she had no past history of mental disorder, staff members at the facility were surprised when one Sunday morning she refused to attend the nondenominational religious services she'd always enjoyed. "The specters, they're cursing the Lord," she remarked of phantasms hovering near the ceiling that no one else could see. She claimed that the "shade" of a resident who had recently died lurked in the chapel, sometimes shaking his finger at her. At lunch, she refused to eat her poached salmon; she insisted that the cook, a Native American woman who worked on weekends, had "poisoned" the fish in retaliation for centuries of mistreatment at the hands of the government.

Her doctor recommended an antipsychotic drug, which she refused to take. But she did consent to magnetic resonance imaging, which showed that she had had a small stroke beneath the surface of the left side of her brain. Other than elevated blood pressure (190/115), her exam was normal. Over the next week she improved, and a month later she ate with good appetite. In a column about her experience, she wrote that her previous ideas had been "peculiar, at best."

Sal

Directly out of high school, Sal had entered the military, where he had served a tour in the first Gulf War. A brave and loyal soldier, he tried to re-enlist after his 4-year tour, but was forestalled by his history of occasional outbursts of rage, sometimes directed toward his sergeants. These never quite rose to the point of disciplinary action, but, coupled with a nagging depression, they caused the Army to reject him for further service. He subsequently worked for a variety of pest extermination companies.

When Sal was 27, his increasingly erratic behavior prompted admission to a VA hospital. He had been found one weekend on the riverfront, running along the levee and screaming about "Star Trekkers" who were threatening to disrupt his visitation with his 4-year-old daughter. He hadn't been hallucinating, exactly. He did say that he might have heard threatening sounds, though they could have been in his head—perhaps put there by the Trekkers. Since his admission, they hadn't bothered him, but he kept trying to alert the FBI to a possible invasion. His doctors first wondered whether he had inhaled toxic chemicals from his job, but a review of his history revealed that he specialized in bat exclusion, which involved caulking, not killing.

Family mythology held that when Sal was a baby, his mother had "run off with the gypsies" and hadn't been heard from since. Sal had been reared by his father and, later, stepmother. The only other family history he knew was that a cousin had died in an institution and might have had Huntington's disease. A copy of his military mental health evaluation revealed that he had a persistent twitching of his mouth, interpreted as a sign of nervousness that further substantiated his unfitness for duty.

Sal improved with antipsychotic drugs, and his doctors diagnosed him as having psychotic disorder NOS. Followed in the outpatient clinic, he continued on his medication and did well for 2 years. Then he began to show distinctive writhing movements of his arms, and problems with his memory were noted. On reevaluation, his diagnosis was changed to psychosis due to Huntington's disease.

Arley

Abandoned by his family when he was 5, Arley had been reared in a succession of foster families. After a disastrous academic career—including repeated fights with students, poor grades and even altercations with teachers—he left school for good when he was 15. For a time he lived on the streets, supporting himself by petty theft and running drugs for a gang. He began using a variety of street drugs—especially amphetamines, but later heroin as well. By the time he was 20 he was using needles to inject himself; often he was careless about sterility.

When Arley was 25, he was admitted to a hospital with pneumocystis pneumonia. That was the first time he had tested HIV-positive, and it led to treatment with a cocktail of drugs that at first kept his symptoms under control. Living on the streets, he was fearful of being robbed or molested ("Whatever else, I'm no prostitute," he had told his doctor). Because his medicines made him drowsy, he decreased the dose so that he could stay vigilant, even when sleeping. Gradually he stopped taking them altogether. Within 6 months, he was back at the hospital complaining of persistent sore throat, which turned out to be due to candidiasis. He was diagnosed with full-blown AIDS and admitted.

Arley couldn't state the exact date, though he knew who and where he was. His speech wandered off into descriptions of scenes he claimed to see—a valley full of bodies bathed in blood; a crowd of young people waving stumps where their arms should be. When he was examined at admission, he worried that his penis had been cut off. He kept looking down inside his pants, which appeared to reassure him only for a few moments. Within days he became mute, staring at the wall next to his bed, and threatening to strike out when anyone approached. His diagnosis was psychosis secondary to AIDS.

Trudy

Off and on for years, Trudy had been treated for psychosis. Always rather easily upset, she would fly into a rage without much provocation. When she was 23, she had her first incident of severe abdominal pain; she carried on so dramatically in the hospital's urgent care center that she was diagnosed as hysterical, despite the fact that she developed nausea and vomiting. She was discharged the following day, but later that afternoon an ambulance returned her to the emergency room.

Curled up on a gurney, Trudy remained completely mute until she was given an injection of Valium. When she gradually began to speak, she claimed that she was dead already, and that the pains she had had signaled the onset of her torture in "the spirit world." However, she denied having hallucinations. Days later, her psychosis had once again yielded to antipsychotic drugs; her clinician attributed her lingering muscle weakness to a side effect of medication.

Between episodes of her illness, Trudy faithfully took the antipsychotic medication she was prescribed—right up to the next attack. They occurred every 4 or 5 years, each time resulting in renewed pain, weakness, and hospitalization. When she was 38, a technician noticed that a urine specimen of hers had darkened after standing in sunlight on a laboratory bench. This prompted further investigation and the eventual diagnosis of acute intermittent porphyria.

Analyses

Once we know that a medical condition exists, the analysis of each of these patients is trivial. It's the knowing, or not knowing, that can trip us up. Most such cases will have features that should draw our attention away from schizophrenia and toward a physical cause: a sudden beginning (Sal), onset in very old age (Edwina), or existence of a prior medical condition (Arley). Trudy was misdiagnosed and treated for schizophrenia for years, but she shouldn't have been, because she didn't have a full enough spectrum of psychotic symptoms—only hallucinations, and only visual ones (the type often encountered in mental disorders associated with physical illness). Chalk up another plea for diagnostic principles that urge us to look for more symptoms and typical symptoms of a disorder. And then there's the issue of *atypical* features: Physical symptoms, such as headache or red urine, strongly hint that we should consider medical disorders for a diagnosis. At least two of these patients experienced periods of confusion, which are also atypical for schizophrenia.

Comment

In the case of Sal, keep in mind that the family history didn't confer risk of mental illness; only the Huntington's gene itself could produce the illness. Also, an occasional medically ill patient will have a psychosis that seems typical of schizophrenia, with few if any features that would tip you off to the organic etiology. The only solution is never to be completely comfortable with a diagnosis that is as fraught with peril as schizophrenia. With apologies to Thomas Jefferson, the price of accurate diagnosis is eternal vigilance.

Substance-Related Psychoses

You often read that substance use can present as a psychosis that closely resembles schizophrenia, but how many of us have actually encountered it?

The data aren't very clear, though it probably happens more often than we realize.

Aileen

Aileen sold televisions for a discount retail chain. Lately she had noticed that the people shown on the sets around the store had begun to watch her—almost to follow her around as she moved from one aisle to the next. At first, she thought it funny and mentioned it to a customer, who quickly left the store. Later she was offended when she noticed that the characters on TV were also discussing her sex life with her boyfriend. She talked to another sales rep, who stood and watched a high-definition monitor with her for quite a while, then ventured that "there was nothing going on at all." Later that day, Aileen was discovered in a back room where there were no televisions, trying to hide inside a side-by-side refrigerator, from which she had removed all the racks. She screamed all the way to the emergency room.

After she was admitted to a locked psychiatry ward, she stopped talking. Several clinicians tried to question her, but each time she would gaze intently at the person, then physically turn away until all they could see was the back of her head. Her boyfriend, Geoff, with whom she had lived for 2 years, was away on a business trip, but a coworker had the telephone number of Aileen's mother, who had to drive in from a neighboring county. She stated very clearly that there had never been a similar episode, and that Aileen had never used street drugs: "In all her 28 years, she's been a real straight arrow—she doesn't even drink." Her mother did note that on the telephone several days ago, Aileen had talked rather fast, and at lunch a few days earlier, she had spoken rapidly and was full of plans for buying a house and renovating it.

There had been no family history of any mental illness, though Aileen's twin brother had smoked pot when he was a teenager. A call to her family practitioner confirmed her excellent physical health; she was taking no prescribed medications, not even birth control pills. She'd fought a weight problem all her life; currently, she was on a low-carbohydrate diet.

When Geoff returned home the following day, he first said she had been "disgustingly healthy," but he later recalled that she had seemed unusually energetic for the past week or two. Then he mentioned that a couple of weeks ago, after her most recent diet had let her down, she had tried some tablets from a bottle given to her by a friend. For at least a week, she'd been downing several a day. Later he brought in a bottle that was labeled *"ma huang."*

Analysis

We'll try to determine the cause of Aileen's delusions and other strange behaviors at two times: when she was first admitted to the hospital, and after her doctor obtained information from her boyfriend. Based only on the collateral information of sudden onset and episode of fast talking from Aileen's mother and her friend at work, we might entertain a mood disorder diagnosis, though we wouldn't go quite all the way and say that she had a bipolar disorder. Why? Just after admission, she showed some atypical features, such as muteness and negativism—hardly the stuff of mania— and there just weren't enough symptoms to make any diagnosis. At that point I'd use the diagnostic principle concerning *undiagnosed*, partly because at age 28 she had had no previous mood episodes, and partly because there just wasn't enough recent history to go on.

Once Geoff returned, further collateral history brought the diagnosis immediately into focus. Although he knew of no physical problems, she had been taking a drug that contains ephedrine, a stimulant that is well known for its ability to produce manic-like symptoms and psychosis. The journey to the diagnosis is a short one, lasting just two steps in Figure 13.1.

Comment

What usually comes to mind when you consider substances that cause mental symptoms? Alcohol and street drugs. However, a wide variety of medications can also precipitate psychosis. After ephedrine caused a number of deaths, the U.S. Food and Drug Administration banned its use in pharmaceuticals, thereby curtailing its opportunities for mischief. However, it can still be found in traditional medicines and imported drugs. The symptoms of psychosis that ephedrine causes are a lot like those of other stimulant drugs, such as cocaine and amphetamine which—unfortunately, are still abundant.

Vern

One of the pitfalls of a major diagnosis like schizophrenia is that its symptoms are so blatant and overwhelming that, once we've identified it, we may be tempted to rest on our laurels.

Vern's emotional symptoms had been gathering for several years; now, at 27, he was finally diagnosed with schizophrenia. Since then, he had been successfully treated with long-acting intramuscular Haldol, which he tolerated well. He liked his therapist at the mental health clinic. "You're my only friend," he had said more than once.

So 6 years down the road, the therapist noted with some surprise that Vern had once again begun to complain of persecution. Poachers were stealing the flank steaks he had bought for his mother's birthday bash; though he'd been born in Baltimore, monks from a local commune had been collecting money to have him deported to Sudan. The delusions grew over a couple of weeks, during which he became increasingly agitated and belligerent, until auditory hallucinations once again required his hospitalization.

There could be no question that Vern was taking his antipsychotic medication; it was planted right there in his hip every 4 weeks. And close questioning couldn't dislodge him from his story that he had used neither alcohol nor street drugs. A call to his mother, however, revealed that Vern had finally found a friend—a substance-using patient with a long and checkered history. Sure enough, when directly questioned, Vern admitted that he and George had frequently smoked crack together for about as long as he'd been having a recurrence of his psychosis.

Analysis

The use of Figure 13.1 is almost superfluous; you might want to check Table 9.3 to see what other symptoms of cocaine use Vern might be subject to. And Table 15.1 lists the types of substances that can cause psychosis and other mental syndromes during intoxication or withdrawal. I'd arrange Vern's two diagnoses—schizophrenia and cocaine-induced psychosis—in reverse order, to indicate which needs immediate treatment.

Comment

The tip-off here is the recurrence of Vern's psychosis despite his continuing use of medication—the effects of which, because it was injected, he could not escape. Of course, even without street drugs as a stimulus, a patient with schizophrenia could develop renewed symptoms. But the safe course is to suspect that something else has occurred to interfere. Dual diagnosis is far too common a finding.

Studies have shown that even when tobacco is excluded, 40% or more of patients with schizophrenia will misuse substances at some time; most popular is alcohol, then marijuana and cocaine. Substance use is associated with aggression, violence, and relapse of psychosis, and it often persists despite adequate treatment for schizophrenia. Substance use can lead to homelessness and incarceration, and it increases hospital admissions and costs of treatment. Even marijuana raises these patients' psychopathology scores on standard tests. Although it has often been suggested that patients with schizophrenia use drugs and alcohol to cope with their psychotic symptoms, at least one study has failed to support this "self-medication" hypothesis.

Other Psychotic Disorders and Comorbidity

I have abstracted this description of a patient known only as S. R. from a classic 1933 paper in the *American Journal of Psychiatry*.

S. R.

An active, ambitious young woman who liked to go dancing, S. R. met her policeman husband when she was 18 and married him just 6 months later. Within a year they were the parents of a son. When the child was 5, they moved to a "fixer-upper" house that troubled S. R.: The furnace wasn't working well, and she thought she could smell gas. She felt bad, had trouble sleeping, and lost her appetite; several times she vomited. Cross and irritable, she brooded about how coarse her husband was and how the 11-year difference in their ages thwarted her desire to mix with people and go out dancing.

When another policeman in their neighborhood committed suicide early in February, her husband remarked that his line of work could make anyone feel suicidal. Subsequently S. R. became depressed, blaming it on interference from his parents, who had never taken to her. Feeling oppressed by his sexual demands, she wished that he would leave her alone. She said that she had a bad heart and would soon die.

One night in mid-February, she impulsively asked to go to the home of her parents; there, she accused them of trying to turn her husband against her. Still sleepless the next night, she accused her brother of planning to poison her husband. Then she called the police and asked to be rescued; ultimately she was hospitalized. Five days after admission, her rectal temperature was elevated at 102°F, and her white blood count was 15,200.

S. R. complained of peculiar noises and of the other patients talking about her; she also suspected that her husband had been unfaithful, had begun to use drugs, and would try to steal her son from her. Other patients, in voices that were somehow "rayed" to her from another room by a person in a trance, said that her husband was of "mixed blood." When he visited her in the hospital, his eyes stared and held a glassy look. She complained of physical sensations that she attributed to poison. She lost her appetite, couldn't sleep, and cried a great deal. She smelled many different odors while in the hospital, and she heard her name broadcast over the paging system.

Whereas she had initially been depressed, after several weeks she appeared happy and was able to laugh. She felt that all of her troubles were due to "radio hypnotism." After 6 weeks of hospitalization, she was discharged home with the diagnosis of dementia praecox. On follow-up 20 months later, she had recovered and completely returned to her old self.

Analysis

With no evidence of a significant medical condition, a substance use problem, or delirium, we move swiftly through steps 1–4 of Figure 13.1 to step 5, which richly deserves a "yes" answer. At the time of her first hospitalization, S. R.'s psychotic symptoms were associated with serious depressive symptoms. This leads us through step 9 to step 12, which asks about length of the depressive symptoms. That's a very good question! What, exactly, is *brief*? Because there's no scientific definition of *brief*, the best I can do is an example. Vern, just described in the preceding section, had been ill with schizophrenia for 6 years; if for a month he now became depressed, that would be brief relative to the overall length of his illness. S. R. had also been depressed for several weeks, but in a far briefer context. As compared with her entire illness, her depression was not brief but "substantial" (as the manuals prescribe). Our decision moves us along to step 13. Her psychotic symptoms apparently persisted long after her mood reverted to normal, bringing us finally to consider the diagnosis of schizoaffective disorder.

Comment

Whew! This has been about as tortured a trip through a decision tree as we'll encounter in our quest for any diagnosis. Was all that work worth the effort? A diagnosis with ever-changing criteria, schizoaffective disorder was controversial almost from its first description. Of the five patients fully described in Jacob Kasanin's original 1933 article, none would fully qualify for such a diagnosis according to the criteria in use today. S. R. was the Kasanin patient who came closest to meeting today's criteria.

Some authors point out that interrater reliability in schizoaffective disorder is unsatisfactory. Other studies use statistical manipulations to suggest that schizoaffective disorder as now described is only a variant of schizophrenia, and that its prognosis resembles schizophrenia—the direct opposite of Kasanin's conclusions. Indeed, the criteria we use are in such flux that schizoaffective disorder is one of the few whose requirements have changed in each of the three major revisions to the DSM (in 1980, DSM-III cannily avoided proposing any criteria at all).

What is the diagnosis of schizoaffective disorder supposed to accomplish? Researchers have long sought a middle ground somewhere between schizophrenia and the mood disorders—a sort of mental health Northwest Passage. If one existed, it would be very much like this disorder. That's why the symptoms have to be so carefully drawn: There must be a substantial period of mood problems accompanied by psychosis, but on the other hand, there must also be a time when there is psychosis without either mania or depression. Otherwise, there would be nothing to differentiate the condition from, say, depression with psychosis.

In my opinion, the diagnosis of schizoaffective disorder is a confused muddle. Its scientific support is weak, and it's used as a "wastebasket" for difficult-to-diagnose patients. In 2003, one clinician even wrote that because so many of his patients had both mood and psychotic symptoms and gave such poor histories, schizoaffective disorder was one of his most frequent diagnoses. Whereas many studies of psychotic patients lump together schizophrenia and schizoaffective disorder, few publish enough details to determine which diagnosis the clinical features fully support, by any set of criteria. Some authors note that depression is fairly common in patients with schizophrenia, especially those who are older, and that it is correlated with the positive symptoms of hallucinations and delusions. At least one writer suggests that we should distinguish two forms of schizoaffective disorder: *concurrent* and *sequential*. That would require yet another revision of the criteria—yet another resetting of the target while clinicians and researchers alike are still trying to adjust their sights to its present location.

Camille

The early 20th-century French sculptor Camille Claudel developed a lifelong psychosis that is diagnosable even through the long-distance lens of biography.

> With little formal education, Camille Claudel went far. The muse, long-term mistress, and sometimes collaborator of the great Auguste Rodin,

she contributed entire figures to some of his works. Though by the age of 30 she was recognized as a talented artist in her own right, at about that time something happened that gradually drew her away from Rodin, her art, and ultimately the world.

Camille had begun to suspect that others, women included, were against her. In fits of anger, she expressed her distrust of Rodin—whom she ultimately accused of deceiving her "by crafty and false character," as she wrote in a letter when she was 38. She became convinced that she knew who was responsible for "depredations committed in the Louvre," and she sent letters containing cat feces to an art inspector. She increasingly withdrew from her friends, and gradually ceased producing works of art at all; she even smashed some of her own works. Poverty-stricken, she was reported to be living in filth, scrounging food from garbage cans. Despite the ample evidence of delusions, nowhere do her biographers ever note evidence of hallucinations or sustained depression.

As the years rolled on, she came to the ecumenical conviction that the Jews, Protestants, and Freemasons were plotting to poison her. Ultimately, at age 49, she was placed in a mental hospital where, in her imagination, even the nurses had joined the plot. For the balance of her life, she lived in asylums. Although she would have been provided with art materials, and the income from her work could have helped her live far more comfortably, she refused to sculpt even in institutions for fear that her work would be stolen from her. To avert the poisoning she felt was imminent, she would eat only raw eggs and unpeeled potatoes, or whatever cooked food she could prepare herself. By the age of 62 she was still able to write letters, which were completely coherent as long as she avoided the objects of her delusions. At 66 she wrote that "the Jewish gang is holding me here" because more than three decades earlier, she had refused to sign a petition at the time of the notorious Dreyfus affair.

Although Camille complained of physical illness from time to time throughout her life, there is no record of a disease that could account for her psychosis. She remained lucid until near the end, when she drifted into senility, still convinced that Rodin was the "odious character" who had ruined her life.

Analysis

The history of Camille Claudel is quite clear: For decades, she had delusions but no hallucinations. Therefore, we must answer "no" at step 5 of Figure 13.1. None of her acquaintances (except possibly her fellow inmates) shared her paranoid vision of her world, so we must say "no" again at step 6. Her ideas, though false, were not bizarre; poisonings and thefts are things that could reasonably happen to someone (step 7), and she was able to function well outside her delusions (step 11). These factors bring us to consider delusional disorder as her diagnosis. Of course, because historical diagnoses rely almost exclusively on collateral information, they can never be more than tentative.

Comment

Patients who have delusions but no hallucinations or other features of psychosis (see the list at the start of this chapter) don't meet criteria for schizophrenia; we say that they have delusional disorder. They usually become ill later in life than is the case in schizophrenia, and their functioning is less impaired. The delusions can be of several sorts, but the *persecutory* type, in which the patient is somehow being cheated, followed, slandered, or drugged, is the most common. Other types include *erotomanic* (someone, often of high station, is in love with the patient); *grandiose* (the patient has a special talent, power, or relation to someone famous); *jealous* (a spouse or lover has been unfaithful); and *somatic* (physical sensations, such as insects crawling on the skin or a foul body odor, imply a medical condition or physical defect). Some patients have features of two or more of these types.

Encountered only about 1-30th as often as schizophrenia, delusional disorder has received publicity far in excess of its numbers. There are a couple of reasons. There is the notoriety that attends instances of stalking, which is sometimes due to the erotomanic form of delusional disorder (the Glenn Close character in the movie *Fatal Attraction* suggests such a person). Then there is our fascination with John Hinckley, Jr. Hinckley, who famously stalked and shot Ronald Reagan in 1981, has been described as having delusional disorder, though there are real doubts as to his correct diagnosis. Of course, like those with schizophrenia, the vast majority of patients with delusional disorder do not kill or harm other people. Those few who do so attract an inordinate amount of attention, fear, and rage.

Ted

The symptoms of psychosis are so striking that they can obscure other important aspects of the history and MSE. It's a mistake to allow that to happen, because a second illness can complicate—and a second diagnosis can facilitate—treatment.

Short and solidly built, Ted vaguely resembled the water heaters and dishwashers he delivered every day for his employer, a major home appliance chain in a West Coast city. He had served honorably in the Army, including a tour in Iraq during the first Gulf War, but after an 8-year enlistment he'd resigned rather than attend the alcohol rehabilitation program mandated by a couple of civilian arrests for public intoxication. After that, he bounced from job to job until a divorce finally persuaded him to join AA. He then obtained his present position, which he had held for well over 5 years. He had settled down, had married for a second time, and was engaged in raising his year-old twin daughters.

As he was maneuvering an electric stove onto his dolly one afternoon, he paused when he heard something strange—a voice that seemed to come from inside the crate. "Ted, drop it," the voice commanded. He was so surprised that he did just that, and the box popped open. Looking inside, he saw nothing but a mute kitchen range. After a few moments, he rode it down the lift on the back of his truck and rolled it into the house. Later that afternoon, he heard two voices coming from a carton of microwaves he had picked up at the warehouse. They were discussing him, calling him a failure, a drunk, and an asshole. He tore the carton completely to shreds before bolting from work to down his first beer in nearly a decade.

Over the next week, a swelling chorus from his crates and boxes had Ted nearly in tears. The following Thursday, he entered his boss's office to try to learn what was going on. The office was empty, but he observed some papers on the desk. "They were carefully lined up with the edge of the desk," as he told the clinician when he checked himself into the urgent care center days later, "and suddenly I *knew* it meant that everything was lined up against me." He noticed that his wife "looked funny" at him, which proved to him that she was in cahoots with his boss.

Ted tried his best to avoid further recourse to alcohol, but lost. Even when drinking, he heard the voices, which grew louder and more insistent. After 2 weeks of heavy drinking, he heard an Air America radio announcer say, "Ted's got to learn." At that point, he made the decision to seek help.

Analysis

Sorting out Ted's psychosis requires some attention to the calendar. It makes a lot of difference that Ted had been psychotic for only a few weeks. This fact, his hallucinations, and his delusions move us to step 10, where a "no" answer brings us to consider the diagnosis of schizophreniform disorder. Although we should always consider prognosis for every patient, schizophreniform psychosis is the only psychotic diagnosis that specifically encourages us to rate how likely the patient is to recover (see the sidebar "Prognosis and Schizophreniform Diagnosis" on page 194). Fortunately for him, a remission to his psychosis is foretold by several of Ted's symptoms: excellent affect, symptoms of psychosis almost from the beginning of his disorder, and very good social and work adjustment prior to the onset of his illness.

We must also discuss his substance use. Ted's alcohol use had been quiescent for years; now that he had become psychotic, his drinking had flared up again. How should we regard it? If we used strict diagnostic criteria (not inevitably the best practice), we might be hard pressed to make a diagnosis of alcohol dependence, but it would be vital to note his recent difficulty with alcohol. Regardless of the number and severity of symptoms he has been having during this episode, I would diagnose alcohol dependence. You can add verbiage to indicate that it is recurrent and of short duration, if you like. The idea with diagnoses is to convey as much information as possible, and Ted's clinicians need to know that they must contend with more than just psychosis. Of course, the alcohol diagnosis would be listed second; whenever psychosis is a factor, it will usually be the first thing to address.

Comment

Half or more of psychotic patients will have additional diagnoses. The problem is that psychosis is so dramatic that we sometimes forget to address any leftover symptoms. Besides substance misuse, you'll need to be alert for indications of depression, panic disorder, and several personality disorders.

Jeannie

Depression can be hard to sort out in the context of psychosis. There are at least three different constructs to think about—psychotic depression, schizophrenia with depression, and schizoaffective disorder. I've put the information into a table (see Table 13.2).

Years ago, I evaluated a very bright woman who had an MBA and worked in her city's financial district. Always in perfect health, now she had been admitted for her first mental hospitalization ever because of a suicide attempt. After several weeks there, she was still completely miserable.

A little over a year earlier, just after her 26th birthday, Jeannie had

TABLE 13.2. Mood Symptoms in Psychosis

	Psychotic symptoms	Psychosis duration	Mood symptoms
Schizophrenia	Two types required	6 months or more	Not significant
Schizophreniform disorder	Two types required	Under 6 months	Not significant
Schizoaffective disorder	Two types required	1 month or more	Prominent, but psychosis alone for 2 weeks
Mood disorder with psychosis	One type required	No lower limit	Always present
Delusional disorder	One type required	1 month or more	Not significant
Two disorders: mood and psychosis	Two types required	Depends on diagnosis	Always present

begun to suspect that someone at work was spying on her. She had no idea why this would happen, but she had noticed telltale signs—the handset on her desk telephone was replaced pointing the wrong way, and the files she maintained on her customers seemed in disarray. Becoming afraid, she drew inward; to keep an eye on her desk, she stopped going out to lunch with other workers in the office.

Even so, the signs kept cropping up. Soon, she knew she was being followed: She repeatedly caught sight of the same car in her rear-view mirror, and when she was out walking, passers-by would wink or wave a folded newspaper to let her pursuers know which way she had gone. For several months she had also been hearing sounds. These began with creaking noises—"like a hangman's rope swinging a body," she explained—but lately she had perceived that there were words and now, sentences. "Mad, mad, mad," they mocked her, "Jeannie's gone forever mad."

After her initial diagnosis of schizophrenia, she had done a great deal of reading about her illness. What she had learned had caused her to become despondent. She knew that she had a chronic illness; that it could be treated, but that it could nonetheless interfere with her work; and that it might even prevent her from marrying and having children. These thoughts had haunted her for weeks; now she had a full-blown depression.

"I'm a chronic schizophrenic," she told me. Tears streamed down her face, which was becoming lined from worry, sleeplessness, and loss of weight. "I'm going to spend my life shut up in a hospital, fouling myself and talking to phantoms. I'm hopeless. I'll be glad when I'm dead."

Analysis

Confirming Jeannie's principal diagnosis is our first order of business. Once past steps 1–4 of Figure 13.1, we can agree right away that she had both delusions and hallucinations that lasted considerably beyond the required 6 months. Although she had developed significant depressive symptoms, they weren't present when her psychosis began. (If we tried hard, we might persuade ourselves that she had schizoaffective disorder, but that's only because some clinicians have the knack of forcing patients into a favorite diagnosis. To me, her mood symptoms seemed relatively brief, compared to the duration of the psychosis.) This analysis takes us through steps 5, 9, 12, and 10, where a "yes" answer affirms Jeannie's diagnosis.

Pursuit of her depression sends us through the Figure 11.1 decision tree, where we encounter a problem: It directs us through steps 5, 9, and 10 to consider schizoaffective disorder, which we've already discarded in the previous analysis. What gives? We've learned a valuable lesson—that there are limitations to the decision tree method. We can agree that without a doubt, Jeannie had a lengthy psychosis and mood symptoms. But determining how these two concepts are related is problematic; it makes a real difference whether you regard mood symptoms or psychosis as your best point of departure. In Jeannie's case, the dilemma would be best resolved by diagnosing two comorbid disorders, schizophrenia and depression. This would allow a simplified view of her two sets of symptoms, each with its own treatment and prognosis. Jeannie's schizophrenia would be listed first, because its treatment was central: I believed that once it was adequately addressed, her perspective on the rest of her life would improve, and her depression might lift. In the event, that's what happened, though other patients have experienced different outcomes.

Comment

Depression in schizophrenia is poorly understood and inadequately studied. Postpsychotic depression has often been diagnosed when a bipolar depressive episode might be appropriate, but even that leaves many depressions to explain. Some patients with schizophrenia experience anhedonia; others have medication effects (especially from the older antipsychotics) that are experienced as depression. However, still others develop deep depression that persist even after their psychotic symptoms have resolved. The fact that about 10% of patients with schizophrenia ultimately kill themselves—a rate second only to that found in the mood disorders—should prompt every clinician to watch carefully for developing depression in every such patient.

Differentiating Schizophrenia from Other Psychoses

I thought it would be useful to collect in one place the characteristics that we use to decide when a patient may have schizophrenia, as compared to other causes of psychosis. Of course, none of the characteristics I have mentioned is absolute. For example, a patient could be young, have a gradual onset, have a positive family history, and *still* turn out to have a psychosis due to the use of cocaine. But on the whole, these are the factors that we should look at in our evaluation of psychosis.

- *Age.* Schizophrenia tends to develop in teenagers and young adults.
- *Marital status.* Patients with schizophrenia are often unmarried.
- *Onset.* Schizophrenia develops slowly; other psychoses are often more rapid.
- *Family history.* As you'd expect, patients with schizophrenia are more likely than average to have relatives with schizophrenia.
- *Drug/alcohol history.* Such a history is less likely in schizophrenia (though these patients may well use drugs and alcohol later on).
- *Confusion.* Perplexity and confusion are associated with eventual recovery in patients with schizophreniform disorder.
- *Premorbid personality.* Some patients with schizophrenia have schizoid or schizotypal personalities before they become ill.
- *Affect.* Affect that is neither flat nor blunted is sometimes found in patients who recover from their psychoses.
- *Hallucinations.* Patients with schizophrenia tend to have auditory hallucinations; hallucinations of other senses suggest a diagnosis other than schizophrenia.
- *Delusions.* Bizarre delusions (things that couldn't really happen, such as being able to direct the world's air traffic by thought waves) suggest schizophrenia; mood-congruent delusions (guilt during depression, grandiosity during mania) suggest mood disorder.

Brief Psychotic Disorder

For a few patients, psychosis is fleeting—a sort of mini-schizophreniform disorder. Over the decades, such illnesses have received a variety of different names, including *brief reactive psychosis* (changed because clinicians couldn't agree on what was an appropriate precipitant). The category now incorporates postpartum psychosis (but not postpartum mood disorder with psychosis—keep that straight if you can). Just one psychotic symptom can qualify a person for brief psychotic disorder, but recovery must occur within 1 month. Because of the requirement for ultimate recovery, this is not a diagnosis you can make prospectively. If the patient has been ill a month, it is already too late for this diagnosis. Read a case history in *DSM-IV Made Easy*. With both schizophreniform disorder and brief psychotic disorder, what's important is that the patient's prognosis is better than the prognosis for schizophrenia.

Shared Psychotic Disorder

Sometimes called *folie á deux*, shared psychotic disorder is a condition so rare that it still elicits case reports in journals. These people are not psychotic in their own right. They only develop delusions in the context of close association with someone else (such as a parent or spouse) who is independently psychotic with, say, schizophrenia or delusional disorder. Then the patient with the shared psychotic disorder also becomes psychotic, pretty much buying into the symptoms of the first person. To an extent, the devotees of religious cults occupy this same boat, believing often impossible stories fed them by leaders. Some of these leaders may be psychotic, as was probably true of Marshall Applewhite, who founded the Heaven's Gate cult. In 1997, seeking to shed their earthly husks and follow the trail of the Hale–Bopp comet, 38 followers of Applewhite killed themselves with poisoned pudding in tiny Rancho Santa Fe, California, launching that community's suicide rate into the stratosphere. (The cultists ultimate destination remains in doubt.) Other leaders may have personality disorders or other mental problems. Some writers believe that shared psychotic disorder isn't really a specific illness at all, but a phenomenon in some way attached to psychotic illnesses.

Whether it's a phenomenon or a mental illness, the belief can only be maintained when the two people involved are relatively isolated from others. Once they are forced to live apart from one another, the independently ill person continues to maintain the psychotic symptoms, whereas the second develops insight that the beliefs were untrue all along. Although for completeness I have included shared psychotic disorder in Figure 13.1, don't expect to encounter it often. If you find one, look for comorbid mental retardation, dementia, or depression in the second person. You can read a case history in *DSM-IV Made Easy.*

14 Diagnosing Problems of Memory and Thinking

When you think logically about it, there's a lot that's illogical about thinking. We often block out thoughts inconvenient to our line of argument; go off on tangents; allow the intrusion of irrelevancies and rude images; and adhere to prejudices and ill-formed rules rather than to reason. Read the verbatim transcript of, say, a politician speaking off the cuff, and just try to count the verbal blind alleys, untangle the twisted syntax, and nail down the indefinite relative pronouns. Yet none of the myriad infelicities of everyday speech indicates much in the way of psychopathology—beyond talking too fast while thinking too little.

Cognition refers to the processes we use to involve all of our perceptions and sensations in planning. A person with a cognitive disorder could have problems in several areas, including judgment, memory, orientation, problem solving, language, interpersonal relationships, and *praxis* (doing things). We've already seen how abnormalities in the content of thought—hallucinations, delusions, and phobias, for example—can point to a wide variety of mental illnesses. Although a disturbance in the process of thinking occasionally occurs in schizophrenia or mania, more often it points to a cognitive disorder: delirium, dementia, and their variants. (Newcomers to the sometimes arcane world of mental health nomenclature will have to learn specific definitions of terms that many employ in a far more generic sense. For nearly 400 years, *delirium* has been used to mean a state of wild frenzy or excitement; *demented* has been long understood to describe someone who is crazed, mad, or infatuated.) Table 14.1 presents the differential diagnosis for disorders of memory and thinking.

The term *cognitive* often implies some sort of testing, but we need to be able to recognize a disorder on clinical grounds. Very often, the first symptoms that show up are abrupt changes in personality, interest, or

TABLE 14.1. Differential Diagnosis with Brief Definitions for Disorders of Cognition

---

- *Delirium.* Substance use or physical illness causes a rapidly developing, fluctuating state of reduced awareness.

- *Dementia.* Substance use or medical illness leads gradually to impaired memory plus other cognitive dysfunctions, including impaired ability to use language as symbols (*aphasia*); perform motor tasks (*apraxia*); recognize familiar objects (*agnosia*); and plan, organize, sequence, or abstract information (*executive functioning*).

- *Amnestic disorder.* Substance use or medical illness causes a profound loss of memory, especially the ability to form new memories. Remaining intact are the patient's general intelligence, ability to focus attention, and ability to learn new tasks (though not new events, ideas, and words).

- *Depression with pseudodementia.* A person develops depression so severe as to have apparent (though reversible) problems with memory and thinking.

- *Dissociative disorders.* Profound, though temporary, loss of memory can occur in people who have dissociative amnesia, dissociative fugue, or dissociative identity disorder.

- *Posttraumatic stress disorder (PTSD).* Amnesia for important features of a horrific traumatic event can affect these patients, who repeatedly relive the event and experience avoidance and hyperarousal.

- *Postconcussional disorder.* For days or weeks after a head injury that produces loss or alteration of consciousness, a person experiences deficits of memory or attention, plus such symptoms as headache, dizziness, fatigue, mood shifts, personality change, sleep disturbance, and loss of spontaneity.

- *Blackout.* Heavy alcohol drinking produces subsequent loss of memory for the time the person was intoxicated but awake.

- *Age-related cognitive decline (ARCD).* An older patient worries about trouble remembering things when memory ability, upon testing, is not pathological but perfectly normal for current age.

---

behavior. Circumstances can enhance our recognition: We suspect dementia in hospital or nursing home patients or in those who are older; we look for delirium in postoperative patients and those who drink or use drugs. Among the terminally ill, the *majority* will have a delirium at some time!

Whatever the circumstances, whichever symptoms you have to evaluate, you should ideally observe the patient on multiple occasions to learn whether the condition fluctuates, as with delirium, or is constant, as with dementia. Your persistence will pay off if you can ameliorate even in some small way the potential havoc wreaked by disorders of cognition, which substitute confusion for clarity and randomness for reason, while reducing what was once personhood to a shell of humanity.

Delirium and Dementia

It is sometimes hard even to identify a cognitive syndrome, let alone to determine its cause. We clinicians must keep in mind a whole range of possible diagnoses, including even multiple diagnoses from a differential list.

Bobby

When Bobby was first admitted as an emergency case, they didn't even know his name. Two police officers had found him wandering on the street, talking to himself and breathing heavily. He didn't seem to know where he was. Because his face was swollen and he seemed feverish, they coaxed him into the back of their squad car.

At first, the emergency room personnel had no history at all; he'd apparently lost his wallet, and the envelope they found in his shirt pocket must have belonged to someone else. The doctor didn't think he'd been mugged, because he had no bruises or bleeding, and the physical exam showed no evidence of a blow to the head. His temperature was nearly 104°F; once in a while he coughed, but didn't bring up much sputum.

Bobby was put into isolation and given some intravenous fluids. Although his gaze wandered as he spoke, after a few hours he could talk sensibly enough to give them the name of his workplace; a call established his identity and a home phone number. Clint, his roommate, came right down. By the time he got there, Bobby was conversing quietly with two women in clown suits whom no one else could see.

Bobby had no history of head injury. In fact, just a couple of days earlier, he had seemed a healthy gay man who always took precautions; he and Clint had both repeatedly tested negative for HIV. The following day, however, microscopic examination of a tracheal washing sample revealed *Pneumocystis carinii*. Bobby had pneumonia, probably due to AIDS.

Once the crisis passed and his cough resolved, Bobby was started on the drug AZT, which was all that was available at that time. His T4 cells were low, but his vital signs were normal; he could now walk and exercise without panting. However, Clint noted that Bobby just wasn't himself. He never returned to work but sat at home, watching TV ("He always hated it before"). He had always been attentive and loving; now, his interest lackluster, he was more or less constantly idle and didn't seem to care. He even wore the same socks several days in a row. "He said he'd forgotten where he kept his clean pairs. He's always been so fastidious."

Clint became seriously alarmed when he noted that his friend complained of feeling weak and had trouble tying his shoes; this prompted his final hospitalization.

Analysis

For the first few hours after admission, before the lab results were in and a history could be obtained, Bobby's diagnosis should have been an undiagnosed mental disorder. Once the data were available, however, his history would suggest two sets of symptoms, approximately demarcated by the time of his hospital discharge. During the first, acute episode, he appeared terribly ill and confused. His gaze shifted around the room, and he was alternately alert enough to give vital information and so sick he saw phantom clowns. These symptoms are classic for a delirium (step 1 of Figure 14.1, the decision tree for a patient with cognitive problems), at which point the problem becomes one of determining cause. Because he neither drank alcohol nor used street drugs, substance use seemed unlikely, but the clinician would have been right to get blood and urine samples for toxicology. In time, testing would yield the answer.

The testing and hospital stay resolved his immediate difficulties, but Bobby's troubles had only begun. His subsequent history requires us to travel the decision tree once again. Bobby had no history of alcohol use, which gets us past step 3, but wait a minute! What about step 2? Couldn't some of his symptoms, such as reduced interest and activity, be construed as depression? Of course, and at some point his clinician might need to evaluate him for depression secondary to a medical condition. But here Occam's razor is a bust: A mood disorder wouldn't begin to explain the breadth of his symptoms. If we start through either of the mood disorder decision trees (Figures 11.1 and 11.2), we immediately confront the question of significant medical condition.

With no history of head injury, we can bypass step 4. His developing memory problems were not just for personal information, such as his name or stressful events in his life; he also had trouble with finding his socks, which carries us past step 5. Bobby clearly had difficulty learning new information *and* recalling previously learned material (step 6 yields a "yes" response for either), so at step 11 we have to consider whether there were symptoms other than loss of memory. He had developed weakness and difficulty tying his shoes, which should move us to consider a dementia. The most likely underlying cause would be his HIV. However, before making any final diagnosis of dementia, we should ob-

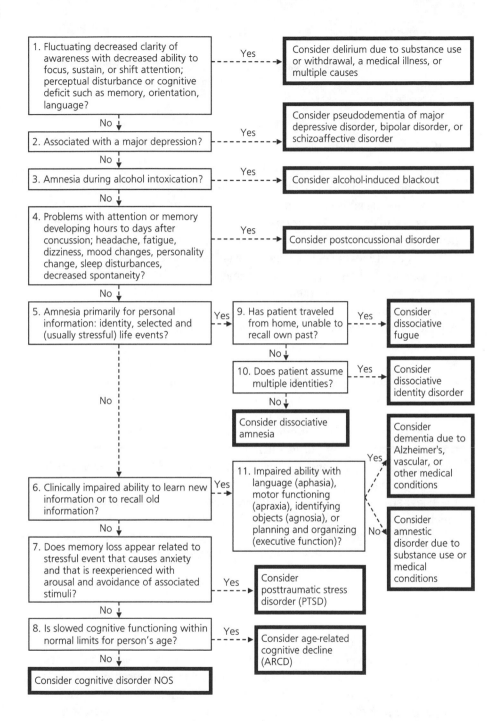

FIGURE 14.1. Decision tree for a patient who has problems with attention or memory loss.

tain a careful neurological evaluation. We'd also want a baseline MMSE, in order to follow the progress of the disease. (See the sidebar "Do I Need Scales?" on page 220).

Comment on Delirium

Acute onset (often over just a few hours), wandering attention, and fluctuating levels of awareness amply suggest delirium. When they occur, hallucinations are usually visual and often quite frightening, though Bobby's only preoccupied him. A delirious person's mood may also change rapidly from depressed to anxious, irritable, fearful, or even euphoric. Whereas Bobby's activity level declined and he was quiet, other patients with delirium become loud and hyperactive. It may actually be easier to diagnose them correctly, because their noise and intrusiveness call attention to themselves, and greater effort may thus be put toward making a diagnosis. A patient may show both states at different points in an illness—another demonstration of the fluctuation that defines delirium. You can see why a single assessment often isn't sufficient to make the diagnosis, and why clinicians often miss it. Delirium can be especially difficult to diagnose when it exists in a context of dementia. Information from relatives or nursing staff may improve the rate of early diagnosis.

Delirium affects 10% or more of medical inpatients, and perhaps three times that many acutely ill geriatric patients. It is a disorder with many causes: brain tumors and trauma; intracranial infections (besides HIV, there's meningitis and encephalitis, among others); infections elsewhere in the body; strokes; nutritional and vitamin deficiencies, and endocrine malfunctions. Besides alcohol and street drug intoxication or withdrawal (remember the classical delirium tremens of alcohol withdrawal), a number of medication types (see Table 9.2) can produce delirium, especially in older patients.

Comment on Dementia

Diagnosing dementia is fraught with error, and there are many ways to go wrong. Early on, you can stumble over those everyday *normal* annoyances we all experience—forgetting appointments and trouble recalling a familiar name, to name two foremost in my own experience. Many such experiences are a part of age-related cognitive decline (ARCD, discussed later in this chapter), in which an older person complains of how long it takes to process information. If other cognitive processes (such as attention, verbal fluency and other language functions, memory, and ability to make decisions) remain minimally affected, it isn't dementia setting in, but just one more spice in the stew of advancing age.

Truly demented persons don't often spontaneously express feelings of marked unhappiness, but had we asked Bobby if he felt depressed, he might have agreed (though perhaps just to cooperate). If you learn from caregivers that the main complaints are apathy, reduced energy, and poor concentration, but the person doesn't actually seem to feel sad, the symptoms may well be due solely to dementia. Apathy or depression is fairly common among patients with dementia resulting from Parkinson's, Huntington's, and Wilson's diseases—and AIDS. These disorders are called *subcortical dementias*, because the site of their pathology is far beneath the cerebral cortex. (In Alzheimer's, a *cortical dementia*, depression is less common.)

Although language ability may be intact, the personalities of patients with subcortical dementia may change, especially as apathy, inertia, and decreased spontaneity set in. Often these changes in behavior and personality are what bring demented patients to clinical attention. Whether you make a separate diagnosis of personality change in the context of a dementia is a matter of judgment; you might if the personality change is obvious and clinically important, as when a patient becomes markedly hostile toward minorities or loses sexual inhibitions.

Here are a couple of additional points in the differential diagnosis of dementia. Patients with schizophrenia can have difficulty thinking (recall that the old name for schizophrenia was dementia praecox, because of its early onset)—either in the acute throes of an episode or after months or years of illness—and many demented patients develop delusions or hallucinations. The age of onset, the presence or absence of a medical cause, and the fact that demented patients usually don't become psychotic until well along in the course of their disease should clarify the differential. Although the cognitive functioning of people with mental retardation is subnormal, there should hardly ever be confusion with dementia, which begins far later in life and involves *deterioration* of cognitive ability rather than a relatively fixed, lifelong incapacity.

Curley

Some patients with serious cognitive difficulties at first appear quite intact. If you only spoke with them for a few minutes, you might not even realize there was something wrong.

"Oh, hi, come on in." With a big smile, the middle-aged man in hospital pajamas welcomed the small group into his room. The students knew that Curley had been a sailor for much of his adult life, but that drink and the devil had caught up with him at last. For nearly 5 years, a cognitive disorder had rendered him unable either to work or even to care for himself. The teacher challenged the students to guess—better, to reason—which cognitive disorder he had. "I'll give you a clue," the teacher finished, just before knocking at Curley's door. "He hasn't hit his head."

The teacher and Curley chatted for a few minutes. They seemed on pretty good terms, for they spoke about a number of things that touched the lives of each. Just when they seemed deep in conversation, the teacher led the group back out into the hallway. After a few minutes, he knocked at the door again, and all reentered.

"Hello! Come on in!" Curley beamed and started to shake hands all around.

"Do you remember these people?" the instructor asked, gesturing to the class.

Do I Need Scales?

Flounders and flutists require scales; for those at other evolutionary stages, the need is relative.

When I was in training, Rorschach inkblots and the Minnesota Multiphasic Personality Inventory represented the bulk of the tests available, and we used almost no scales at all. Then came the Beck and Hamilton depression inventories, and mental health was off to the races. Now you can find an objective measure for just about any aberration of thought, behavior, or emotion you can imagine. If you used them all, you'd spend most of your working life filling out scales.

Of course, if you're doing clinical research, scales provide the numbers with which you determine the effectiveness of your treatments. But most of them don't do much more than formalize the MSE. For many clinical tasks, we can accomplish about the same thing by asking our patients to rate their own discomfort or progress on a 10-point scale from "none" (or "very mild") to "maximum."

However, scales occasionally have great value. For example, many cognitively impaired patients cannot reliably judge how they are feeling, or how impaired they are. The Mini-Mental State Exam (MMSE) developed by Folstein and colleagues (and available as Appendix C of *DSM-IV Made Easy*) provides evidence of how these patients are doing, so that we can follow them over time.

"No, I don't think so—wait! It was last night, down in the piano lounge, wasn't it? We all had some drinks, right?" Curley rubbed his hands and looked thoughtful. "We were drinking Michelob." He continued to chat for a while, describing the band, the grumpy waitress, the beer that had gone a little flat. Nothing in his tone or facial expression suggested that he was putting them on.

Curley maintained good eye contact, and he seemed to focus well on the conversation. When the clinician recited a list of three objects, he immediately repeated them all flawlessly. Minutes later, he couldn't recall any of them.

Analysis

Although Curley's ability to retain new memories was at rock bottom, he could maintain his attention on the conversation, and he seemed perfectly aware of his surroundings as he entertained visitors. That carries us past step 1 of Figure 14.1. With no hint of depression, no head injury, and no recent alcohol intoxication (he'd been hospitalized for weeks), we can reject depression, alcohol blackout, and concussion (steps 2, 3, and 4). At step 5 we note that his difficulty was with learning new information, whereas patients with a dissociative disorder have difficulty recalling material that has already been learned. Step 6, a definite "yes," skips us along to step 11: Curley's cognitive functions other than memory seemed OK, encouraging us to consider the diagnosis of amnestic disorder. The diagnostic principle that substance use should always be considered is vindicated.

Comment

Let's first get past one misunderstanding. The criteria commonly used for amnestic disorder refer to impaired ability to learn new information *or* recall old information. But read the fine print: The problems with learning new material (anterograde amnesia) are always present, whereas trouble recalling past events is variable—recent past tends to be more affected than the remote past. The person's ability to recall material immediately after hearing it should be intact. If not, suspect instead a problem with attention, possibly due to delirium, in which case you wouldn't diagnose amnestic disorder.

What sets amnestic disorder apart from dementia is the relative lack of other cognitive problems: *agnosia* (difficulty recognizing the meaning of stimuli, including people, objects, and spatial relationships); *aphasia* (problems understanding or using language); *apraxia* (inability to perform voluntary motor acts, despite having neither paralysis nor sensory deficit); and problems with *executive functioning* (the planning, problem solving, and perseverance needed to pursue a task). I have used the word *relative* just above, because there isn't always a sharp line between dementia and amnestic disorder. Although Curley had no obvious defect of language symbolism or motor behavior, testing might have revealed more subtle difficulties with planning or carrying out complex behaviors if he had to prepare his own food, shop, and so forth. The take-home message: Amnestic disorder's defining feature is a profound inability to form new memories.

Amnestic disorder is caused by damage within the brain's limbic system—the structure responsible for new learning that lies curled beneath the cerebral cortex, somewhat like a hand clutching a golf ball. The damage is done by thiamine deficiency or oxygen deprivation, perhaps due to carbon monoxide poisoning or surgical misadventure, or any number of the other usual suspects: traumatic brain injury, strokes, tumors, alcohol, or sedative/hypnotics such as benzodiazepines and barbiturates.

When Curley told those stories about drinking in the bar the night before, he was trying to compensate for some of the holes in his memory; perhaps they worried him. In any event, such behavior, called *confabulation*, isn't lying (Curley believed what he said), and it isn't delusional (it tends to come and go, evoked by the needs of the moment). Confabulation isn't specific to the amnestic disorders. Probably caused by frontal lobe brain damage, it is just a way that people who cannot remember things sometimes paper over their difficulties. With time, it tends to melt away. Indeed, for some patients whose limbic systems are only temporarily (so to speak) out on a limb, memory may gradually return if they embrace good nutrition and avoid the drugs or alcohol that initially caused the amnesia.

Other Cognitive Disorders and Comorbidity

Making a diagnosis when there are symptoms of only one disorder can be relatively easy. It is at least as easy to make the wrong diagnosis when a patient has symptoms and signs of more than one illness. Then the differential diagnosis and the decision tree serve an especially vital function, though you need familiarity with the features of both (or all) diagnoses.

Aunt Betty

A few weeks before Betty's 80th birthday, her niece, Gail, brought her to a family practitioner for an evaluation. Betty had lived with her older brother until his death a month earlier. Almost from that day, she had been "failing," had lost interest in her hobby (she loved to decorate cakes), and had complained that she "just couldn't do anything any more." The doctor talked to her for a few minutes, asked her the date (she said she didn't know) and the name of his long-time nurse (she didn't respond); and prescribed 5 mg/day of donepezil. She was becoming senile, he told Gail. The medication, specific for Alzheimer's dementia, might help to slow it, though nothing could alter the eventual outcome. Because Betty also complained bitterly of feeling sad, she was started on amitriptyline 50 mg at bedtime.

Over the next 3 weeks, things went from bad to worse. Aunt Betty retreated even further into herself; several times her niece found her lying on her bed, crying. She neglected her appearance and needed help tying the high-top, lace-up shoes she had worn since she was a teenager. Because she was still having trouble getting to sleep, her doctor doubled the antidepressant. Gail learned that the troubles with buttons and shoes were *apraxias*, symptoms of increasing dementia. A fortnight later, Betty was still sleepless, but now she was also agitated—plucking at her clothing, mumbling something about beetles and wasps, and unable to give coherent answers to questions.

That afternoon, Gail checked Betty into the mental health clinic for a second opinion. There, after 2 hours of assessment and after consultation with her family practitioner, she was taken off all of her medications. Three days later, a calmer Aunt Betty was examined again. At first she had a hard time with the MMSE, several times stating that she couldn't do the task, but with the clinician's patience and encouragement she eventually scored 26 out of 30. When asked if she could tie her shoe, she again claimed at first that she couldn't do it. With encouragement, however, she managed just fine.

Analysis

As with Bobby, we need to consider Betty's diagnosis at several points in time. "But," you might argue, "with any patient, what we want to know is the diagnosis *now*." Very true, but that often means sifting through information that hails from different time periods and may indicate different diagnoses. Nowhere is this more true than for someone who has symptoms of both dementia and depression.

When she came to the mental health clinic, Betty's condition had deteriorated. Her loss of concentration and her problems with language (mumbling) and perception (picking bugs off her clothing) strongly suggest a delirium (step 1 of Figure 14.1), which was probably due to the amitriptyline—a tricyclic antidepressant notorious for this complication in elderly patients. But what about her diagnosis just before she was treated? For that, we need another quick trip to the tree—where step 2 warns us to give precedence to the depression (of which she had many symptoms) and to consider that her symptoms might indicate a pseudodementia.

Off medication, Betty's delirium improved. By this time, her depression had continued longer than her clinicians would expect for uncomplicated bereavement, and she was started on an SSRI. Within a few weeks, she was once again cheerfully decorating cakes for her neighbors. Her final diagnosis was major depressive disorder.

Comment

Pseudodementia is a slight misnomer: The dementia is real, though it's reversible. It is a diagnosis that is often made only in retrospect—a great tragedy if some other dementia is diagnosed by error. Because dementia resides at or near the bottom of the safety hierarchy, it is vital to defer this diagnosis until all the data are in.

Depressive pseudodementia is rather common; it occurs in perhaps 10% of demented older patients, by one estimate. They may complain of memory loss (not typical of most dementias) and may even emphasize it, while tests show no signs. They may be distractible, may be slow to respond to stimuli, and may have short attention spans. "I don't know" and "Can't remember" responses are common, though it isn't clear whether such answers are found more often in depressive pseudodementia than in other forms of dementia. Risk factors for pseudodementia include a previous history of clinical mood disorder, recent bereavement, and family history of mood disorder. Therefore, getting information from relatives can be enormously helpful in making the diagnosis. The onset is relatively rapid (weeks or a few months), and patients complain of guilt, suicidal ideas, vegetative symptoms, and poor memory. Patients with pseudodementia are especially prone to problems with decreased libido, early morning awakening, and anxiety, whereas demented patients will have more disorientation to time, trouble finding their way around the streets, and problems dressing. Table 14.2 lists some of the other features that can help discriminate dementia from depression.

TABLE 14.2. **Features of Dementia Versus Depression with Pseudodementia**

	Dementia	Pseudodementia
Onset	Months–years	Weeks–months
Time of day when illness tends to be worse	Evening	Morning
EEG, brain scans	Abnormal	Normal
Family history of mood disorder	Less likely	More likely
Past personal history of depression	Less often	More often
Social skills intact	No	Yes
Self-blame	No	Yes
Shows concern or distress	No	Yes
Makes good effort at tasks	Yes	No
Cognitive disability	Hides	Emphasizes
Memory improves with coaching	No	Yes
Orientation intact	No	Variable

An even more difficult conundrum is the patient who has both an organic ("real") dementia and clinical depression. This will often be the case; perhaps 10–20% of demented people have some degree of depression. You might recognize depression in a demented person on the basis of a rapid decline with precipitous loss of interest, vegetative symptoms (such as insomnia, appetite and weight loss), ideas of worthlessness, and psychomotor slowing that is even greater than that in organic dementia.

There's a moral here: Depression and dementia aren't mutually exclusive; we must pursue each one independently. An older patient who has symptoms of either depression or dementia should be screened for both. You need to search for symptoms of depression, even in the face of cognitive disorder.

Wilma

The following vignette illustrates how important it is to ask carefully about each patient's history of medical problems, including illnesses, operations, allergies, and injuries.

When Wilma finally saw her doctor, she had been suffering for several weeks, and her mother had been suffering right along with her. Wilma complained that she couldn't sleep, and when she arose in the morning, she was almost unbearably grouchy. "It's a real change for her," said her mother with a sigh. "For her first 17 years, she was the sweetest-tempered thing you could imagine. All my friends with teenage daughters were envious. Now *I'm* the envious one—you'd think she'd had a personality transplant."

For Wilma, the main difficulty was headache, which bothered her pretty much the whole day. Combined with the dizziness and persistent tiredness, it was trashing her concentration for schoolwork. She was sure she wasn't depressed; they'd studied that in the health class she'd taken the previous semester. However, her memory had been "pretty bummed—I couldn't even remember my teacher's name when I went for my piano lesson."

"Have you had any other problems with your health?" the mental health clinician wanted to know.

She had. Several months earlier, against her mother's wishes, Wilma had gone motorcycle riding with her boyfriend—Frank, that was it. She had done so before and knew he was a safe driver, but they hadn't reckoned on the patch of black ice at the sharp curve on the mountain road. She'd worn a helmet, but not Frank, an enthusiastic member of the local anti-helmet-law association. He wouldn't be attending meetings for a while, she agreed, at least until he emerged from his coma.

After the crash, Wilma had been unconscious for nearly an hour. She never could recall riding with Frank that day, and her memories of waking up on the gurney, unsure where she was, were forever tinged with feelings of nausea.

Analysis

If only her mother's initial impressions had been considered, Wilma might have been subjected to a battery of personality tests. Fortunately, her clinician recognized the need for a complete history. Because we don't think that Wilma had a severe depression, and she wasn't currently delirious (though she could have been immediately after the accident), we can quickly bypass steps 1–3. That brings us to the all-important step 4, which encourages us to consider a diagnosis of postconcussional disorder.

Comment

About 5% of adults report a lifetime history of concussion—a blow to the brain that results in unconsciousness or other dysfunction. Mostly the damage is to the frontal lobes, caused when the front of the brain slams against the inside of its hard protective carrying case. Motor vehicle accidents account for a large percentage, but it is also found in football players, shaken babies, and people who fall from ladders. The vast majority of concussions are mild—a brief lapse of awareness or a passing state of altered consciousness when things just don't seem right (the stars and planets of the cartoon pratfall).

Concussion almost always produces some degree of amnesia, though it may last only moments. Generally, the return to normal is rapid and complete. Many people aren't even hospitalized; those who are may be off work for a few days, with the vast majority back in 3 months. But for weeks or months, a few will continue to have symptoms that constitute postconcussional disorder. Although it hasn't yet been given the full sanction of recognition, I think it will be; there are an awful lot of sufferers out there. They all have problems with memory or attention, often accompanied by headache, nausea, dizziness, and tiredness. Apathy, insomnia, irritability, anxiety and (rarely) psychosis can occur. Personality change may be rather mild, like Wilma's, but increased sexuality or other socially inappropriate behavior may also occur. Unlike Wilma, 20% or more experience depression, especially if they use alcohol or drugs, haven't had much education, or have an unstable preinjury work history. If the depression is severe enough to diagnose independently, regard it as you would any other mood disorder.

Postconcussional disorder usually resolves spontaneously. After 3 months of continuing symptoms, we would need to worry about a possible subdural hematoma. Of course, the other cognitive disorder in the differential list is dementia, which requires the severe injury of motor vehicle accidents or boxing and usually includes neurological abnormalities such as hemiplegia or aphasia.

Cognitive Problems That Are Not Disorders

Usually, differential diagnosis is a matter of deciding among competing illnesses. We sometimes forget to consider another important boundary.

Reggie

Not long after Ronald Reagan's 1994 announcement that he was entering "the journey that will lead me into the sunset of my life," Reggie went to see his family practitioner. "I've noticed some things that worry me," he announced. "A lot. I'm afraid I could be getting Alzheimer's."

Although he'd had a raise and advancement to a new level of responsibility just a couple of months earlier, at 63 he was secretly planning to retire the following year. Reggie admitted that he had begun to slow down a bit. "A lot," he corrected himself.

He had always been a little forgetful of where he had put things. But now it seemed to happen more often. When he was deep in thought about his work, it sometimes took a moment or two to shift gears after an interruption, and it also seemed to take him forever to dredge up the names of people he'd known for years. "My wife says I'm as sharp as ever," he conceded, "but she could be just trying to, um . . . " He broke off, searching for the word he wanted.

"Reassure you?" offered the interviewer.

"That's it. You see, that's what I've been experiencing for months."

Although Reggie felt "pretty anxious" at times about his memory, he'd had no panic attacks, and he denied depression or worry related to other issues. Aside from the indignities of getting older, his health had always been good and he'd had no injuries. He did drink a glass of wine nearly every day "to help keep up the good cholesterol." A physical exam was completely normal, and he scored a perfect 30 on the MMSE.

Analysis

Mental health professionals would be likely to suspect a disorder of depression or anxiety, but trips with Reggie through Figures 11.1 and 12.1 prove pretty fruitless. And so it would seem at first with Figure 14.1: Reggie showed no evidence of fluctuating levels of consciousness that would suggest a delirium, no depression, and no evidence of either head injury or alcohol misuse. Of course, his clinician should attempt to obtain collateral information on each of these points, but he would seem to be all clear through step 4. His memory lapses didn't rise to the level of amnesia, and they weren't limited to personal information. In fact, we wouldn't say that he had much of any problem learning new information. With no history of mental stressors (absent the aging process itself, I can promise you), we're just about out of options at step 8. The results of the MMSE were comforting, and with his age and history, Reggie's doctor would have the information necessary to offer the simple reassurance necessary: nothing more than ARCD, mentioned earlier in this chapter. In other words, we've just applied the diagnostic principle encouraging us to consider that a person we are evaluating might just be normal (see the sidebar "How Many Ways Can We Say Normal?").

Comment

ARCD sounds worse than it is. It doesn't even involve, to any important degree, multiple areas of our thinking mechanism. The ability to recognize people and objects, to identify concepts, to perform motor functions, to use language—all these important areas are preserved. The main difficulty is that as we age, and regardless of how smart or how educated we are, the rate at which we process information tends to flag.

ARCD is a statement of normality. Because it isn't a disorder, there can be no criteria; it is a diagnosis of exclusion. You must rule out everything else by taking into consideration not only the person's age, but lifelong capacities, educational achievement, general health status, and culture. Here's the good news: It means that nothing is really wrong, and that the person isn't necessarily headed for senescence. Here's the bad news: It probably won't improve, and it may get worse.

Jen

Some symptoms point the way to a mental health diagnosis; others do not. In determining which is which, we must evaluate all symptoms in the context of the total patient. Loss of memory is such a symptom. We must take care not to jump to conclusions about its importance.

> The phone call that morning was peremptory: "You've got to fit her in today—she's beside herself." That was Jen's mother. When she'd entered Jen's room that morning, she had found her sobbing. "She thinks she's destroyed her mind."
>
> Jen was just 19, a sophomore at an Eastern university that had only recently begun admitting women. She lived at home, but recently had stayed many nights with friends on campus—female friends, her mother had hoped. The previous night, however, Jen had attended an off-campus party thrown by a student she hardly knew. The mob of young people had consumed oceans of alcohol, both beer and hard liquor. Jen had just come off a punishing week of final exams, and, "ready to party," she'd downed several drinks within minutes of arrival. That was almost the last thing

How Many Ways Can We Say Normal?

ARCD is one way of saying *normal*, in the context of a patient's complaint that something seems abnormal. As mental health professionals, we face this sort of situation every day, but how often do we realize it?

Too frequently when we evaluate patients for psychological complaints, we feel obliged to "give them their money's worth"—in short, to make a diagnosis. It is better, and far more satisfying, to tell someone straight out, "There's nothing really wrong with you. You have a problem that we can work on together, but your mental health is fundamentally sound." Of course, we can always let it go at "no mental diagnosis," but that wastes information and does an injustice to the myriad people who come to us every day with problems of living. There are better ways.

A number of situations qualify as troubled but normal. Take relational problems, for example, in which members of a unit have trouble getting along with one another. Of course, the cause could be someone's mental illness, but many relational problems exist wholly without any diagnosable mental pathology. The relationships affected are about as varied as you can imagine: child–parent, friend, sibling, spousal, employee–supervisor, workmates. Another normal, if troubled, state is bereavement, a reaction to the death of someone we love. I've discussed it in Chapter 11 (page 160).

A couple of other terms that indicate normality are less benign. *Borderline intellectual functioning* indicates an IQ somewhere south of the mid-80s, though outside the range of mental retardation and without the problems of living typically encountered by developmentally disabled individuals. *Malingering*, a dangerous term I rarely use, identifies individuals who intentionally concoct or exaggerate symptoms either to avoid something (work, punishment, or military service) or to obtain something (usually drugs or money, as from lawsuits). Such tangible motives are quite different from those of patients with *factitious disorder*, who will feign illness in order to receive medical care. I wouldn't dignify malingering by calling it normal, but neither is it a mental disorder.

For otherwise normal persons with academic, occupational, spiritual, or identity problems, or with difficulty in acclimatizing themselves to a different culture, you can use one of those terms (with *problem* tacked on) to give a label that doesn't carry the stigma of an actual mental disorder. For example, someone who's troubled by doubts about the choice of a career might be described as having an *academic problem*. Finally, there's even a diagnosis for criminals who don't qualify for a personality disorder or other diagnosis: *adult antisocial behavior*. Think Tony Soprano.

she remembered until the next morning, when she awoke, naked and incredibly hung over, in a strange bed with a strange man and an even stranger woman. "I've never done anything like that before," Jen cried when she spoke with the therapist. "I know you can damage your brain with alcohol. I read about it in the psychology class I took last semester."

She hadn't felt depressed or anxious before, "but I sure am now." Jen also didn't think she had hit her head; though it hurt like hell, she couldn't feel any lumps or tenderness. She scored a perfect 30 on the MMSE, and apart from the crying, everything else about her seemed unremarkable.

Jen admitted that she was "pretty upset" by what she might have done while intoxicated: "I've had some experience, but I'm always safe. And discriminating, I always thought." She cried some more, then added, "I'm just so scared I've done something really awful to my brain."

Analysis

Jen's clinician would have to make sure that she hadn't sustained a concussion—common enough in alcoholism, but something to think about in anyone who has suffered a period of amnesia. Her MMSE and her focused attention during the interview ruled out delirium, and there was no evidence of dementia or a depression so deep as to suggest pseudodementia. In fact, the history fixes the diagnosis as an alcohol-induced blackout (step 3 of Figure 14.1). Although not an actual mental disorder, blackout is a rather commonplace experience that sometimes requires clinical evaluation.

Before leaving the figure, drop down to step 5. Could Jen's experience have been a dissociative phenomenon that was anxiety-driven? On the surface, this might seem to fit the definition of dissociative amnesia, but we must rule out more obvious, physical causes first before falling back on what some clinicians consider a faith-based diagnosis (see the next section).

Comment

While blacked out, a person may continue to behave quite normally; it's just that the following day, when the person is sober, little or no memory of behavior remains. People who experience blackouts are reported to engage in a wide range of activities during them, including events as banal as ordinary conversations, as dangerous as driving, and as intrinsically memorable as sexual intercourse. Blackouts result from the effects of alcohol on the region of the limbic system (see page 222) called the hippocampus. Though established memories remain unaffected, the formation of new memories is blocked. Blackouts can be partial or total; the greater the alcohol consumption, especially within a short period of time, the more severely is memory impaired. However, there is no evidence that an isolated blackout implies anything permanently wrong.

When I was in school, we were taught that blackouts were symptomatic of alcoholism, but in recent decades science has determined otherwise. In fact, studies now find that they are common among those who drink socially, even among those drinking for the first time. Perhaps 40% of college students who drink at all have had at least one blackout related to alcohol use. Women may be especially vulnerable to them; a strong minority of young people who drink (especially women) are frightened enough by blackouts that they change their drinking behavior. And that's not a bad thing: Despite their apparent benignity, blackouts can foreshadow later difficulties with alcohol, and so Jen's experience should serve her as a literal wake-up call to reevaluate her recreational choices.

Amnesia and Dissociation

Dissociation is a break in the connection between mental processes that are normally found together. The result is an abrupt, though usually temporary, change in the person's awareness, behavior, or identity, often with amnesia for the episode once it has ended. My dictionary gives *amnesia* as a synonym for forgetfulness or loss of memory. Of course, there is also loss of memory in dementia, but then the defect is global and usually permanent. The amnesia of dissociation implies a gap that, like our hopes for the pothole at the corner, will one day be filled in. Indeed, this is the usual outcome of dissociation—temporary loss of memory that will recover within a period of days or weeks.

Quite frankly, I struggled for days about how to present this topic. Here is my quandary with this set of vexed diagnoses: Dissociation is nearly everywhere, yet it is almost nowhere. It is everywhere, in that it embraces the normal, everyday experiences we all have had, such as daydreaming or becoming so immersed in a magazine article or television program that we lose track of time. Hypnosis is a sort of dissociation often used to assist the treatment of surgical, dental, medical, and psychotherapy patients. Abnormal dissociation, on the other hand, has been identified in the affective blunting of schizophrenia and the numbing of sensation that patients with PTSD develop toward their traumatic experiences. It is also found free-standing, as in *depersonalization* (the sensation of being detached from your body) and *derealization* (the feeling that the world has changed or is not real).

Yet dissociation is also nowhere—almost. In over 30 years as a psychiatrist, I have rarely encountered someone with an unequivocal dissociative disorder. Some writers question the value of these disorders, which they claim cannot be reliably diagnosed and may be manufactured by credulous enthusiasts. Large series of dissociative patients tend to collect in centers that specialize in their treatment or in the clinics of individual practitioners who have written extensively about them. Like everyone else, clinicians tend to find what they expect.

It can be hard indeed to resist the allure of the fascinating diagnosis. An attractive patient who wanders into urgent care, suddenly unable to remember vital material from the past, is ready-made for drama. The patient may be highly suggestible; perhaps there is a history of stress-induced pathology. Precipitated by physical, sexual, or other emotional trauma, the amnesia wipes out recall of specific events or time periods, whereas new learning is unaffected. The amnesia often departs as suddenly as it began—the happy Hollywood ending.

It is clear to me that, as outlined in Figure 14.1, some patients do lose memory functions temporarily due to dissociative disorders, but many clinicians have only read about them. In 2006 *The New Yorker* profiled such a patient, Doug Bruce, who after 2 years had still not regained his memory. Recent studies have reported that these patients may be underdiagnosed among mental health and general medical patients, and so I have mentioned the categories here. But scrutinize your data and your conclusions with a gimlet eye.

Because few patients spontaneously report dissociative experiences, clinicians must ask: "Have you found yourself someplace and not known how you got there? Have you ever not recognized family or friends? Been unable to recall a span of your childhood or adult life? What about finding unfamiliar items among your belongings, or documents you must have written but cannot remember?" Of course, this line of questioning risks suggesting symptoms to susceptible people. Carrying the error a step further, clinicians sometimes identify dissociation and then try to persuade the patient that abuse, which theoretically caused it, occurred during childhood.

At least one authority advises ensuring that the patient's symptoms are genuine as a first diagnostic step. (Remember Tony [Chapter 4, page

36], the patient known for periodically being at odds with the truth, who claimed to have experienced a fugue state.) Although I hate to diagnose malingering, it is only right to point out that amnesia is the mental illness symptom most often malingered. You might want to review what I've written about it in Chapter 4. Oh, yes, and no one—well, hardly anyone—ever thinks to check the patient for somatization disorder.

15 Diagnosing Substance Misuse and Other Addictions

Let me get something off my chest. We are sometimes warned against the term *addiction*, because it doesn't have a scientific definition. Although this is true, the same can be said for so much of the mental health nomenclature that if we were to avoid all inexact terms, we'd find ourselves essentially tongue-tied. Depression, paranoia, phobia, anxiety, mania, schizophrenia—on the street and in the popular press, all have meanings rather different from their strict scientific usage.

The word *addiction* comes down from Roman law, where it meant "surrender to a master." How appropriate to use such a term for the behaviors we associate today with substance misuse and other compulsions! This compact word conveys a clear sense of loss of control and harm to the individual and to society. Other than lack of scientific rigor, its principal drawback is a connotation of reproach that we in the mental health field would rather avoid. (*Habit,* a term applied to the use of addictive drugs for over 100 years, has never been much favored by professionals, either.)

Substance Misuse

Dependence, which has appeared in the context of substance misuse only since the late 1960s, includes two principal features:

1. The person will be affected physiologically. This means that the drinking or other substance use has been heavy and prolonged enough to cause *tolerance,* which is the need for an increasing amount to satisfy craving, or *withdrawal,* in which symptoms develop when the person abruptly decreases its intake. Sometimes there is both tolerance and withdrawal.

2. Loss of control is the other constant feature of dependence. It is shown by using more than the person intends, repeated failure to control the use, preferring use to important activities such as family life, and persistent use despite the knowledge that it is harmful.

Although craving is not mentioned in official criteria, it is nonetheless an important part of the substance use experience. I wouldn't get too hung up over the exact number of criteria a person needs for dependence, because it has been found that so-called diagnostic orphans (those who have some symptoms of dependence, but not enough to meet full criteria) are likely to have substance use problems later on. Nor do I generally belabor the distinction made in the DSMs between substance dependence and substance abuse, except that it is necessary for an official diagnosis and is sometimes useful in deciding on a course of treatment (see the sidebar "What about Substance *Abuse?*" on page 239).

Samuel

How we assess substance dependence is based on two sorts of criteria—the loss of control, and the consequences of use (including social, legal, financial, work, family, and physical/medical). Even though our current diagnostic tools have been forged in comparatively recent times, with them we can mine the past to illuminate the perils of the present.

Every student of English literature knows that as a young man, Samuel Taylor Coleridge wrote "The Rime of the Ancient Mariner." Somewhat less well known is that his personal history traces the route of an almost lifelong dependence on opium.

In the waning years of the 18th century, when Samuel's use began, morphine, codeine, and heroin had not been derived, and opium was usually swallowed in an alcohol tincture called *laudanum*. Samuel used this intermittently from his mid-20s, to enable sleep and ease both worry and pain. At that time the concept of addiction was unknown, and anyone with a few shillings could readily purchase narcotics without prescription from a pharmacist. As an all-purpose remedy for homesickness, exhaustion, and the stress of public performance, Samuel used up to a pint of laudanum per day—a whopping amount by the standards of any era. He also consumed large amounts of alcohol.

Samuel's first serious addiction to opium arose in his late 20s. Although he composed his mystical poem "Kubla Khan" largely while under the influence of laudanum, on balance the drug caused him to spend far more time daydreaming of literary glory than working to attain it.

The physical symptoms that result from using opium are numerous and well documented. For Samuel, one of the worst was constipation—"violent stomach pains and humiliating flatulence" that caused him agony. For relief, he would resort time and again to enemas and other embarrassments that he regarded as punishment for his vice. With his mood swinging from elation to despair, he would awaken screaming from terrifying dreams. During a sea voyage, he hallucinated "yellow faces" in the curtain around his bunk, and he had the illusion that the flapping sails were fish flopping about on deck.

In his notebooks, he also noted symptoms that we recognize today as withdrawal: joint pains, sweating brow, "windy sickness at the stomach," diarrhea, fever, and despair. However many times he promised himself that he would quit, in the end he always returned to opium's "hideous bondage" (in the words of one friend), which left him brooding, lying, and neglecting his work and family. Guilt made him try to conceal the amount he used. In later life he wrote self-pitying letters to friends, whom he accused of misunderstanding him, and he suffered from depression that would suddenly well up and overwhelm him. At one time, he entertained ideas of suicide.

In later years, Samuel's usage was eventually controlled when a physician put him on a prescription, but he sought an additional supply anyway. His druggist allowed him this—but in amounts so tiny that he could live and once again even work effectively.

Analysis

With a little effort, we can compare the symptoms Samuel showed over 200 years ago to today's criteria for substance use disorders. In Table 9.3, you'll note the symptoms of intoxication Samuel recorded. Next, we'll use the definition of dependence provided at the beginning of the chapter to verify that he was in fact dependent on opium. From the amount of laudanum he consumed, we know that he tolerated quantities far greater than an individual unaccustomed to its use could have handled, and of course he suffered severely from withdrawal symptoms. His use began when he was a young man and persisted throughout his life; along the way, we can find ample evidence of lack of control. From his own notes and letters, we can see how he craved the drug; he used it despite the evidence of its physical effects, allowed it to displace his work and social responsibilities, and continued using it despite repeated efforts to curtail its use. Even at over two centuries' remove, he fully meets modern criteria for opioid dependence.

The use of multiple substances is common, and today, after a suitable in-depth interview, Samuel would probably be diagnosed as having both opioid and alcohol dependence. But should we also diagnose a mood disorder? The profound gloom he experienced from time to time was severe enough that he had suicidal ideas; yet, because it seems entirely consequent to his use of opium, I wouldn't call it an independent mental disorder (shaved by Occam's razor). Instead, Figure 11.1 points us to a step 3 diagnosis of substance-induced depression.

Comment

One problem with assessment of substance misuse is the reliability of the informant, as with Samuel, who worked hard to hide the true extent of his addiction. Here's where the diagnostic principle regarding collateral history is especially useful. I always want to trust my patients, but whenever I know that one may be tempted to defer, shade, or otherwise alter the truth, I look for help from informants who care about the patient and from objective measures such as laboratory tests. These are luxuries that were not available 200 years ago.

Substance misuse is often the story of comorbidity. Various studies have found that a third to a half of those who use substances have another mental diagnosis, whereas nearly 30% of patients with other mental disorders meet criteria at one time or another for a substance use disorder. Samuel's depression was related to his substance use, which is the usual case. In fact, nearly every class of mental disorder you can think of is more common in a substance-dependent person. Only infrequently, however, is the disorder one that they would have suffered anyway, regardless of their experience with alcohol or drugs. But these secondary disorders can closely mimic independent mental or emotional illnesses. In most cases, with time and abstinence, the secondary symptoms will abate.

Chuck

In the throes of evaluating substance use, it can be very difficult to decide whether a person's symptoms are all pursuant to the substance or indicate another, independent disorder. If the former, they should disappear once the addiction, dependence, or abuse has been brought under control.

At 38, Chuck sought care because of depression. "Life isn't very good, Doc," was his chief complaint. A tradesman who made good money when he worked, often Chuck didn't. Between marriages once again, he lived with his girlfriend. Although June was the financial mainstay of their little household, she was a bartender who too often tasted her own wares. June had sent along a note in a sealed envelope that bore evidence of clumsy steaming and resealing; she complained in it that with Chuck she had had little or no sex. He admitted that he had read a lot about alcohol and sexual problems; he tried Viagra, but realized that drinking had clobbered his sex drive. "Something to do with testosterone levels, Doc," he informed me. "You can read about it on the 'net at . . ." From memory, he recited a URL full of dots and slashes.

What about Substance *Abuse*?

Substance abuse is an official category of misuse that huddles uncomfortably between casual (recreational) usage and outright dependence. It isn't exactly addiction; the person remains in control of the amount consumed, with no compulsion to use and no physiological symptoms that suggest tolerance or withdrawal. But there will be *recurring* problems, nonetheless. These relate to dangerousness (use while driving and operating heavy machinery are the prime examples) and social difficulties such as disruption of interpersonal relationships (use despite the objections of family or friends). Persons with substance abuse may also have legal peccadilloes such as arrests for driving under the influence, and they'll use instead of fulfilling important personal obligations, leading to poor work performance, absences from school, or neglect of housekeeping or child care duties.

It doesn't take all that much effort to earn a substance abuse diagnosis. Within a year, a person must have had at least two instances of problematic use, which could be the same problem repeated. And the person must *never* have had enough problems with that substance to be diagnosed as dependent. So defined, nearly half of those with substance abuse, according to one study, continued to have some symptoms of drug involvement; a few of these individuals went on to develop substance dependence.

In this chapter, I tend not to emphasize the official terms. Either *dependence* or *abuse* suggests that a person uses more than is good—for the individual or for society. The principal advantage of the distinction is that it helps identify those patients who may need more vigorous and varied approaches to problematic behavior.

Over the years, I've treated a lot of smart patients, but Chuck is the only one who'd actually passed the test and joined Mensa. However, he had never finished high school; after some suspensions (two for theft and one for assault on a teacher), he'd been kicked out, and he said the Mensa card made him feel that he "had substance." After leaving school, he kicked around quite a lot, and then washed out of the Army after setting a boot camp record for going AWOL. Next he tried his hand at violent crime. Though he was pretty good at planning, he wasn't so good at execution. After he and a partner robbed a 7-Eleven that netted them $84 and several 6-packs, they were nabbed just around the corner as they consumed the proceeds of their evening's work. After his release from prison, he wrote a few bad checks and ripped off several employers for some valuable tools, but for none of this was he ever caught.

By this time Chuck was 27, and his drinking, which had started during his brief Army career, had picked up speed. He was downing nearly a 12-pack of beer each evening, and he carried that practice to a series of jobs, none of which lasted longer than a month or two. Then he got married—twice, without bothering about a divorce in between. His first wife's complaints of nonsupport led to information about his other activities, which landed him "back in the can" for another few months. But with his second marriage came a dowry of sorts—a father-in-law who was a big official in the union for one of the construction trades. After a brief apprenticeship, Chuck seemed set for life with a job that paid well and carried enormous benefits. Currently, however, he was drinking more than he was working—at anything; even June was complaining.

Chuck told me that the feelings of depression had come on gradually, worsening over the past half year or so. Fueled by his drinking, he fought with June "whenever I was sober enough," and his appetite was almost nil. His weight had begun to drop, and his sleep had long since gone south.

After an especially hard drinking bout that lasted many weeks, Chuck needed hospitalization. During the admission process, he was unsteady on his feet and even had trouble writing his name. "I'm fine, I'm just terrific," he kept saying, but he slurred his words in a way that said he wasn't really. The next morning on rounds, I was sure of it. After a sleepless night, Chuck's problem with coordination had progressed to a coarse tremor that made him grip his juice glass with both hands.

By the following day, he was in full-blown withdrawal—sweating, pacing (when he wasn't falling down), and vomiting. He also complained about tiny cats "the size of mice" that wore bells and off and on danced on the sill of his window. He thought that he was in a lock-down at the county jail. While still recovering, he talked about another time he'd been like this, when he was jailed after assaulting an undercover federal narcotics officer who was trying to track a suitcase full of powdered cocaine. "Do I have any regrets? Sure, I'm real sorry I got caught. Or 'really,' as we say in Mensa. But I don't feel guilty, if that's what you mean. Guilt is for suckers."

Analysis

In addition to his drinking and problems with the law, Chuck had three mental problems that requiring analysis—depression, psychosis, and disorientation. Figures 11.1, 13.1, and 14.1 direct us to consider a disorder induced by substances. That would square with some of what we know about alcoholism: People who drink heavily often have depression, and alcohol-dependent individuals in the throes of withdrawal will sometimes suffer from delirium tremens, during which they become disoriented and have visual hallucinations. In the vast majority, the depression disappears once the drinking stops without further treatment. This was why, though I always give high priority to the diagnosis of depression, I elected not to treat Chuck for depression right away.

What about Chuck's criminal behavior, and what did it say about his personality structure? Whereas I'd hesitate to offer an early diagnosis for most personality disorders, antisocial personality disorder rests firmly on objective facts that can be obtained from those who know the patient well. Chuck's long history of difficulties with authority and the law (dating to his early teen years), along with his callous lack of guilt, provided a strong basis for this diagnosis.

All things considered, I'd list Chuck's various diagnoses in the order they needed to be treated:

Delirium due to alcohol withdrawal (delirium tremens)
Alcohol dependence
Depression due to alcohol use
Antisocial personality disorder

Because Chuck was in the middle of his withdrawal symptoms, listing the delirium first underscores the importance of focusing first on this potentially life-threatening condition. Because I believed that drinking had directly caused his depression, I felt that it should diminish once he got clear of alcohol.

Comment

Just over half of those who misuse alcohol, street drugs, or prescription medications will have one or more additional mental disorders. Some conditions are more or less independent, but often (perhaps usually), the substance use disorder will bring on depression, psychosis, or an anxiety disorder; as such, they are not *truly* comorbid, only co-occurring. (See the sidebar "Independent Mental Disorder or Substance-Related?" on page 244) We need to know which is which, because our treatment for mental disorders that arise only during substance use will be different than for those that arise independently. Outcome for the dependent disorders may be better or worse than for the independent ones, depending on how effectively we deal with the substance use itself.

Disorders Associated with Substance Misuse

Whether or not they represent independent diagnoses, some other disorders are commonly associated with substance use. Table 15.1 summarizes some of this discussion.

TABLE 15.1. Classes of Mental Disorders That Can Occur during Intoxication (I) or Withdrawal (W)

	Delirium	Dementia[a]	Psychosis	Mood	Anxiety
Alcohol	I/W	Yes	I/W	I/W	I/W
Amphetamines	I		I	I/W	I
Caffeine					I
Marijuana	I		I		I
Cocaine	I		I	I/W	I/W
Hallucinogens	I		I	I	I
Inhalants	I	Yes	I	I	I
Opioids	I		I	I	
Phencyclidine (PCP)	I		I	I	I
Sedatives	I/W	Yes	I/W	I/W	W

[a]Because dementia is associated with long-term, heavy substance use, it scores only a "yes."

• *Antisocial personality disorder.* This is one of the few co-occurring conditions that is *not* caused by the substance misuse. Over three-fourths of patients with antisocial personality disorder also misuse substances, and 10–20% of males and about 5% of females with alcoholism have this personality disorder. Some studies find that an especially heavy history of severe substance use carries a stronger likelihood of comorbidity, especially with antisocial personality disorder.

• *Cognitive disorders.* Delirium is found during intoxication with all substance groups except caffeine; alcohol and the sedatives also produce delirium upon withdrawal. A form of dementia can result from heavy and prolonged use of inhalants, and the amnestic disorder known as *Korsakov's psychosis* is classic for heavy, prolonged alcohol use with chronic thiamine insufficiency.

• *Psychosis.* You expect the hallucinogens to produce psychosis (sometimes delusional disorder), and they do; occasionally they produce prolonged visual disturbances that don't rise to the level of psychosis. These are flashbacks, during which the person will falsely perceive movement at the periphery of vision, or other visual distortions such as trails, geometric shapes, colors that are too intense ("over-Photoshopped," someone once put it), or objects appearing smaller or bigger than normal. When psychosis occurs with phencyclidine (PCP) use, it usually abates after a few hours; sometimes, however, patients will retain symptoms of catatonia or paranoid psychoses for weeks. Here are two problems that can complicate the diagnostic picture: (1) Some patients may not be aware that they've been given PCP; and (2) even if they know what they have ingested, others have no insight that their symptoms are caused by the drug. Over half of those who use amphetamine (especially methamphetamine) develop delusions, and some also have hallucinations. Too often, they become violent. Whereas about 3% of those with alcoholism experience psychosis during heavy drinking or withdrawal, marijuana rarely produces psychosis; it creates its mischief by worsening the symptoms of actual schizophrenia.

• *Depression.* Over 75% of individuals with alcoholism develop depression, the symptoms of which can mimic other clinical depressions. However, for the vast majority (about 95% of men, perhaps 75% of women) the depression improves rapidly after cessation of alcohol use. Mood disorder, especially depression, is also associated with most other drugs of misuse, including marijuana (dysthymia tends to predominate), opioids, and the hallucinogens. Depression also develops during withdrawal from amphetamine or cocaine.

• *Anxiety.* About three-fourths of those with alcoholism have panic attacks during withdrawal, and a social avoidance similar to agoraphobia is also common during first few weeks of sobriety. Panic attacks may also occur during withdrawal from sedative/hypnotics and intoxication with amphetamines. Marijuana users, especially novices, commonly experience panic attacks, and anxiety disorders are also associated with hallucinogen use.

• *Substance use.* No, I'm not being facetious. Although some individuals who use alcohol disdain other drugs, and vice versa, many patients are equal-opportunity users. Furthermore, we must always take great care to consider all of the "big four" drug sources: alcohol, street, prescription, and over-the counter.

Independent Mental Disorder or Substance-Related?

In deciding whether a patient's mental disorder is substance-related or independent, I consider several issues:

1. If the non-substance-related mental illness started first, I would lean heavily toward independence—that is, a disorder *not* caused by the substance use. Antisocial personality disorder, bipolar disorder, and schizophrenia are the conditions most likely to start before substance use.

2. If it isn't clear which started first, I'd apply the diagnostic principle concerning *undiagnosed* and use either that label or *NOS*, then carefully follow to see what happens once the substance use has been dealt with.

3. A substance-related mental disorder should diminish or disappear within a month. If the symptoms persist (perhaps even increase) after detoxification, I'd probably diagnose an independent mental disorder.

4. For an independent mental disorder, I like to see more symptoms rather than fewer, so as to fully meet (or exceed) diagnostic criteria for the illness in question.

5. I search for atypical symptoms. For example, the sudden onset of hallucinations, unusual for schizophrenia, suggests a psychosis cause that is related to other medical disorders or substance use. Visual, tactile, or olfactory hallucinations similarly suggest a nonschizophrenia psychosis.

Other Addictions

We tend to speak loosely and sometimes humorously of many behavioral addictions, among them eating chocolate, watching TV, and buying things on eBay. However, several disorders that involve difficulty controlling impulses to engage in harmful behavior bear striking similarities to substance misuse. Because few of them represent much of a diagnostic challenge, I'll discuss them here in less than excruciating detail.

Pathological Gambling

People who gamble to the point that they harm themselves and others will have symptoms resembling those of both substance dependence and substance abuse (in the strict diagnostic sense; see the sidebar "What about Substance *Abuse?*" on page 239). For example, symptoms like those of dependence can include the need to put increasing amounts of money into play (tolerance) and discomfort when attempting to stop gambling (withdrawal). Symptoms similar to substance abuse include illegal acts to obtain money for gambling and the disruption of personal relationships. Gambling is also one of the nonsubstance-related behaviors (another is overeating) that are often effectively managed through Twelve-Step programs.

Pyromania, Trichotillomania, Kleptomania

For hundreds of years, the Greek word *mania* ("madness") has been used to mean "to have a passion." For over 100 years, the term has been largely coopted for the "up" phase of bipolar I disorder, but the older usage survives in three contemporary behaviors that fulfill the general qualities of an addiction: pyromania (fire setting), trichotillomania (hair pulling), and kleptomania (stealing), each of which serves as a "master" to which the individual feels compelled to surrender. Often beginning in childhood or adolescence, these disorders entail behaviors that can become chronic and last well into adulthood. Despite the aspect of surrender, they are *ego-syntonic*. That is, they are carried out in accord with the person's conscious wishes—not in response to, for example, hallucinations.

Unlike gambling and substance misuse, these conditions are not defined by lists of behaviors that cause the person to run afoul of society. Instead, each behavior begins with a rising tension or excitement that finds release only as the match is struck, the hair strand tweaked, or the un-needed (and unpaid-for) item swept into a coat pocket. The tension may be described as "itching" of the scalp in hair pulling, restlessness, or a combi-nation of pleasure and fear (as in kleptomania).

All three disorders entail secrecy—two because they are illegal, the third because it causes the person to look funny and feel ashamed. How-ever, once you've twigged to the conduct, you're almost home; setting fires and stealing don't require much diagnostic finesse. What they do require is your attention to fistfuls of exceptions. The problem is that these two be-haviors are far more common outside the context of mental disorder. In fact, people who steal or set fires with other motives in mind may try to claim falsely that they suffer from the mental disorder. That's why we have to consider the rather long lists of circumstances in which the diagnoses should *not* be made. For pyromania, the fire setting must not be due to poor judgment (as in mental retardation, intoxication, or dementia) or done for profit, revenge, crime concealment, out of anger, or in response to psycho-sis. For kleptomania, the items must not be stolen in response to anger, delusions, or command hallucinations. In neither disorder can schizophre-nia, mania, or a personality disorder better explain the behavior. For trichotillomania, the restrictions are less severe, though the criterion of clinical distress/impaired functioning would exclude ordinary cosmetic eyebrow tweezing and depilation.

For consistency with the foregoing chapters of Part III, I provide a de-cision tree for a patient who has problems with addiction in Figure 15.1. However, you should have no particular trouble making these diagnoses. The greater diagnostic challenges, as I have described throughout this chapter, lie in determining the independent versus dependent status of co-occurring disorders (in the case of substance misuse) and in determining whether particular behaviors may be related to other disorders or motiva-tions altogether (in the case of some of the other addictions).

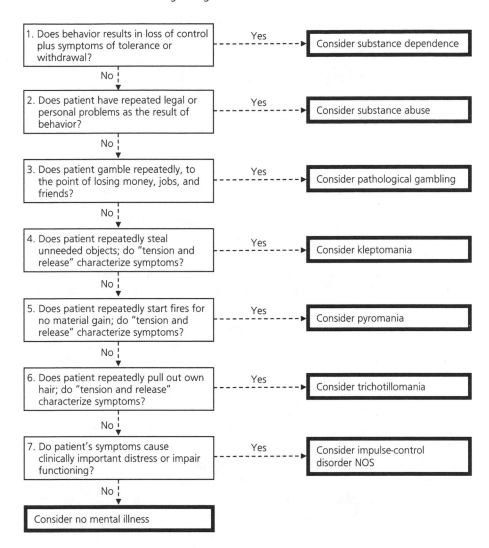

FIGURE 15.1. (Rather boring) decision tree for a patient who has problems with addiction.

16 Diagnosing Personality and Relationship Problems

Personality disorders (abbreviated in this chapter as PDs) primarily involve problems relating to oneself and to other people. They are lasting patterns that can show up in the realms of thought, feelings, behavior, and motivation; they affect interpersonal relationships and the control of impulses. Nearly 10% of the general population and about half of mental patients are said to have disordered personalities. In the latter, it will often seem an afterthought in someone whose main problem is a major Axis I mental disorder of the sort described in the preceding chapters of Part III. Your realization that a PD is present may only develop slowly, after several interviews with a given patient.

Unhappily, with this chapter we approach the limits of science and certainty as regards our ability to characterize and diagnose mental disorders accurately. Our current descriptions of PDs are categorical, which means that we count symptoms until we have enough to cry "Aha!" One result is that there is no limit to the number of personality types we might declare disordered. (At a lecture some years ago, an expert in the field claimed that there may be as many as 2,000 personality disorders. I later told him—in jest, of course—that any one who believed that must have "multiple personality disorder disorder.") Another result is that many patients qualify for two or more PDs; this confuses everyone. Perhaps the biggest problem of all is that categorical systems depend so heavily on interpretation that we are tempted to slip confusing patients into a convenient PD (some would say "wastebasket") category.

Other classification systems rate people along a handful of dimensions that attempt to measure how we regard ourselves and adapt to different circumstances. For example, the popular five-factor model uses the dimensions of neuroticism, extroversion, openness to experience, agreeableness, and conscientiousness. Other systems employ up to a score or more of dimensions. Dimensional models eliminate the possibility of multiple PDs for an individual, but they also increase the amount of effort needed to determine where anyone belongs on each of these ranges.

Defining a PD Diagnosis

Whereas most diagnoses represent a change in a person's usual thinking and behavior (the few exceptions are early childhood conditions such as autism, ADHD, and mental retardation), PDs start early and continue more or less forever. This fact requires a big shift in our diagnostic method. With most other disorders, we need to notice what has changed about a person; when discerning the pattern of a PD, however, we must instead pay attention to the lifelong background of attitudes and behaviors. We must tread carefully the path to diagnosis, scrupulously adhering to the several requirements for assessing PDs. Table 16.1 presents the differential diagnosis for PDs and other personality or relational problems.

Characteristics of PDs

- The symptoms of a PD must be present throughout the person's adult life, at least since late adolescence.

> Bruce was secretive, and in the half dozen years he'd lived just down the street from the crisis residential house, he seemed to be getting worse. His long hair was now unwashed and uncombed; his nails had grown long and dirty. No one liked him, especially the kids he repeatedly chased from his front yard, which was unfenced and nearly as scruffy as its owner. "Personality disorder, schizoid type" was the guess of the mental health specialists who encountered him nearly every day, though they admitted they couldn't be sure without an interview. So it was with surprise and, ultimately, sorrow that after he died suddenly one rainy Saturday afternoon, they read his obituary. Years earlier, Bruce had been a rising star in the summer comedy circuit in the Catskills. Then, inexplicably, he'd dropped completely out of sight. He was only 54 when he died of a slow-growing meningioma, which could have been treated if only he'd been appropriately diagnosed.

Already, you can see this isn't going to be easy. *Accurately* defining a PD requires a lot more detective work than some other conditions, where most of the relevant symptoms are low-hanging fruit.

**TABLE 16.1. Differential Diagnosis with Brief Definitions
for Personality Disorders (PDs) and Other Personality
or Relational Problems**

- *General description of a PD.* A lasting, inflexible pattern of "inner experience and behavior" different from cultural expectations that presents problems in two or more of these areas: thinking, emotions, interpersonal relationships, and impulse control. This begins at an early age and manifests itself in a variety of work, social, and interpersonal situations.

- *Paranoid PD.* These persons distrust and suspect others, whose motives they interpret as malevolent.

- *Schizoid PD.* Isolation from social relationships and restricted emotional range in interpersonal settings characterize these patients.

- *Schizotypal PD.* Here you'll find isolation and discomfort with social relationships, as well as cognitive or perceptual distortions and peculiar behavior.

- *Antisocial PD.* Before age 15, these people repeatedly violated rules, age-appropriate societal norms, or the rights of others (i.e., they qualified for a diagnosis of conduct disorder). After age 15, they show disregard for the rights of others in a variety of situations.

- *Borderline PD.* This is a complicated pattern of unstable impulse control, interpersonal relationships, moodiness, and self-image.

- *Histrionic PD.* Emotional excess and attention-seeking behaviors are typical.

- *Narcissistic PD.* These people will have grandiosity (fantasized or actual), lack of empathy, and need for admiration.

- *Avoidant PD.* Look for social inhibition, hypersensitivity to criticism, and feelings of inadequacy.

- *Dependent PD.* A need to be taken care of leads to clinging, submissive behavior, and fears of separation.

- *Obsessive–compulsive PD.* Preoccupation with control, orderliness, and perfection overshadow qualities of efficiency, flexibility, and candor.

- *Personality traits.* A person exhibits lasting patterns of experiencing self and the environment, but these don't add up to a clear diagnosis.

These three can start later in life:

- *Relational problem.* Two or more individuals interact so as to impair functioning or produce clinical symptoms.

- *Personality change due to a medical condition.* After a physical illness or injury, there is a lasting change in a patient's established personality.

- *Intermittent explosive disorder.* Without other demonstrable pathology, these individuals have episodes during which they act out aggressively, causing physical harm or destroying property.

• Can other disorders, physical or mental, better account for the symptoms?

> For as long as anyone could remember, Max had been the grouchiest postal worker in the history of his branch office. His nasty disposition was the subject of many performance reviews, but his work was so meticulous that no supervisor had the stomach to try to fire him. At home, he was "a bear to live with," as attested by three ex-wives and a flock of angry stepchildren. For his part, Max could never remember feeling anything since his high school days but "lonely and sad"—feelings that he'd declined to share with any of the three mental health clinicians who had tried to help him over the years. "Borderline personality disorder" was what at least a couple of them wrote into his chart.
>
> To the joy of his coworkers, Max retired when he was 55 and took a job managing, of all things, the office of a mental health clinic. After a few weeks, one of the clinicians suggested that he try medication for dysthymia. Within weeks, Max's "personality disorder" disappeared. In a special ceremony the following year, fellow employees feted him as "Mr. Personality."

Before patients are diagnosed with a PD, they should be scrutinized for a variety of other conditions. For example, dysthymia can create dependency; mania may underlie belligerence; and long-term substance use often sets up impulsivity. Also, don't confuse with illness issues such as patients' trouble fitting into cultures or subcultures different from the ones in which they were reared.

• The pattern must be stable. I know that "stable instability" is a bit of a contradiction in terms, but you get the idea: It's the pattern that's stable, even if the behavior wobbles a bit. Consider a counterexample—a person who displays antisocial behavior only when intoxicated or in the throes of a manic episode. Also, you can identify antisocial traits in lots of adolescents, many of whom will straighten out with time. Although official criteria allow you to diagnose a PD in an adolescent whose symptoms have been present for at least 1 year, I think it's safer to wait until the person has fully matured. A PD is serious stuff; once one is diagnosed, the label tends to follow a person around forever. I know I wouldn't want to be responsible for such a label unless it's fully deserved.

• PDs affect several of the features that contribute to a person's character: affect, cognition, impulse control, and interpersonal functioning. If, say, only mood is affected, you should focus your diagnostic interest on a bipolar disorder or dysthymia—but probably not a PD. Or if mood is stable and the only trouble is controlling the impulse to steal, you might first consider kleptomania.

- A PD must cause distress or disturb one or more important life areas, such as work, social, sexual, and family life. I can cite no better example than that of Chuck (see Chapter 15, page 239), whose antisocial behavior wreaked general havoc.

Table 16.2 presents a brief assessment of personality-related problems that may help detect PDs in mental health patients. The 2003 publication in which this assessment appeared reported that a mental patient who answers *yes* to three or more of the eight questions has an excellent chance of having a PD. Note that it is not for use as a diagnostic tool for specific disorders, and it should not be used in screening a general population— only if you already suspect that a patient may have a PD. That way, the person already has passed the requirement of distress or disruption of life areas.

Recognizing a PD

Many experienced clinicians claim that they can sense when a patient has a PD. What they are really doing is (1) matching what they observe against the

TABLE 16.2. Assessing Personality Disorder in Mental Health Patients

1. In general, do you have difficulty making and keeping friends?

2. Would you normally describe yourself as a loner?

3. In general, do you trust other people?

4. Do you normally lose your temper easily?

5. Are you normally an impulsive sort of person?

6. Are you normally a worrier?

7. In general, do you depend on others a lot?

8. In general, are you a perfectionist?

Note. From "Standardised Assessment of Personality—Abbreviated Scale (SAPAS): Preliminary Validation of a Brief Screen for Personality Disorder" by Paul Moran, Morven Leese, Tennyson Lee, Paul Walters, Graham Thornicroft, and Anthony Mann, 2003, *British Journal of Psychiatry, 183,* 228–232. Copyright 2003 by the Royal College of Psychiatrists. Reprinted by permission.

countless patients they have evaluated in the past; (2) noting certain behaviors and items of history that are typically associated with a PD; and (3) identifying discrepancies. I can't help you with the first of these—only time can confer that sort of experience—but I can cast a few pearls from groups 2 and 3. Unhappily, without a reliable history, in some cases there is essentially nothing that will tip you off. For example, it will be nearly impossible to recognize an antisocial person like Ted Bundy, the personally charming butcher of over a dozen young women in the 1970s. In that sense, the diagnosis of antisocial PD demonstrates the value of third-party informants.

Note that no one behavior is diagnostic of a PD, so you can't take any of these items to the bank; all must be evaluated in the context of all else you know about this person. The items are meant as flags, not criteria. What you observe may not be a PD at all, but just personality traits, which we all possess to some degree. Sometimes the clues you spot may mean another diagnosable disorder entirely.

Information from the History

Some items will be obvious from the history, even when the patient is your only informant.

- In particular, problematic behaviors that recur—for example, repeatedly firing a clinician (operationally, three or more times; there are plenty of legitimate reasons to change medical care providers). Other examples include repeated legal difficulties (especially incarcerations), mental hospitalizations (in the absence of a confirmed diagnosis of a bipolar disorder or schizophrenia), or changes of spouses or jobs (neither of which carries quite the stigma it once did). I'd also include patterns such as hoarding, making suicide attempts after disappointments, and repeatedly running away after fighting with a relative.
- Multiple suicide attempts, though PD shouldn't be your first diagnosis in this instance.
- Exclusive emphasis on any one aspect of life: workaholism, partying, sex, playing bridge, or other hobbies. For example, I'd worry about a college student who does nothing but study, partaking in no extracurricular activities or social life.
- Obviously false answers (e.g., 2 + 2 = 5) or a vague story that keeps changing.
- A family history of PD (such as antisocial or histrionic).

- Childhood history of sexual abuse, or being reared by parents with long-time, heavy substance use.
- Certain diagnoses with a strong likelihood of associated PD: eating disorders, dissociative disorders, somatization disorder, social phobia (often found with avoidant PD), schizophrenia (often linked with schizotypal PD), and substance misuse.
- Chronic difficulty working with others.
- Lack of friends and close relationships, especially with no apparent need for any.

The Patient's Affects and Attitudes

Certain affects and attitudes may be manifest even during the initial interview. Here are a few from a list you will eventually expand from your own experience:

- Negative affects and attitudes without apparent embarrassment. Examples include expressions of violence, arrogance (often found in narcissistic PD), and conscienceless lack of remorse and empathy (for example, bragging about criminal exploits or indifference to suffering).
- Disregard for one's own suffering, long associated with histrionic PD.
- In the absence of dementia, mania, or schizophrenia, discrepancies or inconsistencies between affect and stated mood, or mood and content of thought.
- Perplexity when asked to describe feelings of others.
- Excessive rigidity, as shown by inability to "get along by going along" in the workplace or family.
- Attitudes of chronic victimization (someone else was at fault, "I didn't do it," "I was framed").

Behaviors Observed Over Time

Often, only after you begin work with a patient do you learn enough to diagnose a PD. Some key behaviors include the following:

- Glancing toward the window or door in a show of enhanced vigilance.
- Repeated suicide gestures or episodes of self-mutilation (such as wrist cutting).

- Excessive dependence—chronically stating, in effect, "I want you to decide."
- Demanding something, then rejecting it. Examples include hospitalization, followed by against-advice discharge; medication, which the patient then refuses to take.
- Repeated failure of therapeutic measures normally effective for your current Axis I diagnosis.
- Paying more attention to clothing and grooming than to relationships.
- Impulsivity, including extravagant gestures such as setting one's hair on fire or other modes of self-injury.
- Extreme reactions to events, such as attempting suicide upon learning that a relative has cancer.
- Evidence of consistently faulty judgment: multiple instances of not following medical advice, promiscuity that results in rejection or disease, repeated legal troubles (especially criminality).

The Therapeutic Relationship

Again, some issues in the therapeutic relationship will become apparent quickly; others may take a while to emerge.

- Initial extravagant praise for your abilities as the clinician, with disparagement of the patient's previous therapist, followed later by complaints and devaluation.
- Negative affects directed toward you, including dysphoria, anxiety, anger, and belligerence. Then there are overt acts of hostility, such as kicking in an office building wall or letting the air out of your tires. (Ask me about those sometime.)
- Seductive, self-dramatizing, whining approaches to you and others.
- Manipulative behaviors: requesting a hospital pass from one caregiver when another won't allow it; demanding a certain favored hour for therapy; implying disaster if medication isn't forthcoming; repeatedly inquiring about your personal life; asking to be held, massaged, kissed, and more; attempting to smoke in the office; using your first name despite requests to do otherwise; making repeated telephone calls on weekends; changing appointments at the last minute.
- Gift giving—even a Danish and coffee can have strings attached.
- Repeated tardiness for appointments.

- Stalking the clinician, the ultimate clinical nightmare. (Again, you have it from someone who's been there.)
- Neglecting physical symptoms (such as an abscessed tooth)—a worry to any clinician.
- Negative feelings on the part of the clinician: annoyance, fear, distrust, anger, or even, despite misbehavior, attraction. Any of these can suggest that one of you may have a PD.

Recognizing a PD can be a challenge in some patients, though in others it may seem obvious.

Robin

"There are some things I won't talk about," Robin declared on her first visit. With her unlighted cigarette, she gestured toward the scars laddering her left arm. "That's one of them. I saw you looking."

It was now late November, but Robin had a deep tan. Though she looked every day of her 37 years, her burnished auburn hair was pulled back in a long ponytail. "I just don't feel happy," she complained. "Some days I'm depressed, but mostly I'm just out of sorts. I hate my life." Sometimes, she said, she felt bad around the time of her periods, but more often it seemed related to what was going on in her life. "My low-end job sucks, and no one really likes me."

Robin's complaints were legion. Last year at Thanksgiving, she'd accused her mother of favoring her older sister, Alicia; the three hadn't gotten together since. That was only part of the rupture with her family. She'd lost one job when she impulsively danced topless at an office party she'd attended. Over several weeks, she had picked up men from the singles bar she frequented after work. More than once, she had brought one home with her to spend the night—causing no little inconvenience for her sister, with whom she shared a flat. Tempers had flared late one evening when Robin walked through the door with yet another "drunken loser," in her sister's words, "though she never drinks more than a beer or two herself." Now they weren't even on speaking terms, compounding Robin's misery.

With Robin's permission, the therapist called Alicia for some background information. Because they both worked at the same government office, Alicia had a lot of insight into what she called her sister's *modus operandi*. "Ever since she was a little kid, she's been a walking focus of discontent," Alicia reported. Over the telephone, you could almost hear her frown. "She's always suspicious that someone else is saying things to make her look bad, to try to get her in trouble." When she was a senior in high school, Robin had broken off with her best friend, who she thought was trying to steal her boyfriend. "Now I'm certain that this girl was a lesbian—what would she want with *anyone's* boyfriend?" Alicia asked.

She continued, "During the last election, Robin was wild in support of the President. She was always talking politics and passing out campaign literature, even though it's against office policy. But when the White House issued a presidential order she didn't approve of, she said she felt betrayed, and started campaigning for the other side. That's how she is— always blowing hot and cold. Our boss'd love to get rid of her, but you know the government—it would take an act of Congress to fire her."

To a fellow employee, Robin had criticized their boss for the decision not to hire a temp when a coworker took paternity leave. Later Alicia overheard her telling the boss that the choice was solid, because the coworker hadn't been pulling his weight. "When I called her on it, Robin blew up and threatened never to speak to me again. Typical of her, also, that she always comes crawling back. I've never known someone who was so afraid of being alone, but so often shoved other people away."

Analysis

First, we would need to know whether Robin had a major Axis I mental diagnosis (see step 1 of Figure 16.1, the decision tree for a patient with character/interpersonal difficulties). Although the details in this vignette are sketchy, her clinician did learn enough to determine that she probably didn't qualify for an anxiety, mood, or psychotic disorder, and that she didn't drink or use drugs. (Had she qualified, we'd be doubly careful about also diagnosing a PD.) Although more information would be needed about her physical health, Alicia's historical review argued against any recent change (step 2). Robin's challenge early in the interview would alert most experienced clinicians to the possibility of a PD. Robin herself mentioned numerous instances of difficulty getting along with other people, especially those in her own family.

Robin would thus seem to fit the general description of someone with a PD: She had lifelong difficulty controlling her impulses and maintaining her interpersonal relationships; without being psychotic, her thinking was skewed by ideas that others opposed her; and her emotional state was precarious. None of the specific patterns of the recognized PDs (see Table

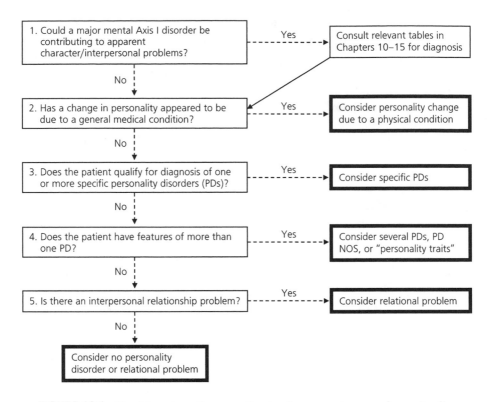

FIGURE 16.1. Decision tree for a patient who experiences character/interpersonal difficulties.

16.1) would adequately define her character, however, so we'd have difficulty giving her a specific PD diagnosis (step 3). She did appear to have several disordered personality traits, including dramatic need for attention (dancing seminude), paranoia (suspicions about her girlfriend), and borderline characteristics (multiple episodes of self-mutilation). At step 4, then, we might well consider her for several personality traits or PD NOS. Although we could theoretically continue on through our decision tree and look for a relational problem in addition, in the face of so many personality traits it seems a bit of a waste.

Comment

The diagnosis of a PD is beset with many problems. Here are just a few of them:

1. Contrary to the impression you might get from a casual reading of diagnostic manuals, most people have mixtures of personality traits and PDs. Yet clinicians tend to diagnose only one PD, even when patients meet criteria for two or more.
2. When more than one PD *is* diagnosed, what does this actually mean? Surely not that the patient has several personalities. And how does this help inform treatment?
3. There is no sharp dividing line between PD and normality.
4. The three PD clusters (odd or aloof; dramatic, impulsive, or erratic; anxious or fearful) currently in use have little basis in objective research.
5. So far, little work has been reported that would pinpoint the cause of PDs.
6. PDs are especially hard to evaluate. Often the patient interview alone doesn't suffice, even when a standardized interview is used; neither does psychological testing. Rather, we need interviews with relatives and others who have known the patient well, at least from late adolescence, to demonstrate that the behaviors in question are both enduring and pervasive.

Some PDs have special issues. Many researchers place schizotypal PD on a continuum with schizophrenia; the *International Classification of Diseases*, 10th revision, even lists it on Axis I. Although we list somatization disorder on Axis I, it so often goes hand in glove with histrionic PD that it's hard to determine where one begins and the other leaves off. Avoidant PD is often found with social phobia. Some clinicians use *borderline* more to express general disapproval than to describe a specific disorder. And fears of abandonment are symptomatic of both borderline and dependent PDs.

We could address some of these issues by describing personality with a dimensional system. For example, on the five-factor model mentioned at the start of this chapter, Robin might score high on neuroticism (vulnerability to self-consciousness and emotional instability); about medium on extroversion (outgoing and warm) and openness (the cognitive tendency to aesthetics and creativity); and low on agreeableness (degree of comfort with social interactions) and conscientiousness (competence and dutifulness). However, the dimensional approach won't save us when data are skewed by the presence of mood or other Axis I disorders.

Although clinicians sometimes focus so strongly on Axis I disorders that they ignore the presence of PDs, the opposite problem also arises: An apparent PD drives away consideration of other, more treatable (and even more dangerous) mental conditions.

> Consider the case of Elizabeth Shin, an enormously bright and talented MIT sophomore. After many months of care related to anxiety and depression, she burned herself to death in her dormitory room. On several occasions she had cut herself, which prompted speculation that she had borderline PD. Did her clinicians pay too much attention to an apparent PD and thus give short shrift to her repeated statements that she wanted to kill herself?

What can we take away from the discussion of PDs and their confounds?

- Maladaptive traits are present in many people who don't meet criteria for a PD.
- Examine all patients for character issues that influence how they do business with the world, whether or not they meet anyone's formal criteria for a disorder.
- Perhaps it is better to use the general PD criteria given earlier. It is certainly *far* better to use these relatively objective standards than to depend on your subjective impressions—a much-ignored diagnostic principle.
- An important function of the PDs is to remind us to look for associated Axis I disorders.

Phineas

In addition to the problem of detecting major mental pathology, you must also be alert for how long the person has had character pathology and how it was acquired.

> One fall day in 1848, Phineas Gage, the foreman of a railway construction gang in Vermont, had just tamped down an explosive charge when all hell broke loose. As a local newspaper reported the following day, an accidental explosion blasted Gage's tamping iron through his left cheekbone and out through the top of his head. The tapered iron was 43 inches long and over an inch in diameter at its widest; it weighed just over 13 pounds. Although most of the left frontal lobe of his brain was destroyed, Phineas may not even have lost consciousness. The following day a newspaper reported that he was "in full possession of his reason, and free from pain." His recovery was so successful that 10 weeks later, he returned home to New Hampshire.

Within a few months he sought to return to work, but as his friends sadly noted, "Gage was no longer Gage." Formerly capable and efficient and possessed of a good business sense, now he was profane, irreverent, obstinate, impatient with others, vacillating, and capricious. Indeed, his personality was so altered that his company would no longer employ him. Unable to plan for the future or hold a job, he died penniless 13 years later. Although his brain was not autopsied, his skull was preserved and can now be viewed at the Warren Anatomical Museum at Harvard Medical School.

Analysis

At step 1 of Figure 16.1, we can conclude from the history that there does not appear to have been a major Axis I mental disorder, such as a mood, psychotic, or substance use disorder. That gets us to step 2, where we can agree that Phineas's change in personality was well accounted for by the horrific injury he sustained. Although relationship problems might have developed later, they do not form part of this particular exercise.

Comment

The obvious difference between a PD and Phineas's personality change is time: The former must be present from a young age. The varieties of personality change are legion, including agitation, passivity, irritability, aggression, labile moods, childishness, irresponsibility, apathy, rigidity, and lack of motivation, reduced empathy, disagreeableness, and diminished conscientiousness. As with PDs, information from informants other than the patient is of critical importance; newspaper accounts are optional.

Personality change is often related to a traumatic brain injury, which when severe is likely to cause symptoms. Personality change can also be caused by diseases such as strokes, Alzheimer's disease, benign or malignant tumors, HIV disease, multiple sclerosis, spinocerebellar ataxia, neurosyphilis, Huntington's disease, cerebral malaria, toxicity, and encephalitis—in fact, just about any disorder that affects the metabolism or structure of the brain. If the personality change is prominent, you can diagnose it even in a patient with dementia; in fact, it may be how dementia first announces itself. Some researchers have found that personality change early in the course of Alzheimer's disease predicts that the functional decline may be more rapid than usual. The obvious conclusion is that any patient whose character structure has changed should receive a full medical workup for possible physical causes.

Diagnosing Relational Problems

In every chapter of this book, we have wrestled with boundary issues between different illnesses. Here is a case that explores a different sort of boundary.

Marcie

Marcie was 32 and the mother of two small children. Although she had abandoned a promising career in marketing when she became pregnant, she loved being a stay-at-home mom. However, for the past several weeks she had been distressed, anxious, and somewhat depressed. Actually, she told the clinician, she felt fine most of the time, but her mood began to slip toward evening, when Ian arrived home from work. She didn't know whether that could have anything to do with it, because "we have a great marriage, and he's a terrific dad." She hesitated. "But, well, we have been fighting a lot."

The clinician probed: "Money? Sex? These are the big issues for most couples." Their battleground was her brother's drinking. Ray lived across town in a rented flat, but he spent much of his time with Marcie and her family. From the garage of her home, Marcie and Ray ran the small mail-order business they had inherited from their mother just a year ago. "On her deathbed Mom begged me to take care of Ray, and I promised I always would. And I never dodge my responsibilities."

Their mother had sheltered Ray, and now Ian was accusing Marcie of behaving just like her. Marcie acknowledged the truth in this claim, but she couldn't let Ray go. "He may be heavy, but he's still my brother," she explained. Ian had long resented the jokes she made to slide away from serious discussions.

Ian didn't dislike Ray. In fact, he rather enjoyed his company, when Ray was sober—which, Marcie admitted, "any more is mostly never." Now she and Ian fought nearly every night, and much of the weekend too. She said that she had no problems with sleep or appetite. In addition, she denied actual panic attacks and death wishes, and she remained passionately interested in her children and her business. Her sex interest was also excellent, she said, "when Ian and I are on, um, speaking terms."

Analysis

Marcie lacked the symptoms for a step 1 Axis I disorder, and there was no evidence of a lifelong PD (step 2). Indeed, she didn't really have enough symptoms to warrant *any* of the usual clinical diagnoses. The fact that she became symptomatic only when her husband was home should move us into other realms.

An adjustment disorder would seem to be a real possibility, but let's think about that diagnosis and its several drawbacks. The criteria are vague: "clinical significance" is required; no other Axis I or II disorder can account for the symptoms; and they require you as the clinician to judge that they occur in response to a stressor (even if your crystal ball is in the shop). Furthermore, any prospective diagnosis must be listed as *provisional*: You can only know that you've made the right diagnosis if the symptoms go away once the stressor lifts.

In Marcie's case, both spouses were apparently contributing to the difficulty, which would make it seem just about perfect for a relational problem. By the way, this diagnosis also suggests a way to deal with the problem, whereas a diagnosis of adjustment disorder depicts a patient as a passive vessel, filled with anxiety and depression until something happens to take away the strain. If you feel strongly that you would want to give Marcie an Axis I or II diagnosis, I'd go with *undiagnosed*—I wouldn't even know what kind of NOS to give her.

Comment

It's a truism that many people consult us not because they are ill, but because they have problems working, living, or just plain getting along with others—their siblings, children, parents, spouses or partners, and even co-workers:

- For a year, a brother and two sisters have fought over their parents' estate.
- A mother and her teenage daughter quarrel about dating; the daughter stays out late, the mother nags. Both are angry.
- Same-sex lovers in a 10-year committed relationship are at odds over whether to adopt a baby.
- A man uses amphetamines and frequently beats his wife, who always refuses to press charges or seek shelter.
- A woman lies in a coma for 15 years while her husband and parents argue about whether she should be allowed to die.

The examples above share several features. The behaviors in question often act as a circle of cause and effect: A mother punishes her daughter for staying out, and the daughter in turn rebels at the perceived overcontrol by staying out later. In other words, the dispute centers upon the way the individuals respond to one another. The pattern involves anguish and sometimes danger, and is relatively constant from one situation to another. It usually isn't just a response to a particular event, and it persists not for days or weeks, but for months or years. It is unresponsive to social or religious suasion, and there is evidence of impact on individuals' health and functioning.

Recognizing Relational Problems

Shelves groan with books that propose to assess couple and family discord, and I promise not to burden them—and you—any further. Instead, here is a brief outline to help you decide whether a relational problem describes your patient's difficulties:

1. You'll probably need collateral input to ascertain that this is an interpersonal issue—that two or more individuals contribute to the conflict. Even if the second person denies it, the behavior you observe may tell another story.
2. The relationship must be important. No matter how heated it is, an argument between travelers who meet on a train doesn't qualify.
3. The conflict itself must be relatively enduring. Most relationships have their ups and downs; we mustn't react with alarm to every lurch on the Ferris wheel of family life.
4. Does an individual's mental diagnosis provide background? If so, it must not be the sole source of the conflict. It probably happens often that a given clinical situation entails both an individual diagnosis and a relationship problem. They may be completely separate, or one may flow from the other, in which case the relationship problem is said to be *embedded*.
5. To identify an impairment of social functioning between the parties, you may find some help in the Global Assessment of Relational Functioning (GARF), which guides clinicians to evaluate the relationship in terms of problem solving, organization, and emotional climate. (The GARF is included in Appendix B of DSM-IV-TR.) Among other symptoms might be sexual dissatisfaction, uncontrolled anger, indifference, and poor communication.

The early years of the 21st century have witnessed a huge debate over whether to include relational problems as a regular part of future diagnostic manuals. As of this writing, the issue hadn't yet been sorted out, but regardless of the degree to which they are formalized in criteria, the problems still exist and must be identified and treated. They represent part of the enormously important aspect to the overall provision of mental health care called *problems of living,* which can include just about anything that isn't an actual mental disorder. The diagnostic manuals place all this psychosocial and environmental stuff on Axis IV, but note that they can be elevated to Axis I if they are the focus for seeking evaluation or treatment. The list of potential problems of living includes the following:

Family (death, divorce, neglect, abuse)
Support group (living alone, being a victim of discrimination, emigrating)
School (difficulties with teachers or classmates, illiteracy)
Workplace (stressful schedule or working conditions, discord with supervisor or coworkers)
Housing (homelessness, unsafe conditions, trouble with neighbors)
Finances
Access to health care (through lack of insurance, geographic isolation)
Legal (being a victim of crime, getting arrested, being involved in litigation)
Other issues, such as problems of acculturation, religion, retirement, and the effects of war or terrorism

Distinguishing Disorder from Normality

And here is yet another sort of boundary to keep in mind.

Horace

After Horace reached his university's mandatory retirement age of 65, he spent his first 20 emeritus years teaching his old subjects as a volunteer. Years later, he told a clinician, "I eventually got too old to get myself there on a regular basis, so I've spent the last 8 years working in my garden, writing letters to the editor, and reading the classics." What brought him to mental health attention was his response to his general physician's news that there was a small cancerous growth in his left kidney. Horace buttoned his shirt and smiled as he said, "Well, good. At 93, I think this is just the right time for me to take my leave. Exit Horace." Subsequently, he refused even to discuss the operation that, if undertaken right away, would almost surely provide a cure.

The mental health consultant learned that Horace sometimes felt down for a few hours ("And who wouldn't? My wife died several years ago, and I've outlived all my old friends"), but he had no other symptoms of a mood disorder. He drank two glasses of wine each day ("It's good for my cholesterol"), but he denied having any difficulty whatsoever interpersonally, financially, or with the law.

Analysis

Several mental health clinicians reviewed Horace's case with his attending doctor. After half a hour of digging for further symptoms, they determined that they couldn't make a case for any Axis I disorder (step 1). They agreed that he regarded his situation with equanimity, spoke dispassionately, and appeared to have made a rational choice. There had been no step 2 personality change. In fact, there was no evidence of any problem with his personality (steps 3 and 4); he had always been a sweet-tempered man, beloved by family, colleagues, and students. Finally, other than the distress felt by Horace's physician, there were no interpersonal problems to merit a diagnosis of a relational problem (step 5). We are apparently left with a person who, with no mental illness, had every right to make what he regarded as a logical, everyday decision about his own health care needs. The consulting committee did encourage the treating physician to discuss again the merits of an operation.

Comment

How often does a clinician wonder, "Could this patient have *no* mental illness?" I suspect it happens rather less often than it should. Indeed, research in this area is apparently entirely lacking—Medline searches for *no mental illness* and similar phrases consistently come up empty. One problem is the absence of a distinct line between normality and illness. Extend Horace's momentary "feeling down" to a few days, and would he then be ill? Add sleeplessness; would he be ill then? What if he lost his appetite? At some point, all would agree that he had a clinical illness, but the grey area leaves much room for dispute.

The follow-up: Horace's physician did press the issue of the kidney operation, emphasizing the pain and loss of control if his cancer were to metastasize. He ultimately relented and speedily recovered from a successful operation.

17 Beyond Diagnosis

Compliance, Suicide, Violence

All clinicians need to keep in mind three issues that are important for evaluation but transcend the boundaries of diagnosis: compliance, suicide, and violence.

Compliance

When I was a student, *noncompliance* meant that the patient didn't follow the clinician's directions. Now an ethos of cooperation—partnership between patient and care provider—has changed how we view this important subject, which some clinicians are beginning to call *adherence*.

Of course, there are degrees of noncompliance/nonadherence. One patient might just disregard a recommended exercise program; another might "forget" many doses of Antabuse, endangering sobriety. In between are myriad opportunities for confusion and error.

Research in this area lags, but still we know a fair amount from controlled studies, though much of it is pretty predictable. For example, noncompliance is greater among outpatients than inpatients. It increases with more time in treatment, a more complicated treatment regimen, and more side effects; you can reduce it with careful supervision, education about the nature of the disease, and a supportive environment. Patients who are satisfied with the course of treatment are much more likely to be compliant than are unhappy ones. Indeed, noncompliance per se may not be the only reason—or may not be the reason at all—why treatment is not working; other factors may need to be considered (see the sidebar "Why Doesn't Treatment Work?").

The effects of noncompliance run from mundane to major. Of course, no treatment can be effective if it isn't utilized, and for some patients, not

Why Doesn't Treatment Work?

The question "Why doesn't treatment work?" has a number of answers, each of which is probably right some of the time.

- *Wrong treatment.* Some patients with depression respond to SSRIs, others to cognitive-behavioral therapy. Still others—for example, those with atypical depression—may require a monoamine oxidase inhibitor.
- *Insufficient time.* Often patients despair of treatment that simply hasn't yet had enough time to work. This is famously true of psychotherapy, as well as most medications.
- *Wrong dosage.* Usually this applies to drug treatment, and usually it means that too little of the medication has been prescribed. Some drugs have a "therapeutic window" of effect, which means that either too little *or* too much can prevent optimal response.
- *Other treatments interfere.* Here's another problem with medication: The use of one can decrease the effectiveness of another.
- *Side effects.* Very often, unwanted effects (another medication issue) cause such grief that patients reduce doses or drop out of treatment altogether.
- *Other compliance issues.* The patient doesn't do the exercises, attend day care, practice the homework assignments for cognitive-behavioral therapy, or take medications as prescribed.
- *Use of substances.* In many ways, the effects of street drugs or alcohol can complicate treatment and its assessment.
- *Wrong diagnosis.* This may be the most common, though least heralded, factor of all those that contribute to the apparent lack of treatment effectiveness. It is also one of the easiest to rectify.

taking the prescribed treatment (say, a course of cognitive-behavioral therapy) may only mean that depression continues without relief. More serious consequences could include repeated episodes of illness and multiple hospitalizations.

When she was in the depressed phase of her bipolar I disorder, Belinda was a model patient who always recovered quickly. But when manic, she would neglect her medication and end up hospitalized over 1,000 miles away, where she grew up. With her fourth or fifth episode, I was called to her house one evening to find her in her front yard, spraying her living room furniture with the garden hose.

Still others may become estranged from family and friends.

Maude had been a champion swimmer, who often won medals and one year came close to qualifying for the U.S. Olympics team. But at 23 she developed schizophrenia, and forever afterward she claimed that her antipsychotics made it difficult to perform in the water. Time and again, she would stop taking her medication and become psychotic. With each hospitalization she refused medication, necessitating a court hearing to determine whether she should be medicated against her will. More than once, the judge was sympathetic to her pleas and discharged her from care. When I last spoke with her, she was in a nursing care facility, so psychotic that she couldn't even feed herself. Eventually her husband divorced her and took the children to live with him.

Sometimes the results are dire, as shown in two more brief reports:

Severe recurrent depression caused Jolene to retire from her job with the post office when she was 44. About every 2 years, she became severely melancholic, couldn't sleep, lost weight, and refused to answer the telephone when her brother called to ask how she was doing. In her despondence she would develop suicidal ideas, but with every episode, she waited so long before calling for help that she couldn't be managed at home and had to be hospitalized. Each time, she stayed in the hospital only long enough to receive four electroconvulsive treatments, then signed out against advice. "I stopped because I felt better" was her usual rationale. She then failed to follow up with outpatient visits or treatment. This pattern went on for more than 20 years. After the last time I saw Jolene, I heard nothing more for about 2 years, until a relative called to say that she had hanged herself.

In December 2005, a distraught Rigoberto Alpizar ran from his plane, which was about to take off from Miami, and onto the jetway. After allegedly yelling something about a bomb, he reached into his carry-on bag as he refused to surrender to the air marshals. They shot him dead. His wife told another passenger that he had a bipolar disorder and had not taken his medication. No bomb was found, and no link to terrorism was ever suggested.

Obviously, identifying compliance issues is important for clinicians and patients alike. Here are some clues and resources you can use to assess the risk of noncompliance in your patients.

- *Ask the patient.* At every visit, I routinely ask each patient to describe each medication and its schedule of use. I frequently learn that the regimen is different from what I have recommended. Routine questioning offers a chance to discuss the issue without sounding critical. Differences from my expectations are easily discussed as a misunderstanding or as the patient's response to side effects; the usual solution is a successful compromise. Similar procedures could apply to diet, schedules of exercise, cognitive-behavioral homework, and more.
- *Ask relatives.* Collateral information from those who know the patient well may turn up problems with compliance.
- *Note lack of improvement.* Noncompliance is a likely factor when patients do not experience the expected response to treatment.
- *Are there side effects?* With drug regimens, *lack* of expected side effects should tip you off that your patient isn't getting enough medication—perhaps none at all.
- *Check environmental factors.* Is there a support system? Does this patient's peer group pride itself on refusing drugs or other treatment modalities?
- *Monitor caregiver factors.* How fully have you educated your patient about the need for treatment? How often are appointments scheduled (monthly or more often will help ensure compliance)? Does the patient perceive your relationship as strongly positive and helpful? Does the patient understand the theoretical reasons behind the treatment approach?
- *Watch for telltale symptoms.* Noncompliance can result from depression (the patient may have an apathetic response to treatment recommendations), euphoria (the patient may feel "too well to be sick"), delusions (the patient may be suspicious of your motives), poor insight (the patient may be unable to understand that an illness requires treatment), or anger (the patient may be acting out).
- *Observe red flags.* Compliance issues are especially relevant to mania, schizophrenia, dementia, personality disorder, and substance use. Patients with both substance use and another major Axis I mental disorder are especially vulnerable.

Suicide

The low base rate of suicide (about 1% of the general population) and the inexact nature of the science make it hard to predict which individuals will attempt suicide and which will succeed. We have to rely on the seemingly numberless studies that try to pinpoint characteristics of suicide risk.

Jay had retired after 30 years of honorable service in the Marine Corps. For a time he'd worked in his brother's machine shop, but now he mostly just sat at home. A couple of years earlier, his wife had died. They'd been childless, and he had never been a particularly social person. Now, in his late 60s, he lived alone on his military pension and Social Security.

No one had heard much from Jay until he was brought to the emergency department after he attempted suicide by carbon monoxide poisoning. He had been discovered unconscious in his garage when a neighbor returned home unexpectedly at lunchtime and heard the purring of an engine. After several touch-and-go hours in intensive care, he recovered enough to speak with a mental health consultant, who learned that he had been drinking heavily to combat a severe melancholia.

Jay was sallow and gaunt. His clothes hung on his 6-foot frame—clearly, he had lost 20 pounds or more. He said that when he awakened about 3 or 4 each morning, he would lie there and brood about the death of a friend with whom he served in Vietnam. "I could have picked up that grenade and heaved it, but I just jumped behind some sandbags." He had lost his interest in hunting, but he still kept two rifles and a pistol locked in a cabinet. He had smoked all his adult life; a doctor had recently told him that a spot on his lung was "suspicious," and that he needed to come in for more tests. Not a religious man, he said that if he learned he had cancer, he wouldn't have it treated, though his father had died a horrible, lingering death from lung cancer. Jay would either move to Oregon and request physician-assisted suicide, or "just do the job myself, in the comfort of my own living room."

From the available information, Jay's clinician felt that there was an extremely high risk of further suicide attempts and placed him on a one-to-one suicide watch. That evening about 10, Jay went into the toilet and closed the door. Five minutes later, the aide attending him called out, and the staff broke down the door. They found him, nearly lifeless, hanging from a loop of bath towel and cut him down.

There are two basic sets of risk factors for suicide: those that pertain to mental illness, and those of a personal or social nature. I've put them into a couple of lists for easy study.

Mental Disorders and Suicide

Like Jay, the vast majority of those who attempt or complete suicide have a diagnosable mental illness. Although suicide and suicide attempts are not tied to any one diagnosis, each is associated with suicide behaviors.

• *Mood disorders.* Major depression and bipolar disorders account for about half of all suicides, mostly because patients haven't been treated adequately for depression. Risk of suicide increases with more severe depression and with the presence of melancholic features (loss of pleasure in usual activities, feeling worse in the mornings, insomnia typified by awakening too early in the morning, loss of appetite or weight, excessive guilt, and a quality of mood that is more profound that typical grief). Recent studies have reported that in either depression or bipolar disorders, treatment with antidepressants or lithium decreases suicide risk—a lot.

• *Schizophrenia.* About 10% of patients with schizophrenia die by suicide, usually in the first few years of illness. Risk is higher in those with paranoia or depressive symptoms, and lower in those with negative symptoms (flat affect, impoverished speech, inability to initiate action). In a person who has made previous attempts, command auditory hallucinations increase risk for another.

• *Substance misuse.* Patients with any type of substance dependence have a risk of suicide 2 to 3 times that of the general population (in those with heroin dependence, it is least 14 times greater). In alcoholism, loss of a close relationship through divorce, separation, death, or interpersonal friction is a common precipitant; risk increases further still if drinking has been recent and heavy.

• *Personality disorder.* The risk of suicide is especially great in antisocial and borderline personality disorders.

• *Others.* Illnesses as different as PTSD and ADHD may also confer an increased risk for suicide. There is even a risk with panic disorder, especially if major depressive disorder or substance use is also involved. Patients with somatization disorder often attempt suicide; although there are few data, I believe that these people also carry an increased risk for completed suicide. And please remember that having more than one mental disorder greatly increases the risk of attempts and completed suicide.

Individual Factors in Suicide

For many years, numerous social and personal characteristics have been known to increase the risk of suicide:

- *Male gender.* Men have four times the risk of women for *completed* suicide, whereas women are three times as likely to *attempt* suicide.
- *Advancing age.* Suicide rates rise throughout the lifespan to peak in the over-85 group.
- *Race.* Whites are far more likely to commit suicide than are people of other races.
- *Employment.* Unemployed and retired persons, and those with long absences from work, may suffer from lower self-esteem and reduced access to support networks—both of which may increase their risk.
- *Marital status.* Being single or divorced (divorced is worse) is a risk factor; married people are less likely to commit suicide.
- *Religion.* The risk for Protestants is higher than that for Catholics and Jews. Risk for Muslims is unclear.
- *Family history.* Suicide in a relative increases individual risk, even beyond the presence of mental disorder.
- *Living alone.* Isolation often breeds despair.
- *Gun ownership or access to lethal means.* And don't forget medications that can be lethal in overdose.
- *Physical disease.* The burden of obstructive lung disease, cancer, epilepsy, chronic pain, and a host of other debilitating conditions predisposes patients to suicide; multiple illnesses greatly increase the risk.
- *Feelings of hopelessness.* An unrelieved gloomy view of the future has been identified as especially predictive of future suicide.
- *Recent mental hospitalization.* The first few days after discharge are the most dangerous.
- *Financial difficulty.* The image of stock market investors leaping from windows during the Great Depression of the 1930s was no myth: The national suicide rate increased by 20%.
- *Heavy gambling losses.* This factor may be mediated by depression, not pathological gambling per se.
- *Talking about suicide.* The saying "Those who talk about it don't do it" is exactly the opposite of fact: Most people who kill themselves have communicated their intent, often to a care provider.
- *Suicide of others.* The death by suicide of a friend, relative, or even a

total stranger can increase the risk—especially in adolescents, for whom the pull of group behavior is especially powerful.

• *Prior suicide attempt.* This is one of the strongest predictors we have. After an attempted suicide, risk for completion persists up to four decades later. In one study, of those who made a medically serious suicide attempt, 9% had died within 5 years, 59% of these by suicide. When evaluating an attempt, it is important to consider both medical and psychological seriousness. A medically serious attempt is one that causes unconsciousness, significant loss of blood, or disruption of parts of the body beneath the skin (tendons and arteries are examples). Psychologically serious attempts are those in which the patient expresses regret at surviving, has made efforts to avoid discovery, or states a determination to make another attempt. An attempt that entails either type of seriousness should put you especially on guard.

A number of scales have been devised to measure the degree of suicidal intent and the seriousness of a prior attempt. The "References and Suggested Reading" section at the end of the book lists some websites that provide information about such scales.

Violence

Mental health clinicians famously fail to predict violent acts accurately— even within the next few hours or days, let alone further in the future. Over the years, lore has accumulated about factors that supposedly relate to violence. Some of this lore is accurate; some is not. Consider two scenarios:

> A few months past her 21st birthday, Brenda drank and used amphetamines. In fact, she cooked methamphetamine in a lab she'd helped her boyfriend construct in his grandmother's basement. From age 11 Brenda had repeatedly run away from home, in part to escape the beatings her stepfather had inflicted for years. Though she was smart, her inattentiveness yielded abysmal grades in school, and she dropped out when she was 15. Since then, she'd been in and out of juvenile hall. At 16, after consuming alcohol and "other stuff" (she wasn't sure what) at a rave, she stabbed and nearly killed another girl. Although Brenda was released from custody when she turned 21, her parole officer noted that she'd recently resumed drinking. Moreover, she had threatened several times to "finish the job" on the girl she stabbed years ago.

Brent, also 21, fell ill during his junior year at university. Always a steady, earnest student, both Brent and his family were surprised at how quickly his grades tumbled once the voices he now heard began telling him he was the Devil. "Academically, he just seemed to wither away," said his aunt, with whom he lived while attending school several hundred miles from where he grew up. After the first few weeks of the fall term, he gradually stopped going to class. He neglected his appearance and refused to go home for Christmas. By the end of April, he wouldn't even leave the house. When questioned, Brent said that he had come to realize that he was the Antichrist, and through him the world would be destroyed. His aunt told the clinician that her husband kept a pistol in an unlocked desk drawer; she didn't know, but she thought it might be loaded.

Many clinicians would probably assess Brent's history of psychosis and the fact that he was a young male with apocalyptic delusions as factors rendering him likely to commit a violent offense. However, over the years, traditional clinical methods have proven unreliable in assessing violence potential. A large part of the difficulty lies in the fact that studies of violence are often based on general population samples, whereas we clinicians want to know how likely *our patient* is to commit an act that will harm another person. To that end, in the past decade researchers have developed actuarial models that rely less on clinical information and judgment, and more on data from records and demographics. Some of the findings may surprise you.

- *Diagnosis.* Traditionally, violence is associated with a number of diagnoses—schizophrenia, mania, sociopathy, conduct disorder (in children and adolescents), intermittent explosive disorder, and substance use disorders (especially on days a person actually uses drugs or alcohol). However, the overwhelming majority of mental patients do not perpetrate violence. In fact, a major Axis I mental disorder such as bipolar I disorder or Brent's schizophrenia carries a lower risk of violence than does personality disorder. A number of physical brain diseases can also lead to violence—head injuries, seizure disorders, Alzheimer's and other dementias, infections, cancer and other mass lesions, toxicity (including drug and alcohol), and metabolic conditions. Always, the comorbid diagnosis of substance misuse is an important predictor of violence.
- *Gender.* Men are traditionally regarded as committing the major share of violence. However, among mental patients, women like Brenda are about as likely to perpetrate violence as men, though their victims may

be less likely to require medical attention. Women's violence is especially likely to occur in the home.

• *Prior violence.* A history of violent behavior is a traditionally strong predictor. Remarkably, assessment of violence isn't usually a problem; patients are often quite willing to admit to prior offenses. Brenda's prior assault and conviction clearly demonstrated her potential.

• *Abuse.* Childhood physical (but not sexual) abuse history is positively associated with later violence.

• *Antisocial personality disorder.* The risk of violence is greatly increased in patients who carry this diagnosis. Although more information would be needed to be sure, Brenda's history should alert us to the possibility of conduct disorder and antisocial personality disorder.

• *Hallucinations.* Command hallucinations that order the person to commit violence increase the risk; other hallucinations are not related. Delusions, such as Brent's ideas about being the Antichrist, do *not* predict violence.

• *Anger and thoughts/fantasies of violence.* Ideas of violence beget violent behavior.

• *Age.* The time of violence, like the time of love and procreation, is youth. No surprises here.

In short, the actuarial model predicts that violent mental patients will tend to be those who are hostile, are young, misuse drugs, and have a history of previous violent behavior. And it would be Brenda, not Brent, who represented the greater risk of the two cases described above. Numerous studies report that discharged mental patients are likely to perpetrate violence only if they use substances. Unfortunately, they are more likely than the general public to misuse substances. When mental patients do reoffend, it usually occurs a relatively short time after discharge from a hospital.

Finally, consider the sobering observation that some of our most notorious violent patients might have slipped past the best of our current predictors: Prosenjit Poddar (who murdered Tatiana Tarasoff, eventually leading to the recognition of a duty to protect known as the *Tarasoff principle*); Mark David Chapman (who killed John Lennon); and John Hinckley, Jr. (who attempted to assassinate Ronald Reagan). Each of these individuals had had intense fantasies, but no prior history of violence. Even with the best in current research and instruments, we can deliver only predictions, not promises.

18 Patients, Patients

With the following case vignettes, you can further explore the methods we've discussed in the previous 17 chapters. I have selected patients varied enough to cover the diagnostic principles and major classes of disorders. Some of these cases are fairly simple; others are remarkably complicated. We'll start off with a simple exercise in forming a differential diagnosis.

John

John Clare was a working-class man from England's North Country who became famous in the early 1800s for lyrical nature poetry that lives in print today. Throughout his adult life, John drank a great deal (mainly beer). His sexual contacts with a variety of young women, some of whom were probably prostitutes, may have prompted mercury treatment for syphilis. As a young man, he suffered from recurrent depressions, and he may have experienced bursts of activity and writing. In his later life, he had many hallucinations and was chronically delusional—believing, for example, that he had two wives simultaneously, that he was Robert Burns and Lord Byron, and that he was the son of King George III.

Analysis

The available (albeit skimpy) facts are enough for us to practice constructing a differential diagnosis based on a safety hierarchy. I may not mention the differential diagnosis in every patient vignette, but still we should honor it by using it—every time. Here's how I think about John's psychosis:

Treatable disorders that can quickly have a profound effect on health:
—Psychosis related to alcohol use
—Psychosis related to syphilis
—Psychosis related to mercury poisoning

Serious disorders, urgent to treat, though the consequences may be less wide-ranging:
—Bipolar I disorder, with psychosis
—Major depressive disorder, recurrent, with psychosis

Disorders that are chronic and tend to have a poor prognosis, regardless of treatment:
—Schizophrenia and schizoaffective disorder (untreatable in the early 1800s)
—Alzheimer's dementia with psychosis

John spent most of the last three decades of his life in asylums, ultimately dying when he was 70. Although a recent biographer has suggested that John suffered from a bipolar disorder, the course of his lengthy, chronic psychosis gives me serious doubts. Several diagnostic principles drive the selection process—among them, and most important, the admonitions always to consider chemical and general medical causes. With no more information than we have, I'd have to invoke the diagnostic principle of choosing the term *undiagnosed* for the rustic poet who could pen such lines as these:

> I am—yet what I am, none cares or knows;
> My friends forsake me like a memory lost:
> I am the self-consumer of my woes . . .

Marian

When Marian appeared for counseling, she felt anxious, and her chronic headaches had worsened. In the course of several weeks, she said, she had managed to worry off about 10 pounds. This was no surprise, since her "appetite had fallen completely off the scale—I haven't eaten a thing for days." She lamented that she worried about everything. Her father's health was declining; her sister's marriage was on the rocks. Her job in the county tax assessor's office paid enough to live on, but she felt dissatisfied that she had too little responsibility for her age and experience. She thought she might quit this job and look elsewhere, as she had done half a dozen other times over the past few years. Now 33 and with her boyfriend scheduled for deployment with the Army Reserves, Marian felt the ticking of her biological clock: "One day I'd like to have a family—only not if I still have this much anxiety." Shoulders slumping, she broke into tears.

While in high school, Marian had had a series of panic attacks. She remembered how, during an algebra midterm exam, her head started to nod uncontrollably and her heart raced as she fought to breathe. Terrified, she'd have gotten up to leave, but her legs felt too weak to support her. Instead, she sat there and suffered, unable to cry or concentrate; she had earned a D on the test. After several repeated attacks, they began to tail off and eventually disappeared altogether, but the empty, sad feeling that was left behind stayed with her throughout her formal education.

Just before Marian graduated from college, her mother died of breast cancer—the same fate as had met her grandmother and an aunt. Feeling abandoned and emptier than ever, she began drinking. Over the next 10 years, alcohol gained and lost her several lovers of varying quality. When Jürgen, her current boyfriend, threatened to leave for good if she didn't quit, she finally did. "I haven't touched a drop in the 8 months since," she explained, with a slight smile and steady gaze at the interviewer.

The depression was what had driven her to this appointment. For weeks, she'd suffered from low mood that was nearly constant; she was also having such difficulty concentrating at work that she was afraid she'd be fired, even if she didn't quit. Of course, the recent downturn in the economy didn't make her feel any more secure in her job. She'd lost most of her interest in sex ("I haven't even hinted at that to Jürgen"), and she had begun wondering at the absence of joy in her life. "I even cried for an hour when my cat coughed up a hairball."

Analysis

In assembling a differential diagnosis, I would invoke the following possibilities: mood or anxiety disorder due to metastatic cancer or other physical condition, substance-induced mood or anxiety disorder, major depression, dysthymia, GAD, panic disorder, alcohol dependence, and a personality disorder. Based on what Marian told the interviewer, you could work your way through the decision trees for mood and anxiety disorders, as I would, to arrive at a consideration of both GAD and some form of clinical depression. But, as it turned out, there was more to Marian's case than she was willing to admit at first.

That evening, Marian started the recommended course of an SSRI. A few nights later, she called her clinician from the emergency room: "I'm in the bag," she moaned. Without prompting, she admitted that she had been drinking right along and, fearful of losing her boyfriend, had lied about it to everyone.

Life has its surprises, especially if you are a mental health professional, and you'll just have to learn how to roll with punches. Of course, the
new information beats the older history; it requires both a complete revision of Marian's diagnosis and a therapeutic sea change.

We might wonder: Should her clinician have more diligently pursued
her claim that she had stopped drinking? Of course, it is important to trust
your patient, as I always try to do. But perhaps the truth process might
have been helped along by a reminder of its importance to her health and
future happiness. I often say something like this: "If you feel you can't talk
honestly about something, just ask, 'Could we skip that subject right
now?' "

It might also help to review the red flags I have mentioned in Chapter
4 (see the sidebar "Recognizing Red Flag Information" there). Is it suspicious that Marian extravagantly claimed to have eaten nothing for days,
that she had symptoms of numerous disorders, or that she'd quit a number
of jobs? Was the interviewer perhaps lulled by her forthright, seemingly
candid manner? How might she have responded to an interviewer's request to meet with Jürgen?

At any rate, the only diagnoses I'd give her at this point would be primary alcohol dependence and secondary depression of some sort. I'd hold
off on any diagnosis of an anxiety disorder until she had had several weeks
of sobriety—this time, for real.

Ingrid

Ingrid had worked as cashier at a comedy club on Portland's east side for
just a few weeks when her boss requested that she seek help. "I was crying all the time, and he said it was bad for business," she said between
sniffles. A few months earlier, after an abusive marriage ended in divorce,
Ingrid had moved from rural central Oregon (where she had grown up) to
her mother's new home in Portland. Despite her mother's presence, for
several months she complained of feeling isolated and "all alone in the
world."

To the interviewer, it wasn't clear whether her depression was due
to the divorce or the move away from the area where she had lived all her
life. Either way, Ingrid replied, she was miserable—unable to sleep or eat,
feeling guilty about everything, thinking she'd be better off dead, sometimes *wishing* she were dead already. "Lately, I've felt as bad as I ever did
on one of those bridges," she said. "Wait a minute," the interviewer interrupted. "What bridges?"

When Ingrid was a high school junior, the car in which she and three friends were riding crashed into an overpass abutment. The boy driving was drunk and he died, as did her best friend in the front passenger seat. Ingrid and the boy in the rear seat miraculously escaped unscathed, and forever after she avoided both drugs and alcohol. With an effort, she forced herself to "get back on the road," and so maintained her ability to drive. Ever since, however, even watching someone else cross a bridge in a movie or on TV caused a tightness in her chest.

Although she was usually healthy and calm, confronting bridges always frightened her, "like the world was coming to an end or something." Usually she had a panic attack—her heart beat too fast, she wanted to run but felt frozen, and she had such shortness of breath she seemed about to suffocate. And she'd *never* ride across a bridge; she would always imagine what would happen if an earthquake struck. ("Remember the 1989 San Francisco quake that collapsed part of the Bay Bridge and a major freeway? It killed dozens.") There had been no problem when she lived in the dry flatlands, where real bridges are unknown. "If someone gave them a bridge, they'd have to dig a hole to put it over," she commented. Portland, however, is both earthquake-prone and studded with bridges. That was why she took the comedy club job—it was the only one she could find on her side of the river.

Ingrid could go shopping just fine (on foot), and though she'd never much cared for heights, she denied having any other real phobias. She denied having panic attacks or other anxiety symptoms, and she'd never had symptoms of mania.

Analysis

The differential diagnosis I'd construct for Ingrid would go as follows: the usual (and terribly important) mood and anxiety disorders due to a (so far, inapparent) medical condition or substance use issue, major depression, dysthymia, somatization disorder, PTSD, GAD, panic disorder, specific phobia, and agoraphobia. Let's start with the depression, because it is more dangerous, more acute, and often more readily treated than many of the others. Absence of mania confines us to Figure 11.1; absence of physical disease and substance use, and a history of general good health, move us along through steps 5 and 9; we determine that we should consider Ingrid for a diagnosis of major depression without psychosis. Note that by using the decision tree, we have avoided the temptation to diagnose an adjustment disorder, for which we could imagine ample justification: a divorce, a move, living with her mom, and a change of jobs.

The anxiety disorder requires a trip through Figure 12.1. We have already rejected the possibilities of any disorder related to physical or chemical causes, but step 7 brings us up short: Ingrid did have a fear of crossing bridges. That moves us on through steps 11 and 12 to step 13, which suggests that we consider a diagnosis of specific phobia.

Now, which diagnosis—mood or anxiety—do we list first? As so often is the case, major depression is the more urgent to treat, so we should mention it first, even though it developed second. Anxiety disorders often go unreported for months or years, until another mental disorder— something even more stressful than anxiety—intervenes.

Kat

When evaluated in her early 30s, Kat had complained of ill health all her life. Her medical history extended to her early high school years, when the pain of "ulcers" (never proven) often prevented her from participating in gym class. At about that time she also began to suffer from severe headaches, which caused her to take to her bed for several days at a time. Although she referred to these headaches as migraines, she had never responded well to the usual migraine prophylaxis or to treatment with sumatriptan.

Her father, a medical doctor, supplied much of her early medical treatment, including a variety of narcotic painkillers. He had never exercised much supervision, however, and she had essentially self-medicated her depression, insomnia, anxiety, and suicidal ideas. When depressed, she would sometimes hit her head against the wall, cut herself with knives or scissors, or scratch her forehead with a piece of broken mirror. Later she claimed not to remember hitting her head. Without a trace of irony, she said, "I must have been bouncing off the walls." She had also taken several antidepressant drugs and at least two mood stabilizers, with little resulting improvement.

Kat's medical history was long and involved. At one time or another, she had experienced aphonia, weakness, heart palpitations, dizziness, hyperventilation, anxiety attacks, marked weight change, nausea, abdominal bloating, constipation, menstrual pain, menstrual irregularity, amenorrhea, menstrual hemorrhaging, lack of interest in sex, inability to experience orgasm, pain on intercourse, pain in extremities, and burning pains in other parts of her body. She had long suffered from premenstrual irritability and said she was allergic to many foods and medications. When she was 26, she talked one surgeon into removing the tip of her coccyx for "persistent butt pain."

When she was barely out of her teens, Kat had married a man several years older than she. He called her by her real name—Katherine—and was more than patient with her. He coped with her difficulties, he said, by smoking marijuana. The couple had two children, who were often cared for by one of their grandmothers while their mother's medical problems were being addressed. Kat's family history included many relatives with emotional problems, including grandparents and great-grandparents with alcoholism and a mother who also had headaches and depressions.

Immature and dependent, Kat was often whiny and petulant. Yet, when she wanted to turn on the charm, she could be attractive, almost seductive, especially in her relationships with men. Her personality had been called "borderline" by at least one of her previous clinicians, "histrionic" by others.

Analysis

Kat's history presents a richness of choice that includes physical, mood, anxiety, substance use, and even cognitive disorders. However, we'd like to make the smallest number of diagnoses possible; Occam's razor lives. Using the decision trees for either mood or anxiety disorders, we quickly come to the question of whether the patient had a long history of many unexplained somatic symptoms. Because Kat did have such a history, we are encouraged to consider somatization disorder.

Of course, somatization disorder does not rule out the possibility of an independent mood disorder. But Kat had been treated (ineffectively) for clinical depression with a great variety of medications. In my experience, patients with somatization disorder usually also have mood or anxiety conditions, but these rarely respond well to medication.

Fritz

A 17-year Navy lifer, Fritz couldn't drink during deployments, and while in port he somehow managed to conceal his intoxication at work. But he spend evenings and weekends at the club or in his basement bar. His wife, Cindy, loyally cleaned up after him, apologized for him, reared their family, paid their bills, and managed their legal affairs. "It always seemed normal—it's the way it was with my own parents," she explained the day she finally got Fritz to counseling.

When he was 40, Fritz developed pancreatitis and almost died. While still recovering, he made friends with an AA member in the next hospital bed and got religion. "Just like the president," he had informed Cindy.

The trouble started during his first few months of sobriety. Despite his drinking, or maybe because of it, he and Cindy had always gotten along well. She didn't nag him much about his drinking, and he let her alone to manage, which she had always done brilliantly. Once he was no longer perennially intoxicated, that deal was off. Now he expressed an opinion about everything, from how to cook a brisket to what school their daughter should attend in the fall. He even enrolled Cindy at a spa to shed some of the weight she'd built up over the years.

"I preferred things the way they used to be," she concluded. "From the time I was 10, I've coped with men who're drunk. But now that I've got one who's sober, *I'm* the one at sea."

Analysis

Fritz's alcohol dependence was beyond question; it had affected his family life for many years. By its absence, it had now contributed to a change in his relationship with his wife (step 1 in Figure 16.1). Although Fritz had just had a major medical illness (pancreatitis), there's no step 2 physiological mechanism through which it could have caused the couple's marital issues. Though the clinician might want to revisit the issue at some point, the brevity of Fritz's change and its nonpervasive nature would speak against a personality disorder as the cause of the current difficulties, so we'll vote "no" at steps 3 and 4. Because Cindy's own upbringing and her acceptance of Fritz's former drinking clearly contributed to the stability their marriage had enjoyed until Fritz's recent reform, we finally arrive at step 5 and the advice to consider a relational problem.

William

While still on active duty, William Minor, a young surgeon for the Union Army in the American Civil War, had begun to imagine that he was being persecuted. He noticed that fellow officers would glance at him suspiciously and mutter about him; he even challenged one of his best friends to a duel. William carried a concealed revolver while off duty, and he was known to visit prostitutes frequently, almost obsessively. Although he had complained of headaches and dizziness, no physical illness was ever diagnosed. This officer, who had served with distinction on the battlefield, was eventually invalided out of the Army due to "nerves."

At age 33, William was hospitalized as homicidal and suicidal. Released several years later, he continued to feel persecuted by men who slipped poison into his mouth while he was sleeping. Ultimately, he went to England to paint and recuperate. There he shot and killed an innocent stranger he imagined was one of the Irishmen who, as he had complained to the police on several occasions, kept sneaking into his room and hiding in the rafters. Found not guilty on grounds of insanity, he was confined to the Broadmoor asylum in England for the next 38 years.

At 40, William remained convinced that intruders tried to get into his cell at night. He reported that he felt something being pumped into him, and that at night he could feel a cold iron being pressed against his teeth. He asked a fellow inmate to cut his throat for him. At age 43, he complained that the marrow of his spine was being pierced, and that instruments of torture were being used to operate on his heart. A year later, he became convinced that electric currents were being passed through him; he also claimed that at night, he would be transported as far as Constantinople, where he was made to "perform lewd acts in public." After the Wrights flew at Kitty Hawk in 1903, he believed that his nocturnal transport took place in flying machines. Only once, when he was about 50, did he ever claim to hear a sound that could be a hallucination; it was of the door of his cell being opened at night.

With ample time, and money to spare from his Army pay, William responded to an advertisement for people to help gather quotations for what eventually became the *Oxford English Dictionary*. Over the course of 20 years, he contributed tens of thousand of quotations, becoming the editor's friend and ultimate resource for many hard-to-document words. When so engaged, he would talk coherently and intelligently, and was often cheerful. Yet he was ultimately so remorseful for his crime that he offered financial help to the family of the man he had killed. For a time the man's widow even served as his courier, bringing to him at the asylum books he had ordered from London shops.

Toward the end of his life, perhaps to combat the sexual urges of which he had grown ashamed, William cut off his own penis with surgical skill and cast it into the fire. As an old man he returned to the United States, where he was diagnosed with dementia praecox.

Analysis

William's undeniable psychosis requires the following differential diagnosis: schizophrenia, delusional disorder, psychotic depression, schizoaffective disorder, and psychosis due to a medical condition. Using Figure 13.1, we can summarily reject a substance use factor. Both dementia and somatization disorder seem terribly remote possibilities for this patient, but we need to think about the possibility of a medical cause for his complaints.

Could a tumor or perhaps an endocrine condition have caused both his paranoid thinking and his headaches and dizziness? Confronted today with such a patient, we'd order numerous laboratory tests. In the case of William, however, the test of time will have to serve as a proxy; decades of psychosis without suggestion of a specific illness allow us to slip beyond step 1.

At step 5, we come upon the nut of the diagnostic problem: Just what symptoms did William have? Of course, his delusions were extensive and enduring, but did he have any other basic symptoms of psychosis that would affirm the diagnosis of the old term for schizophrenia, dementia praecox? His thinking (speech) and his behavior regarding matters that did not pertain to his delusions were unexceptional; rather than showing flattened affect or lack of interest or motivation, if anything, he could be forceful and heated. And nowhere does history suggest that he had pronounced hallucinations, other than one mention that he thought he heard his door opening at night—hardly the sort of auditory hallucination typically experienced by patients with schizophrenia. On the other hand, he did report extensive hallucinations of touch, which are typical of patients with delusional disorder. And that is where we end up, with a patient who functioned so well apart from his delusions (step 11) that he contributed literally thousands of quotations to a dictionary we still use today.

Were William's delusions—such as of being whisked far away at night—nonbizarre, as required by the definition of delusional disorder? This one, though implausible, could have physically happened, though some were more debatable. However, he had many other delusions that were perfectly possible, thereby fulfilling the definition.

A more important issue has to do with the dangers of trying to diagnose a patient one has never met. It is one thing, as an exercise, to use the historical record to attempt a diagnosis for someone long dead. However, clinicians must be extremely careful about offering their opinions on persons who are still alive, unless these opinions are based on interviews plus all the collateral information it is possible to gather.

Scott

Raised in a strongly religious family, Scott had imagined from the age of 6 that Jesus was constantly watching to see whether he would do something naughty. If he should ever be caught, a mark against him would be entered in a long ledger. Consequently, he always sought to make sure that his actions were precise, his behavior perfect.

Little Scott even sought to move and walk "perfectly." He would only cross between rooms by stepping carefully over an imaginary line drawn at the doorway, and he would start climbing any flight of stairs with his left foot; if he forgot, he would have to go back and start again. He would count the number of stairs in a flight, then immediately try to forget it. He was also careful to arrange his schoolbooks and papers with their margins exactly parallel to his desktop edge. When he was very young, none of this seemed out of place, but as a teenager, he felt peculiar and ashamed.

Scott started high school feeling all alone. His father had died rather suddenly the year before, and he and his mother continued to live on their small rural acreage outside town. Their quiet lifestyle left him much time to think. What if the house should catch fire—would the volunteer fire department, located miles away, be able to put it out in time? With farmers growing more and more blueberries, would the water in their well dry up? These thoughts would often intrude on his study time or prevent him from falling asleep at night.

When Scott was 17 and about to graduate from high school, one evening he suddenly "realized" that his life was about to end and that he had nowhere to go. He felt empty, cried to himself, and began to think about suicide. At about that time, stories of students who had murdered teachers and classmates were much in the news, and over the next several days Scott felt increasingly compelled to think about ways of inflicting violent death. He had no gun and didn't think he could buy one, but he had access to all the knives he could possibly need. Whenever his mother asked him to peel a potato or dice a carrot, through his mind would flash a scene in which he was stabbing her to death with the knife. That would make him feel so physically nauseated and shaky that he had to sit on a stool to work at the sink. After high school, he got a job in the print shop of the local weekly newspaper. He never considered moving away from home.

Scott was interested in women, but he had no earthly idea how to approach them. He worried that he would never find the right person and would remain unmarried all his life. At night he would masturbate while thinking about the girl who had sat in front of him in senior English class. With release, he would be flooded with shame and the feeling that he had to atone by reading verses from his Bible. When he doubted that he had read every word, he'd go back over them again several times.

When he was 25, his mother started to show signs of forgetfulness. They sought the help of a specialist, who eventually gave them the diagnosis Scott had feared: Alzheimer's disease. Over the next couple of weeks, his weight dropped as his appetite plummeted, and he stayed up late, feeling guilty and worrying that he might kill himself. On their third visit to the clinician, Scott broke down in tears and confessed that he had purchased a small, single-shot pistol at an antique show the week before.

Analysis

Although the differential list we must consider for Scott seems a lot like the one for many other patients, that doesn't mean it is any less important. Remember always that a wide-ranging differential diagnosis is the bedrock of accurate mental health diagnosis. For Scott, I would include general medical and substance use causes of anxiety and depression, major depressive disorder, dysthymia, bipolar disorders, OCD, GAD, and a personality disorder.

Of course, we list this stuff, only to discard much of it. We find no medical or substance use issues that would trip us up at the first three steps of Figure 12.1. With a clear history of both obsessions and compulsions, we strike pay dirt at step 4, which directs us to consider a diagnosis of OCD. OCD is one of those diagnoses with such remarkable symptoms that clinicians could overlook symptoms of other disorders. However, the diagnostic principle about multiple diagnoses reminds us to ask, "Have we covered all the symptoms?" The answer is "No," for Scott's worries about such varied problems as a dry well, a house afire, and a lonely bachelor life were not explained by OCD. He experienced these ideas not as fears but as worries, they interfered with his sleep and studies, and he had experienced no unusually traumatic event, so at step 6 we must also consider the diagnosis of GAD.

In addition, the step 17 asterisk directs us to carefully consider any symptoms of a mood disorder, and that means a trip through Figure 11.1. Although the information available in the vignette is a bit scanty for a final diagnosis, major depression seems a good possibility—a nice demonstration of our diagnostic principle always to consider a mood disorder.

Which diagnosis should we list first? The mood disorder would be most likely to cause immediate harm, placing major depression at the top of the list for further evaluation and treatment. Next would come OCD, and finally GAD.

Misty

"It rose right up out of the toilet—long, and green, with sharp fangs. I was terrified!" She giggled. "It's still in there, I know—I hear it at night. It sings in Chinese."

During her first interview that fall, Misty spoke slowly, as if she found each word lying in a minefield. She looked older than 23; her nearly black hair was thin and straggly, and the dark circles under her eyes gave her the look of a *Doonesbury* comic strip character. As we spoke, she chipped away with her thumbnail at the dark paint that dotted her right hand. I already knew quite a lot about her from her father, who had spoken to me the week before, just after his son's appointment.

Misty was an artist who had already had one well-reviewed show the year before. Her specialty had been wispy images of guileless children and adolescents that seemed ready to float off the easel. However, her father had noticed a change before Christmas, nearly a year ago, when her work gradually took on heavy lines and her color palette darkened. "Now her images just lie there, brooding on the canvas," he said. "It chills me just to view them."

Earlier that week, her father discovered she'd pulled the wires of her phone out of the wall. He recalled that over the past couple of months, she had installed double bolts on both doors of her flat. When I asked Misty about this, she turned away and mumbled a comment to someone I couldn't see. Then she said, "I was just replacing the old lock—it was broken. And I tripped over the telephone wire."

Always quiet and reclusive, Misty had had only one friend in high school, another artistically inclined girl. Even after graduation, when she had interacted more with other artists at shows, she'd never had a boyfriend. Her older brother had fallen ill years earlier; he was chronically beset by auditory hallucinations that medication could never quite vanquish, and by the persistent delusion that he was being monitored by the CIA. He had been treated for schizophrenia by a series of clinicians.

Analysis

The differential diagnosis we'd construct for Misty's psychosis would include psychosis due to physical disorder or substance use, schizophrenia, schizoaffective disorder, and schizophreniform disorder. Referring to Figure 13.1, we can move past steps 1–4 and agree that she had hallucinations. Moreover, her bland emotional response, despite the giggling, sounded a lot like a negative symptom. These data move us on to steps 9 (where we answer "no") and 10 (also "no"), leaving us to consider schizophreniform psychosis.

But wait a minute: Didn't Misty's father report that he had noticed changes many months earlier? Wouldn't that put her over the 6 months needed for a diagnosis of schizophrenia? And what about her strong family history of schizophrenia? I need to underscore a very important point here: A person who may have a disorder as serious as schizophrenia needs the benefit of all the skepticism we can muster. In this regard, changes in art technique don't mean psychosis, and family history can only suggest a diagnosis, not direct one. We want our information to guide us to our conclusion, not stampede us to premature closure. I'd also point out the two-sided diagnostic principle about typical and atypical symptoms. In this context, Misty's visual hallucination of a green snake is a bit unusual—the sort of finding that might make us worry about a possible (if improbable) organic cause for her psychosis.

Although I'd also agree that the objective sign of her glancing to the side and speaking would beat her denial of hallucinations (yet another diagnostic principle), here's the bottom line: Whereas in my heart of hearts I believe that Misty might well turn out to have schizophrenia, I would still be unwilling to commit to such a high-risk diagnosis without more data.

Leonard

The first thing Leonard said when he appeared for his initial interview was that he'd gotten no help at all from his previous clinician. The second thing, almost, was that he didn't want anyone to contact his previous health care providers.

At 49, Leonard complained he'd had anxiety and depression for much of his adult life. Oh, yes, he might drink as many as five or six beers some days, but entire weeks went by without any drinking at all. He had used Xanax for many years—only a milligram per day on average, though when he was extra stressed he took up to three tablets. He was vague about other possible substance use. He occasionally smoked marijuana, but only when at a party, and it never seemed to bother him. He had tried numerous antidepressants and other psychotropic drugs; nearly all of them caused profound side effects.

Leonard was born in rural Nebraska, where his parents worked a small truck farm when they weren't drinking. His father, bright but with little formal education, had resented having children. When he came home from an evening's tour of their town's three bars, he'd sometimes haul Leonard out to the watering trough behind the house and "jokingly" whip him with a leather belt until he thought he would pass out. His mother also drank heavily and periodically became severely depressed; twice she had attempted suicide. *Her* father had leaped to his death from the top of his small town's highest building when she was a girl.

A skilled artisan, Leonard had been self-employed for the last decade restoring furniture. He had previously worked at a wood joinery, but was fired when he had an affair on company time with his employer's au pair. Although he could make anything with his hands, he had trouble focusing attention on paperwork; consequently, he hadn't paid his taxes for several years. When asked about this, he seemed nonchalant, as though it didn't really matter much at all.

Leonard's anxiety attacks were usually preceded by thinking about his personal problems. Although he described them as feelings of terror, they were never accompanied by physical symptoms such as pounding heart or shortness of breath. He also complained of nearly constant anxiety that didn't seem to be related to a specific worry, problem, or emotion. "I'm just not a worrier," he claimed. He did admit to intermittent suicidal ideas, though never with plans or an attempt; these ideas centered about the concern that he wasn't going anywhere in life. "When I'm 50, if I'm still right where I am now, I'll be a failure. That's when I'd drink the Kool-Aid."

Analysis

Right away, we are concerned that we cannot know enough for a proper diagnosis about anyone who intentionally withholds information from his clinician—the ultimate red flag warning (again, see the sidebar on this topic in Chapter 4) that something is amiss. However, despite his apparent manipulations, we should not leap to the conclusion that the main diagnosis should be a personality disorder. Leonard did present symptoms of depression (his clinician had wondered about bipolar II disorder), anxiety (could he have PTSD or GAD?), and substance misuse—all of which we should enter into his differential diagnosis. And, of course, he could have a personality disorder. In fact, there isn't enough information for a definite diagnosis in any of the areas we've considered. When that's the case, there's only one remedy: *undiagnosed.*

In this case, as in so many others, *undiagnosed* prevents closure and reminds us that we must continue to inquire into the reasons for a patient's symptoms. Often, this means obtaining more information; for example, had Leonard experienced legal difficulties? *Undiagnosed* also discourages us from attempting treatment that is experimental or unusually dangerous. And his clinician might even use the lack of a definitive diagnosis to enlist Leonard's full cooperation with the information-gathering process.

At length, a letter did arrive from a previous physician, who had refused to treat Leonard further with medications because of his drinking.

He had been in a severe auto accident, caused by alcohol-fueled speeding when driving his SUV. The passenger in the other auto had died; the driver was still in a coma. Of course, this information allowed a fuller, more specific diagnosis.

Gilbert

Though *The Ordeal of Gilbert Pinfold* was one of Evelyn Waugh's less weighty creations, it was written from personal experience and thus provides fodder for our diagnostic adventures. An insomniac middle-aged writer with no previous mental illness, Gilbert sought to escape the stresses of his English life by cruising to Ceylon, leaving his sleeping draughts behind. From the very first, he encountered rough sailing: He had trouble understanding a shipping office clerk and the procedures. He dropped things when he first boarded the ship, and he was a little disoriented during the first day out. He kept falling asleep.

Then the hallucinations began. At first, it was just music; then Gilbert heard a dog's feet tripping along the deck, next a clergyman giving a sermon, and then the crew swearing. Finally, he began to overhear lengthy speeches from many voices. They came to him from just outside his door, over a wireless device that was somehow piped into his cabin, or even to his table in the lounge. It became clear to him that he was to play a key role in the resistance to a plot to take over the ship. In a panic he cried out, "Oh, let me not be mad, not mad, sweet heaven."

Stepping onto the deck, Gilbert found it deserted; the voices now told him that the plot had been a hoax. He felt that all the passengers were looking at him and talking about him. The voice of a young woman declared that she loved him and wanted to spend the night with him, but her mother intervened. Gilbert lay awake all night as voices urged him to leap into the ocean. They were, he believed, trying to psychoanalyze him.

By the end of Gilbert's 14-day adventure, he had escaped his hallucinations and delusions. He was neither depressed nor particularly anxious, but he was confused about how long he'd been at sea—and about just what he'd done there. Although he believed he'd sent a dozen telegrams, in reality there was only one.

Analysis

Most clinicians would probably start with a differential diagnosis for psychosis: substance misuse or physical cause of psychosis, mood disorder with psychosis, schizophreniform psychosis, schizoaffective disorder, and schizophrenia. (You can see how truly committed I am to a wide-ranging differential diagnosis; even on first reading, I didn't for a moment believe that Gilbert had schizophrenia.) Of course, knowing the outcome (rapid, complete resolution) makes it easy to travel the first couple of steps in Figure 13.1 to a diagnosis of a psychosis induced by drug withdrawal. We remember that just before becoming ill, Gilbert had discontinued his long-time sleeping medication.

OK, so Gilbert had a drug withdrawal reaction. Did he show any symptoms in addition to those of psychosis? A careful reading of the vignette reveals that he dropped things, was disoriented, and had trouble understanding what a clerk was telling him—all symptoms pointing to a cognitive disorder. Figure 14.1 brings us at once to the definition of delirium, which would fit Gilbert perfectly. The culprits were the sleeping draughts containing chloral and bromine he had been using, unbeknownst to his doctor, who had prescribed additional powerful drugs. Indeed, before Gilbert had left on the voyage he had admitted to his wife that he was "doped to the eyeballs," and he had difficulty writing legibly or even tying his shoelaces. Small wonder that he was having a drug withdrawal delirium—a horse that too many clinicians forget to think about while they are out pursuing zebras.

Norma

"It's a long story," Norma said. "It isn't a happy story." Pieced together from various sources (including a long chat with her grown daughter, Pat), it was a miserable tale indeed.

Norma had a withered leg—a birth defect that had clouded her entire childhood. She wore a brace with a build-up shoe, and when she walked, she had to move her foot forward with a kicking motion. "Running was a joke," she reported with a snort. Her childhood anger was fueled by the fact that her older sister, Arlette, was athletic and extremely popular with boys. Although Norma was smart and quick-witted, throughout her school years she added alienation to her anger, rebelling against authority. With another girl from her high school class, she used to dress provocatively and go down to the naval yard, where they'd welcome sailors home from months at sea. "I had a couple of scares back then," Norma admitted, "and penicillin was my best friend." Her mother, guilt-ridden over the damage she feared was her fault, catered to Norma's frequent demands for extra privileges, while severely limiting Arlette's freedom.

Despite her intelligence, Norma swore she'd never go to college. Instead, from high school she moved to Fairbanks and got a job with a company that supplied groceries and clothing to workers on the Alaska oil pipeline. It paid well, and it left her the time she needed for recreation, much of which involved men. Through three promotions she kept her job, long enough to meet her first husband, Kirk. "I knew right from the first that Kirk was gay," Norma said. "But he was so cute—looked like Tony Perkins—I just had to have him. Chased him all around the Arctic Circle one summer. I think he finally married me to be rid of me. Anyway, the marriage was a disaster—no surprise—and after we had two children, he ran off with a priest."

She then moved to the lower 48, where it was far cheaper to live; rather than finding another job, however, she ran through her savings. She tried hard to get on disability, but was rejected several times. A doctor had gone out of the way to help her, but she turned on him and threatened to blacken his reputation. "I know he lied about me in his report," she complained. "I told him I was going to report him to the medical board."

Eventually, she solved her insolvency by getting married again. "Whenever my second husband drank, he'd treat me like pond scum—blackened my eye several times, even before the wedding," she said. She would call the police when he beat her up, then refuse to press charges. "He always swore he loved me and wouldn't do it again, so we'd have a few beers and make love." When he finally left her for another woman, she was furious; she harassed him by telephone and in person until he got a restraining order. Since her second divorce, she'd had several boyfriends, whom she tended to berate until they abandoned her. Then she'd cry and say how lonely she felt.

Pat and her brother, Danny, had more or less reared themselves while Norma ran a talent agency she started on money she'd borrowed from Arlette. "Mom had lots of energy and creativity," Pat summed up. "But she didn't waste any of it on us."

For months, she'd barely spoken to either of her children. "Seven previous counselors have told me it's the kids' fault we don't get along," Norma complained. Danny had broken with her completely. She had found out he was living with another man, and wrote a letter to several of her relatives, that he'd turned out to be "just as queer as his father." Pat had told her, "You give new meaning to the term *family outing*."

Norma now stayed home and surfed the Internet. "I got tired of people looking funny at my leg, thinking up snide comments." Her retirement plan was to inherit money once her mother died.

Norma finally consented to an evaluation "because I decided I didn't know who I was." Although her appetite had been poor, she had recently gained 5 pounds. At times she felt "depressed and empty," but mostly that was when she stepped on the scales, she admitted with a chuckle. She had never been suicidal: "It's for chumps."

Analysis

Everything we know about Norma (even though it is not nearly enough yet) seems to cry out "personality disorder." Here are the hallmarks, based partly on collateral information from her daughter: Her symptoms were lifelong; they affected her in several ways (mood, thinking, interpersonal functioning, and impulse control); they caused her distress and affected various personal and social situations, such as family relations and work; and the pattern had been stable for a number of years. However, Figure 16.1 (and a diagnostic principle) urges us first to carefully consider other possibilities. From the material we have, her depression appeared to be neither intense nor long-lasting, and it certainly hadn't been present throughout her entire adult life, as it would need to be to explain her behavior. At worst, I'd consider it an adjustment to her changing life circumstances, in part brought on by the way she dealt with people. Norma's short leg had certainly marked her psyche, but it wasn't the sort of step 2 medical problem that would directly cause mental disorders. We'd need to explore further the question of how much she drank, and I'd want to know about anxiety symptoms, too. But here, for once, is someone I'd consider as possibly having no major Axis I mental disorder.

Would Norma fully meet criteria for a named personality disorder? Not on the basis of the current information, though some clinicians might favor a borderline diagnosis. Because her life history is so replete with personality disorder symptoms—which include some borderline, paranoid, histrionic, and perhaps narcissistic features—I would use the term *personality disorder NOS* at step 4.

Raymond

When Raymond was growing up in eastern Washington State, he played baritone horn in the high school band. For a small school, the band played pretty well, so it was often invited to bigger cities for parades and competitions. During their bus trips, Raymond usually played penny-ante blackjack. "I always felt a shudder of excitement when I won," he told his clinician years later. "No matter how often it happened, I never grew bored with it." He had had another fling with gambling—craps—during his early

20s when he served in the Army Reserves, but he'd had the good sense to get out of the military before the first Gulf War: "I wasn't *that* high a roller."

He took a job with a civilian contractor working on toxic Superfund site cleanup. Using a forklift, Raymond had to move huge drums of radioactive waste into a storage facility. The leisurely pace left a lot of time for recreation, so he and some coworkers would play poker. They started at dollar pots, but after a few months, whole paychecks could disappear at the turn of a card. When an Indian casino opened down the street from his work, he first tried video poker. Later he graduated to roulette, and a friend would cover for him as he took increasingly long lunch hours. After work, he often walked home rather than take the bus, to save the $1.50 for gambling.

Gambling gave Raymond a lift when he felt depressed (often about his gambling). Though he maxed out seven credit cards, his wife didn't find out until bill collectors started calling at the house. He tearfully promised her that he would stop, and he did—for a time. At first he attended Gamblers Anonymous meetings, but later he went to the casino instead.

To the intake worker at the mental health clinic, Raymond remarked that his job took courage. "Misjudge the weight, lose your concentration for a second, and boom! You glow in the dark for the rest of your life, all 7 days of it." It had always seemed strange; at the gaming tables, Raymond had nerves of steel. But to move tons of nuclear waste took just a little of what his grandmother had always called "Dutch courage." He tried to limit himself to three or four beers in a day, though several times he operated his forklift when he was high. When he did drink during the day, no one knew except one close friend at work—and the cop who on two occasions had watched him fail field sobriety tests.

Analysis

All those who repeatedly lose more than they can afford have a gambling problem; the question of whether the gambling qualifies as pathological seems almost academic. Much gambling takes place as a social activity with friends; the person is willing to lose up to a specified amount as entertainment, but not to jeopardize the rent or food money in the process. But many of Raymond's gambling behaviors spoke to their addictive nature: gambling by himself, concealing it from his wife, feeling uncomfortable if he couldn't do it (analogous to the withdrawal symptoms of substance addictions), making repeated attempts to control the behavior (he had failed at Gamblers Anonymous), and gambling instead of working. When push came to shove, with his wife doing the pushing, even Raymond seemed to agree he had a problem. You don't really need Figure 15.1 to arrive at a step 3 diagnosis of pathological gambling.

What about Raymond's drinking? With no history of tolerance or withdrawal (step 1), he wouldn't qualify by strict criteria for alcohol dependence. As far as we are aware, he didn't drink all that much, but he had had a couple of problems: two driving while intoxicated arrests and use of alcohol in a dangerous situation. Regardless of whether we call Raymond's problem *dependence* or *abuse*, it still represented substance use that created problems for the patient and society. Raymond's story also provides stark evidence of the similarity between gambling and substance misuse, which are highly comorbid. And by the way, though I have not listed a differential diagnosis for Raymond, from Table 6.1 I would take careful note that major depression also often accompanies both gambling and substance use.

Which diagnosis should we list first? Both conditions would require prompt attention, and they apparently arose more or less together. At least gambling wouldn't be likely to cause Raymond to mishandle a barrel of toxic chemicals, so I'd go with the drinking.

Reynolds

A full professor of chemistry at a Midwestern technical school, at age 57 Reynolds had "never known a sick day," as he later told his interviewer. One afternoon, standing at his workbench looking at a test tube full of crystals he'd just precipitated, he suddenly *knew* that the chairman of his department had marked him for dismissal. The thought caused him to bolt from his lab and carefully collect and burn all of the correspondence in his files.

Within a few hours, out of the corner of his left eye, Reynolds began to see swooping blurs of light that trailed after objects and gradually faded to black. Over the next 2 weeks, these increased to such an extent that he could barely focus on his work. He missed the first two appointments with the family practitioner who had taken care of him for 30 years. "First I didn't remember making an appointment; then I couldn't remember when it was," he later confessed. By the time he finally appeared, he'd been ill for over a month and was so distraught that he cried during the exam. After doing a thorough workup and finding nothing physically wrong, the doctor wrote "Sounds like early schizophrenia" in a letter of referral to a mental health care provider.

Analysis

Even this fragmentary presentation allows us to note several relevant points. Foremost is the importance of not leaping to conclusions based on appearances; instead, historical information should provide the bedrock of our assessments. Reynolds's primary care physician should have constructed a differential diagnosis and safety hierarchy, which would have included the disorders mentioned in Table 13.1. Working through Figure 13.1, we'd first have to wonder whether Reynolds had been exposed to some toxic chemical (step 2). But what if we didn't have access to this history? Then the most extreme diagnosis we could make would be schizophreniform disorder at step 10. Note that Reynolds had visual hallucinations, which are nontypical for schizophrenia, as is his age; at 57, he was far older than the usual patient with schizophrenia.

What can we predict about Reynolds's future with schizophreniform disorder? Of the features that predict a good prognosis (see the sidebar "Prognosis and Schizophreniform Psychosis" in Chapter 13)—confusion, psychotic features early in the course of the illness, good premorbid functioning, and affect that is not blunt or flattened—Reynolds had them all.

Tonya

"I found out that I'm pregnant. That's what got me here. It made me so anxious—joyful, but anxious." Tonya stared straight forward and laughed, in a sort of rapid giggle that she repeated often during the next 45 minutes. Her freckles and tousled auburn hair made her seem younger than her 27 years. "It gives me panicky feelings that I'm at last going to do something worthwhile."

Just what she had been doing previously was a little unclear. Reared in California, Tonya had left school in the ninth grade and run away to join the carnival. When she was 16, she got married and moved with her husband to the South for several years. "He also worked for the carnival, like me. I did pretty much anything. He did cocaine." Another giggle. "Eventually I left him and moved here. This is a great city for the homeless," she added. This last time she'd been homeless for several months, but she had lived on the streets for "pretty much my entire adult life."

"In Georgia, I was jumped by three girls I'd turned in for child molestation," she said. "I ended up hurting one pretty bad; she died, but the police said that it was justifiable homicide, and they didn't hold me." She moistened her lips, but this time she didn't laugh. She admitted that she was happier now, in the hospital, than she'd been ever before. "But I don't think I'm too happy—my mood has been pretty midline the last couple of months. My sleep? Oh, that's probably 8 or 9 hours a night."

A year or two earlier, while hospitalized in Georgia after an overdose, Tonya had been treated with an antidepressant. She thought it had helped her. "I had been drinking some—well, a lot—for a long time. Maybe a pint a day." She said that gin earned her some arrests for DWI and beating up her husband. "I got so drunk I used to wet myself." She admitted to having the shakes, and some mornings she would have to take a "hair of the dog."

Tonya had made two other suicide attempts. Once she cut her wrists; she had also tried hanging, but couldn't get the knot just right. That was when she discovered that she'd been sleeping with her half brother. He had known about the relationship; she had not. When she discovered they had the same father, she felt betrayed. With neither attempt had she done any serious physical damage to herself. "That's when they told me I'm manic–depressive," she explained.

When depressed, Tonya's sleep didn't usually change, and she could focus on reading or watching TV. Her appetite remained mostly unchanged, and she often felt "hyper and restless."

Tonya's mother was mentally abusive, and her father had forced sex on her. "He was a drinker; when I was barely a year old, he did unspeakable thing. I remember it all so clearly, even today." Her father's relatives were all "drinkers" like him; her mother's relatives were all "nervous— they had a lot of anxiety and depression." Despite it all, she remembered her childhood as being basically happy. "I had a good time as a kid. I had a girlfriend, and in the sixth grade we had sex together. Afterwards, I told the other kids at school about it, so I became more or less the class pariah." As an adult, Tonya hadn't had sex with women, but she admitted that when she was with the carnival, she had engaged in prostitution. "Actually, I've been pretty promiscuous most of my life. I have no idea who my baby's father is."

Tonya had also worked as a waitress, at a machine shop, and at a 7-Eleven for 3 years; she had never been fired. As noted earlier, she'd attended school only until the ninth grade, but she later earned a general equivalency diploma. Though always a good student, she described herself as having few friends and "always being a loner, even today." This was one reason she was so glad to be pregnant—now she'd always have a friend. (A slip of paper in the front of her chart noted that her pregnancy test had come back negative, though she hadn't yet been given this information.)

When this interview took place, Tonya had been hospitalized for 3 days with a diagnosis of bipolar I disorder. Throughout the interview, she maintained attention and seemed to connect well with the interviewer. Other than the giggling, which seemed a function of embarrassment, her mood was level and appropriate. Alert and quick, she passed the usual tests for orientation, calculations, and memory without difficulty. She denied having previous anxiety or panic attacks; she didn't feel she was being followed or persecuted, "though a bus once told me, 'Good job!' Yes, it seemed as clear to me as your voice is now. And I wasn't using drugs or alcohol then."

Analysis

In a differential list of possible diagnoses—major depression, bipolar I disorder, panic and other anxiety disorders, psychosis of various sorts, traumatic brain injury, substance use, personality disorder—the one issue that seems pretty clear is Tonya's drinking. By her own admission, she'd been a heavy consumer of alcohol, which had led to a number of difficulties, including driving violations and domestic violence. I would consider her as having alcohol dependence, but the extent to which drinking contributed to her other difficulties would need to be sorted out.

Tonya's current clinicians were treating her for bipolar I disorder. Was this wise? Of course, mood disorders reside near the top of any safety hierarchy, and she said she had previously responded well to treatment for depression; it's a diagnostic principle that could push us toward such a diagnosis, if we were in a mood to be pushed. But a great deal of her history was atypical or contradictory: She remembered abuse when she was a year old; she couldn't get the knot right for hanging; with depression, her energy level increased and her sleep wasn't much changed; though she was admitted for anxiety and depression, her affect during the interview didn't seem especially depressed. And her claim that the police "didn't hold me" after she killed someone seems like fantasy.

Anxiety and even panic symptoms coincided with her "pregnancy," and I don't like to trust information that may be crisis-generated. I would note the voice from the bus, but I would not be pushed very far in the direction of psychosis without more symptoms. Of course, the prostitution and other features of a highly disorganized life would make me consider personality disorder—but, although this seems a good bet, I wouldn't make that diagnosis without a lot more information.

To wrap up, here's another instance where, other than alcohol dependence, the only safe diagnosis at this point would be mental disorder, undiagnosed type.

Appendix: Diagnostic Principles

Throughout this book, I've described the principles that for years have guided me through the evaluation of thousands of mental health patients. Here I've collected them all, arranged into four broad categories. I'll be the first to admit that these 24 principles sometimes overlap and sometimes conflict with one another, and that the four categories I've put them into are a bit fluid. But these maxims provide the bedrock on which for decades I've constructed my mental health diagnoses.

The principles are listed here in the order in which you might want to use them when evaluating a patient; it's a little different from the order in which I've first mentioned them in the text. I've also sometimes shortened the text versions here. Finally, I've added letters (which might make them a little easier to use when you are actually working with a patient) and the page numbers where they are first discussed in the text.

Create a Differential Diagnosis

A. Arrange your differential diagnosis according to a safety hierarchy (page 16).
B. Family history can guide diagnosis, but because you often can't trust reports, clinicians should attempt to rediagnose each family member (page 29).
C. Physical disorders and their treatment can produce or worsen mental symptoms (page 17).
D. Consider somatization disorder whenever symptoms don't jibe or treatments don't work (page 110).
E. Substance use can cause a variety of mental disorders (page 17).
F. Because of their ubiquity, potential for harm, and ready response to treatment, *always* consider mood disorders (page 120).

When Information Sources Conflict

G. History beats current appearance (page 24).
H. Recent history beats ancient history (page 26).

I. Collateral information sometimes beats the patient's own (page 26).

J. Signs beat symptoms (page 27).

K. Be wary when evaluating crisis-generated data (page 28).

L. Objective findings beat subjective judgment (page 28).

M. Use Occam's razor: Choose the simplest explanation (page 30).

N. Horses are more common than zebras; prefer the more frequently encountered diagnosis (page 31).

O. Watch for contradictory information (page 36).

Resolve Uncertainty

P. The best predictor of future behavior is past behavior (page 47).

Q. More symptoms of a disorder increase its likelihood as your diagnosis (page 47).

R. Typical features of a disorder increase its likelihood as your diagnosis; in the presence of nontypical features, look for alternatives (page 47).

S. Previous typical response to treatment for a disorder increases its likelihood as your diagnosis (page 48).

T. Use the word *undiagnosed* whenever you cannot be sure of your diagnosis (page 48).

U. Consider the possibility that this patient should be given no mental diagnosis at all (page 51).

Multiple Diagnoses

V. When symptoms cannot be adequately explained by a single disorder, consider multiple diagnoses (page 61).

W. Avoid personality disorder diagnoses when your patient is acutely ill with an Axis I disorder (page 62).

X. Arrange multiple diagnoses to list first the one that is most urgent, treatable, or specific. Whenever possible, also list diagnoses chronologically (page 64).

References
and Suggested Reading

I've included here citations for a number of studies and papers mentioned throughout the text, as well as some of the important papers written about diagnostic method. One or two of the classic papers date back several decades or more; despite their age, they still have the capacity to teach us. For those interested in learning more about the real-life individuals (both historical and modern) who are mentioned in the text or described in case examples, I provide sources of information on these persons.

General References on Interviewing and Diagnosis

American Psychiatric Association: *Diagnostic and Statistical Manual of Mental Disorders* (4th ed., text rev.). Washington, DC: Author, 2000.—For DSM-IV-TR, a few DSM-IV criteria have received minor face-lifts, and the text has been revised to reflect recent research.

Hales RE, Yudofsky SC: *The American Psychiatric Publishing Textbook of Clinical Psychiatry* (4th ed.). Washington, DC: American Psychiatric Publishing, 2003.—Highly authoritative text, addressing all aspects of mental health diagnosis and treatment in 1,700 pages.

Hersen M, Turner SM: *Adult Psychopathology and Diagnosis* (4th ed.) New York: Wiley, 2003.—Aimed at graduate students in psychology, counseling, and social work, this 700-page text covers the spectrum of diagnostic conditions.

Montgomery K: *How Doctors Think*. New York: Oxford University Press, 2005.—A professor of humanities and medicine (who is not a physician herself) discusses clinical judgment and the practice of medicine.

Morrison J: *DSM-IV Made Easy*. New York: Guilford Press, 1995; revised version, 2001.—This one-volume approach to understanding DSM-IV-TR reflects the revised criteria.

Morrison J: *The First Interview*. New York: Guilford Press, 1995.—An introduction to the art and science of mental health interviewing.

Morrison J: *When Psychological Problems Mask Medical Disorders*. New York:

Guilford Press, 1997.—Provides mental health information concerning 60 medical illnesses.

Nurcombe B, Gallagher RM: *The Clinical Process in Psychiatry*. New York: Cambridge University Press, 1986.—Hefty guide to organizing mental health information and making diagnoses.

Sadock BJ, Sadock VA: *Comprehensive Textbook of Psychiatry* (8th ed.). Philadelphia: Lippincott Williams & Wilkins, 2005.—This 4,000-page behemoth covers all aspects of mental health illness and treatment.

Diagnostic Method

Allen VG, Arocha JF, Patel VL: Evaluating evidence against diagnostic hypotheses in clinical decision making by students, residents and physicians. *Int J Med Informatics* 1998; *51*:91–105.

Andreason NC: Editorial: Vulnerability to mental illness. *Am J Psychiatry* 2005; *162*:211–213.

Coderre S, Mandin H, Harasym PH, Fick GH: Diagnostic reasoning strategies and diagnostic success. *Med Educ* 2003; *37*:695–703.

Faust D, Nurcombe B: Improving the accuracy of clinical judgment. *Psychiatry* 1989; *52*:197–208.

Fava M, Farabaugh AH, Sickinger AH, Wright E, Alpert JE, Sonawalla S, Nierenberg AA, Worthington JJ 3rd: Personality disorders and depression. *Psychol Med* 2002; *32*:1049–1057.

Hall KH: Reviewing intuitive decision-making and uncertainty: The implications for medical education. *Med Educ* 2002; *36*:216–224.

Hall RC, Popkin MK, Devaul RA, Faillace LA, Stickney SK: Physical illness presenting as psychiatric disease. *Arch Gen Psychiatry* 1978; *35*:1315–1320.

Heilig M, Forslund K, Asberg M, Rydberg U: The dual-diagnosis concept used by Swedish social workers: Limited validity upon examination using a structured diagnostic approach. *Eur Psychiatry* 2002; *17*:363–365.

Honig A, Pop P, Tan ES, Philipsen H, Romme MA: Physical illness in chronic psychiatric patients from a community psychiatric unit: The implications for daily practice. *Br J Psychiatry* 1989; *155*:58–64.

Keel PK, Dorer DJ, Eddy KT, Franko D, Charatan DL, Herzog DB: Predictors of mortality in eating disorders. *Arch Gen Psychiatry* 2003; *60*(2):179–183.

Kennedy N, Boydell J, Kalidindi S, Fearon P, Jones PB, van Os J, Murray RM: Gender differences in incidence and age at onset of mania and bipolar disorder over a 35-year period in Camberwell, England. *Am J Psychiatry* 2005; *162*:257–262.

Kessler RC, Berglund P, Demler O, Jin R, Merikangas KR, Walters EE: Lifetime prevalence and age-of-onset distributions of DSM-IV disorders in the National Comorbidity Survey replication. *Arch Gen Psychiatry* 2005; *62*:593–602.

Kessler RC, McGonagle KA, Zhao S, Nelson CB, Hughes M, Eshleman S, Wittchen HU, Kendler KS: Lifetime and 12-month prevalence of DSM-III-R psychiatric disorders in the United States. *Arch Gen Psychiatry* 1994; *51*:8–19.

Koran LM, Sheline Y, Imai K, Kelsey TG, Freedland KE, Mathews J, Moore M: Medical disorders among patients admitted to a public-sector psychiatric inpatient unit. *Psychiatr Serv* 2002; *53*:1623–1625.

Krueger RF: The structure of common mental disorders. *Arch Gen Psychiatry* 1999; *56*:921–926.

Mark DB: Decision-making in clinical medicine. In Kasper DL, Braunwald E, Fauci A, Hauser S, Longo D, Jameson JL (Eds.): *Harrison's Principles of Internal Medicine* (16th ed.). New York: McGraw Hill, 2004.

Roberts B: A look at psychiatric decision making. *Am J Psychiatry* 1978; *135*:1384–1387.

Welner A, Liss JL, Robins E: A systematic approach for making a psychiatric diagnosis. *Arch Gen Psychiatry* 1974; *31*:193–196.

Witztum E, Grinshpoon A, Margolin J, Kron S: The erroneous diagnosis of malingering in a military setting. *Mil Med* 1996; *161*:225–229.

Diagnosing Depression and Mania

Bai YM, Lin CC, Hu PG, Yeh HS: Risk factors for substance use disorders among inpatients with major affective disorders in Taiwan Chinese. *Gen Hosp Psychiatry* 1998; *20*:98–101.

Brockington I: Postpartum psychiatric disorders. *Lancet* 2004; *363*:303–310.

Garvey MJ, Tuason VB: Mania misdiagnosed as schizophrenia. *J Clin Psychiatry* 1980; *41*:75–78.

Ghaemi SN, Sachs GS, Chiou AM, Pandurangi AK, Goodwin K: Is bipolar disorder still underdiagnosed? Are antidepressants overutilized? *J Affect Disord* 1999; *52*:135–144.

Hirschfeld RM, Lewis L, Vornik LA: Perceptions and impact of bipolar disorder: how far have we really come? Results of the National Depressive and Manic–Depressive Association 2000 survey of individuals with bipolar disorder. *J Clin Psychiatry* 2003; *64*:161–174.

McCullough JP Jr., Klein DN, Borian FE, Howland RH, Riso LP, Keller MB, Banks PL: Group comparisons of DSM-IV subtypes of chronic depression: Validity of the distinctions, part 2. *J Abnorm Psychol* 2003; *112*:614–622.

Werth JL Jr., Cobia DC: Empirically based criteria for rational suicide: A survey of psychotherapists. *Suicide Life-Threat Behav* 1995; *25*:231–240.

Diagnosing Anxiety and Fear

Bruce SE, Machan JT, Dyck I, Keller MB.: Infrequency of "pure" GAD: Impact of psychiatric comorbidity on clinical course. *Depress Anxiety* 2001; *14*:219–225.

Fava GA, Rafanelli C, Grandi S, Conti S, Ruini C, Mangelli L, Belluardo P: Long-term outcome of panic disorder with agoraphobia treated by exposure. *Psychol Med* 2001; *31*:891–898.

Lee DO, Helmers SL, Steingard RJ, DeMaso DR: Case study: Seizure disorder presenting as panic disorder with agoraphobia. *J Am Acad Child Adolesc Psychiatry* 1997; *36*:1295–1298.

Zimmerman M: What should the standard of care for psychiatric diagnostic evaluations be? *J Nerv Ment Dis* 2003; *191*:281–286.

Diagnosing Psychosis

Evans JD, Heaton RK, Paulsen JS, McAdams LA, Heaton SC, Jeste DV: Schizoaffective disorder: A form of schizophrenia or affective disorder? *J Clin Psychiatry* 1999; *60*:874–882.

Genova P: Dump the DSM! *Psychiatric Times* 2003; *20*: Issue 4, www.psychiatrictimes.com/p030472.html

Gurland B. Aims, organization, and initial studies of the Cross-National Project. *Int J Aging Hum Dev* 1976; *7*:283–293.

Kasanin J: The acute schizoaffective psychoses. *Am J Psychiatry* 1994; *151(Suppl. 6)*:144–154.—A reprint of a 1933 article in the same journal.

Lammertink M, Lohrer F, Kaiser R, Hambrecht M, Pukrop R: Differences in substance abuse patterns: Multiple drug abuse alone versus schizophrenia with multiple drug abuse. *Acta Psychiatr Scand* 2001; *104*:361–366.

Maj M, Pirozzi R, Formicola AM, Bartoli L, Bucci P: Reliability and validity of the DSM-IV diagnostic category of schizoaffective disorder: Preliminary data. *J Affect Disord* 2000; *57*:95–98.

Marneros A: The schizoaffective phenomenon: The state of the art. *Acta Psychiatr Scand 106(Suppl.* 2003; *418)*:29–33.

Ripoll N, Bronnec M, Bourin M: Nicotinic receptors and schizophrenia. *Curr Med Res Opin* 2004; *20*:1057–1074.

Tsuang D, Coryell W: An 8-year follow-up of patients with DSM-III-R psychotic depression, schizoaffective disorder, and schizophrenia. *Am J Psychiatry* 1993; *150*:1182–1188.

Zisook S, McAdams LA, Kuck J, Harris MJ, Bailey A, Patterson TL, Judd LL, Jeste DV: Depressive symptoms in schizophrenia. *Am J Psychiatry* 1999; *156*:1736–1743.

Diagnosing Problems of Memory and Thinking

Folstein MF, Folstein SE, McHugh PR: Mini-Mental State: A practical method for grading the cognitive state of patients for the clinician. *J Psychiatr Res* 1975; *12*:189–198.

Diagnosing Substance Misuse and Other Addictions

Schuckit MA, Smith TL, Danko GP, Bucholz KK, Reich T, Bierut L: Five-year clinical course associated with DSM-IV alcohol abuse or dependence in a large group of men and women. *Am J Psychiatry* 2001; *158*:1084–1090.

Diagnosing Personality and Relationship Problems

Moran P, Leese M, Lee T, Walters P, Thornicroft G, Mann A: Standardised Assessment of Personality—Abbreviated Scale (SAPAS): Preliminary validation of a brief screen for personality disorder. *Br J Psychiatry* 2003; *183*:228–232.

Suicide and Violence

Beautrais AL: Subsequent mortality in medically serious suicide attempts: A 5 year follow-up. *Aust N Z J Psychiatry* 2003; *37*:595–599.
Gardner W, Lidz CW, Mulvey EP, Shaw EC: Clinical versus actuarial predictions of violence of patients with mental illnesses. *J Counseling Clin Psychol* 1996; *64*:602–609.

Material on suicide intent scales:
www.neurotransmitter.net/suicidescales.html
www.clinical-supervision.com/Pearce%20Suicide%20scale.htm

Information about Real-Life Personages

These entries are placed in alphabetical order by the persons' last names, followed by the chapters in which the persons are mentioned and then by the bibliographical information.

Rigoberto Alpizar (Chapter 17): Goodnough A: Fretful passenger, turmoil on jet and fatal shots. *New York Times*, Dec. 9, 2005.
Marshall Applewhite (Chapter 13): www.rickross.com/groups/heavensgate.html
Kenneth Bianchi (Chapter 4), John Hinckley, Jr. (Chapters 13 and 17), Ted Bundy (Chapter 16), and other mentally disordered criminals: www.crimelibrary.com
Doug Bruce (Chapter 14): *The New Yorker*, Feb. 27, 2006, 27–30.
John Clare (Chapter 18): Bate J: *John Clare: A Biography*. New York: Farrar, Straus & Giroux, 2003.
Ayral-Clause O: *Camille Claudel: A Life*. New York: Abrams, 2002.
Phineas Gage (Chapter 16): www.deakin.edu.au/hbs/psychology/gagepage
Effrain Marrero (Chapter 9): Wilson D: Steroids are blamed in suicide of young athlete. *New York Times* March 10, 2005.
William Minor (Chapter 18): Winchester S: *The Professor and the Madman*. New York: HarperCollins, 1998.
Joe Namath (Chapter 8): http://en.wikipedia.org/wiki/Joe_Namath
Opal Petty (Chapter 7): Lehmann-Haupt C: Opal Petty, 86, patient held 51 years involuntarily in Texas. *New York Times* March 14, 2005, Section C, page 15.
Samuel Taylor Coleridge (Chapter 15): Holmes R: Coleridge: *Early Visions, 1772–1804*. New York: Pantheon, 1999; Holmes R: Coleridge: *Darker Reflections, 1904–1834*. New York: Pantheon, 1989.

Charles Darwin (Chapter 12): Barloon TJ, Noyes R Jr.: Charles Darwin and panic disorder. *JAMA* 1997; *277*:138–141.

Carolyn Heilbrun (Chapter 11): Grigoriadis V: A death of one's own. New York, Dec 8, 2003; www.newyorkmetro.com/nymetro/news/people/n_9589/

Jim Piersall (Chapter 12): Piersall J, Hirshberg A: *Fear Strikes Out: The Jim Piersall Story*. Boston: Little, Brown, 1957; Piersall J, Whittingham R: *The Truth Hurts*. Chicago: Contemporary Books, 1984.

Daniel Paul Schreber (Chapter 13): Freud S: Psycho-analytic notes on an autobiographical account of a case of paranoia (dementia paranoids). In Strachey J (Ed. & Trans.): *The Standard Edition of the Complete Psychological Works of Sigmund Freud* (Vol. 12). London: Hogarth Press, 1958 (orig. pub. 1911).

Elizabeth Shin (Chapter 16): Sontag D: Who was responsible for Elizabeth Shin? *New York Times* June 2, 2002, Section 6, page 10.

Virginia Woolf (Chapter 10): Lee H: *Virginia Woolf*. New York: Knopf, 1997.

Andrea Yates (Chapter 11): O'Malley S: *"Are You There Alone?": The Unspeakable Crime of Andrea Yates*. New York: Simon & Schuster, 2004.

Index

This index indicates definitions by the use of **boldface** and case examples by *italics*. A page number followed by "*t*" indicates a table.

Diagnostic Principles

Create a Differential Diagnosis

A. Arrange your differential diagnosis according to a safety hierarchy (page 16).

B. Family history can guide diagnosis, but because you often can't trust reports, clinicians should attempt to rediagnose each family member (page 29).

C. Physical disorders and their treatment can produce or worsen mental symptoms (page 17).

D. Consider somatization disorder whenever symptoms don't jibe or treatments don't work (page 110).

E. Substance use can cause a variety of mental disorders (page 17).

F. Because of their ubiquity, potential for harm, and ready response to treatment, *always* consider mood disorders (page 120).

When Information Sources Conflict

G. History beats current appearance (page 24).

H. Recent history beats ancient history (page 26).

I. Collateral information sometimes beats the patient's own (page 26).

J. Signs beat symptoms (page 27).

K. Be wary when evaluating crisis-generated data (page 28).

L. Objective findings beat subjective judgment (page 28).

M. Use Occam's razor: Choose the simplest explanation (page 30).

N. Horses are more common than zebras; prefer the more frequently encountered diagnosis (page 31).

O. Watch for contradictory information (page 36).

Resolve Uncertainty

P. The best predictor of future behavior is past behavior (page 47).

Q. More symptoms of a disorder increase its likelihood as your diagnosis (page 47).

R. Typical features of a disorder increase its likelihood as your diagnosis; in the presence of nontypical features, look for alternatives (page 47).

S. Previous typical response to treatment for a disorder increases its likelihood as your diagnosis (page 48).

T. Use the word *undiagnosed* whenever you cannot be sure of your diagnosis (page 48).

U. Consider the possibility that this patient should be given no mental diagnosis at all (page 51).

Multiple Diagnoses

V. When symptoms cannot be adequately explained by a single disorder, consider multiple diagnoses (page 61).

W. Avoid personality disorder diagnoses when your patient is acutely ill with an Axis I disorder (page 62).

X. Arrange multiple diagnoses to list first the one that is most urgent, treatable, or specific. Whenever possible, also list diagnoses chronologically (page 64).